THE PHARMACOLOGICAL BASIS OF MIGRAINE THERAPY

Edited by

Willem K Amery, MD PhD
Jan M Van Nueten, Dr Sc
Albert Wauquier, PhD

PITMAN

First Published 1984

Catalogue Number 21.0036.81

Pitman Publishing Ltd
128 Long Acre
London WC2E 9AN

Associated Companies
Pitman Publishing Pty Ltd, Melbourne
Pitman Publishing New Zealand Ltd, Wellington

British Library Cataloguing in Publication Data

ISBN 0-272-79782-0

Printed and bound in Great Britain
at The Pitman Press, Bath

FOREWORD

In September 1983 Janssen Pharmaceutica in Beerse hosted an international symposium on migraine, where clinicians and basic scientists from different disciplines, discussed past achievements and present advances in our understanding of the pathophysiology of migraine and of the pharmacological approach to migraine therapeutics. The subject was studied from a broad angle covering many diverse but interrelated aspects. Since the introduction of antiserotonergics, which were shown to be beneficial in a number of patients, the discovery of new ways of treatment has been significantly hindered by the lack of understanding of the processes involved in migraine. The role of serotonin as one of the mediators of vasospasm and its antagonism by antiserotonergic compounds has for a long time dominated scientific thinking in this area. There can be little doubt that the occurrence of vasospasm is but one of the phenomena possibly occurring during a migraine attack. A recent hypothesis proposes focal brain hypoxia as a pivotal event in migraine, giving rise to a cortical spreading depression wave as well as to the headache. Another recent theory highlights the possible role of neuropeptides of the opioid type in migraine. New hypotheses will hopefully give a new impetus to this field. Experimental research is currently going on and may lead to the discovery of better migraine drugs.

The papers in this book were presented at the meeting held on 19–20 September 1983. We believe it to be the first book covering the many facets of our current understanding of the multifactorial migraine process and of the pharmacological basis of its treatment.

The symposium would not have been possible without the continuous stimulating interest of Dr Paul A J Janssen. The editors are indebted to a number of persons who actively contributed to the organisation of the meeting. To all those not mentioned by name, we offer our apologies. We especially thank Mr M Debroye and Mrs D De Bruyn for being actively engaged in a large number of practical matters; we thank Mrs R Lauryssen-De Keuster and Miss K Mertens for carrying the secretarial burden; we also thank Mr T Marr for his significant help in brushing-up the style of the present contributions.

It is our hope that this publication will contribute to the understanding of the aetiology and treatment of migraine and that it will provide a useful reference work for those who have a teaching task covering migraine or pharmacology, and that it will stimulate the development of new therapies for migraine.

Willem K Amery MD PhD
Jan M Van Nueten DrSc
Albert Wauquier PhD

LIST OF CONTRIBUTORS

W K Amery
MD PhD
Department of Clinical Research, Janssen Pharmaceutica N.V., 2340 Beerse, Belgium

M C Arne-Bès
MD
Department of Neurology, University Paul-Sabatier, CHU Rangueil, 31504 Toulouse, France

D Ashton
Dr Sc
Department of Neuropharmacology, Janssen Pharmaceutica N.V., 2340 Beerse, Belgium

A Bès
Prof MD
Department of Neurology, University Paul-Sabatier, CHU Rangueil, 31504 Toulouse, France

M J Biggs
BSc M Phil
Research Assistant, Department of Pharmacology, King's College, Strand, London, WC2R 2LS, United Kingdom

M Boccuni
Dz MD
University Institute of Internal Medicine and Clinical Pharmacology, Florence, Italy

G W Bruyn
Prof MD
Department of Neurology, Academisch Ziekenhuis Leiden, 2333 AA Leiden, The Netherlands

L I Caers
PhD
Department of Clinical Research, Janseen Pharmaceutica N.V., 2340 Beerse, Belgium

F Cangi
MD
University Institute of Internal Medicine and Clinical Pharmacology, Florence, Italy

F Clifford Rose
FRCP
Physician in Charge, Princess Margaret Migraine Clinic, Department of Neurology, Charing Cross Hospital, London, United Kingdom

B Comet
MD Dr Sc
Department of Neurology, University Paul-Sabatier, CHU Rangueil, 31504 Toulouse, France

J L David
MD

Département de Clinique et de Séméiologie Médicale, Hopital de Bavière, Université de Liège, 4020 Liège, Belgium

F De Clerck
Dr Sc

Department of Pharmacology and Laboratory of Haematology, Janssen Pharmaceutica N.V., 2340 Beerse, Belgium

Ph Dupui
MD

Department of Neurology, University Paul-Sabatier, CHU Rangueil, 31504 Toulouse, France

H L Edmonds
Prof PhD

Department of Anaesthesiology, University of Louisville, USA

L Edvinsson
MD PhD

Department of Clinical Pharmacology, University Hospital, S-22185 Lund, Sweden

M Fanciullacci
Prof MD

Associate Professor of Clinical Pharmacology, University Institute of Internal Medicine and Clinical Pharmacology, Florence, Italy

G Gatto
MD

University Institute of Internal Medicine and Clinical Pharmacology, Florence, Italy

G Géraud
Prof MD

Department of Neurology, University Paul-Sabatier, CHU Rangueil, 31504 Toulouse, France

K Ghose
MB BS PhD MRCP

Department of Geriatric Medicine, University Hospital of South Manchester, Manchester M20 8LR, United Kingdom

W Gommeren

Department of Biochemical Pharmacology, Janssen Pharmaceutica N.V., 2340 Beerse, Belgium

A Guell
MD

Department of Neurology, University Paul-Sabatier, CHU Rangueil, 31504 Toulouse, France

A J Hansen
MD PhD

Department of Medical Physiology A, The Panum Institute, University of Copenhagen, 2200 Copenhagen, Denmark

E S Johnson
PhD BSc MB BS

Reader, Department of Pharmacology, King's College, Strand, London, WC2R 2LS, United Kingdom

M Lauritzen
MD

Department of Medical Physiology A, The Panum Institute, University of Copenhagen, 2200 Copenhagen, Denmark

J E Leysen
Dr Sc

Department of Biochemical Pharmacology, Janssen Pharmaceutica N.V., 2340 Beerse, Belgium

J Olesen
MD

Department of Neurology, Gentofte University Hospital, 2900 Hellerup, Denmark

W J Oosterveld
Prof MD

Academisch Medisch Centrum, Vestibular Department, 1105 AZ Amsterdam, The Netherlands

A Panconesi
MD

University Institute of Internal Medicine and Clinical Pharmacology, Florence, Italy

U Pietrini
MD

University Institute of Internal Medicine and Clinical Pharmacology, Florence, Italy

P R Saxena
Prof MD

Department of Pharmacology, Erasmus University, 3000 DR Rotterdam, The Netherlands

F Sicuteri
Prof MD

Professor of Clinical Pharmacology, Director of the University Institute of Internal Medicine and Clinical Pharmacology, Florence, Italy

M G Spillantini
PhD

University Institute of Internal Medicine and Clinical Pharmacology, Florence, Italy

E L H Spierings
MD PhD

Department of Neurology, University Hospital 'Dijkzigt', 3015 GD Rotterdam, The Netherlands

P Tfelt-Hansen
MD

Rigshospitalet, University of Copenhagen, 2200 Copenhagen, Denmark

J M Van Nueten
Dr Sc

Department of Pharmacology, Janssen Pharmaceutica N.V., 2340 Beerse, Belgium

A Wauquier
PhD

Department of Pharmacology, Janssen Pharmaceutica N.V., 2340 Beerse, Belgium

ACKNOWLEDGMENTS

Table I on page 39 has been reproduced with the kind permission of the Editor of *Headache 1979 19:* 397–399.

Figure 1 on page 108 and Figure 2 on page 109 have been reproduced with kind permission from *Brain Research 1976; 115:* 377–393.

Figure 3 on page 112 has been reproduced with kind permission of the Editor-in-Chief of *Cephalalgia 1983* (in press).

CONTENTS

INTRODUCTION

W K Amery

When assembling a series of contributions on the pharmacological basis of migraine therapy, one is immediately confronted with the enigmatic nature of this disease. It is safe to say that, even today, the pathogenesis of migraine, a disease reputedly known for up to 50 centuries, is far from being understood. Nonetheless, research into the pathophysiology of the disease and its treatment has gradually given rise to a series of hypotheses regarding the pathogenesis of migraine, to the development of new drugs based upon such theories and to the clinical evaluation of newer and older agents by means of well-designed controlled clinical trials. We have thus at our disposal not only a series of very interesting hypotheses, but also a variety of effective drugs, which, however, sometimes seem to have very little (if anything) in common, apart from having a beneficial effect in migraineurs.

There is no generally accepted concept explaining the pathogenesis of migraine and, although a series of effective drugs for the treatment of this condition is available, their mechanism of action is, at best, poorly understood. What is agreed, however, is that migraine is a type of paroxysmal headache, and this headache is bound to have a certain pathogenesis.

At least some theories of the pathophysiology of migraine have, however, proved useful in designing effective drug treatments and the mere existence of such treatments provides a valid platform for an in-depth reflection on the pharmacological basis of migraine therapy. Many factors are hampering migraine research and a rapid and successful elucidation of the pathophysiology of migraine and the mechanism of action of migraine treatments cannot be expected in the near future. In view of this, the most appropriate way to proceed is probably the compilation of an inventory, and this has been the aim of the editors of this book. In addition, since, ultimately, the most suitable species for studying human disease states is man, this volume would not have been complete without a chapter on clinical pharmacology.

1

All of this should not make us forget, however, that there are two specific difficulties that are major obstacles in migraine research. Perhaps, it is only when these obstacles have been removed that we shall be in a position to understand migraine and its treatment. On the other hand, one must not underestimate the role which new concepts and new drugs can play in unravelling the migraine enigma. What, then, are these difficulties?

a) One lies on the experimental side. There is no reliable animal model of migraine available. Researchers may, for example, dream of finding a model (Figure 1) of a rat that clutches its head (because of headache) during or subsequent to an episode of cortical spreading depression. Unfortunately, there is an enormous gap between such a dream and today's reality and we are still very far away from a reliable experimental model of migraine.

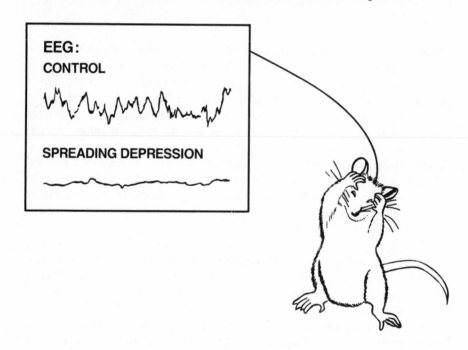

Figure 1. Theoretical experimental model of migraine

b) The other difficulty is a clinical one. The diagnosis of migraine is made on clinical grounds, especially on the patient history. Criteria for the classification of headache and the definition of migraine have been proposed and have actually gained wide acceptance. Yet, the scientific community continues to feel unsure as to whether migraine is one, two or even more diseases. In addition, whereas the clinical diagnosis of classical migraine is usually rather

2

straightforward, the border between common migraine and some other types of headache — especially tension headache — is often blurred. It is especially in the latter context that a pathognomonic marker of migraine, be it a laboratory or other measurement, would be more than welcome in confirming (or rejecting) the diagnosis.

The conclusion of this introduction, then, is a plea not only for continuing our efforts to establish a firm pharmacological basis of migraine therapy, but also for refining our diagnostic methods for this disease, whose social impact is all too often underestimated.

Part I

**PATHOPHYSIOLOGY OF MIGRAINE AND
ANIMAL PHARMACOLOGY**

1

THE ROLE OF VASOCONSTRICTION
IN THE PATHOGENESIS OF MIGRAINE

J Olesen, M Lauritzen

Migraine is traditionally regarded as a disease caused by abnormal vascular reactions in the brain and/or extracerebral tissues. This idea originates mostly from the pulsating nature of the migraine pain but is also supported by many older studies, mainly by the Wolff group [1]. Most of these studies were done with techniques which at best, can be regarded as qualitative. They were also done before medical science realised the necessity of statistical calculations, control groups etc. They consequently need re-examination, but in this review we shall not try to analyse them. The important evidence in relation to vasospasm/vasoconstriction/ischaemia arises from modern studies of cerebral blood flow.

Physiology of cerebral vasoconstriction

Vasospasm

To understand the following review of previous literature it is necessary to keep in mind exactly what happens when an artery to the brain constricts for reasons unrelated to metabolism of its area of supply, e.g. by sympathetic nervous activity, by circulating or locally released vasoconstrictors. Brain arterioles have a tremendous capacity for dilatation as illustrated by the autoregulatory response, i.e. constancy of cerebral blood flow despite reduction of arterial blood pressure [2]. Usually arterial blood pressure can be dropped to about 60 per cent of normal values before blood flow begins to decrease. The constancy of blood flow is maintained because of progressing arteriolar dilatation. If blood pressure is further decreased, blood flow also decreases, but oxygen uptake and cerebral metabolism continues undisturbed because the brain can increase its extraction of oxygen, in other words, the arteriovenous oxygen difference in that brain region will increase. Finally, when the brain cannot increase the oxygen extraction any more, a further decrease in blood pressure will result in impaired cerebral metabolism and function. The same series of events may be observed if an artery

7

to the brain gradually constricts. With a modest constriction, arterioles will dilate and maintain constancy of regional cerebral blood flow. Actually the lumen of the artery must be reduced by 80 to 90 per cent before blood flow in the supplied area decreases. Further constriction now results in reduced cerebral blood flow and gradually increased arteriovenous oxygen difference until finally cerebral function and metabolism is impaired.

What are the most sensitive methods used to disclose such vasoconstriction? In the early phase when arterial constriction is compensated for by arteriolar dilatation, only an increase in regional cerebral blood volume can be observed. As constriction increases and cerebral blood flow begins to fall, measurements of regional cerebral blood flow are of value, although sometimes difficult to interpret (see below). A better indicator in this phase is an increased arterio-venous oxygen difference or a reduced cerebral venous pO_2 from the affected area. Finally in the phase with reduced cerebral blood flow and reduced metabolism, measurements of cerebral blood flow, metabolism and arteriovenous oxygen difference or cerebral venous pO_2 are all valuable.

Spasm and ischaemia or functional depression of regional cerebral blood flow (rCBF)

Brain blood flow is closely linked to metabolism, which again is linked to cerebral function. Reduced function caused for example by intoxication or dementia results in decreased metabolism and cerebral blood flow. The coupling between blood flow, metabolism and function is very close and can be demonstrated globally as well as within regions and even within single columns of cerebral cortex [3]. We are thus faced with a problem when recording globally or focally reduced cerebral blood flow. Is the reduction due to vasospasm? Or is it a natural adaptation to decreased function and reduced metabolic needs? Modern PET-scanning techniques can answer the question but have not yet been applied to migraine patients during attacks.

Conventional [133] Xenon methods can only indicate whether a reduced CBF is due to spasm or metabolic depression:

1 Reduced blood flow secondary to vasospasm is likely to be located within one or more regions of supply of large cerebral arteries.

2 In order to elicit clinical symptoms vasospastic CBF reduction must be marked (see above), whereas a primary metabolic disturbance may cause symptoms with lesser CBF reduction.

3 In an ischaemic area autoregulation, i.e. the ability of the brain to keep blood flow constant despite variations in blood pressure, is usually lost. Only more severe ischaemia will result in abnormal reactivity to changes in arterial pCO_2. Normal regulation or different patterns of disturbance suggest non-ischaemic mechanisms.

8

Methods for studying cerebral vasoconstriction

Cerebral blood volume

This is a relatively easy measurement to take. A gamma emitting tracer which remains intravascularly is injected, the concentration of tracer in the blood is determined and gamma irradiation from various parts of the head are recorded. Before the advent of tomography the method was hampered by superposition of extracerebral tissues and a necessity to measure from truncated cones of brain tissue in the whole depth of the hemisphere. With single photon or positron emitting tomography measurements should be more accurate, but these techniques have not yet been applied to migraine [4].

Arteriovenous oxygen difference/cerebral venous pO_2

These two measurements can only be performed with access to cerebral venous blood. Usually samples have been taken from the internal jugular vein, which gives an average estimate of brain arteriovenous oxygen difference/brain venous pO_2, but no regional information. With positron emission tomography (PET) it is possible to obtain regional determination of the oxygen extraction fraction, i.e. the fraction of oxygen extracted from the blood in a particular area [5]. None of the methods has been used during migraine attacks.

Regional cerebral blood flow

For many years intra-arterial injection of a gamma emitting diffusible tracer was the dominating method. The only tracer of significance has been [133] Xenon. The principle of the method is that a bolus of this inert radioactive gas is delivered into one internal carotid artery. It is distributed to the carotid artery territory and immediate diffusion equilibrium is established. Wash-out of radioactivity is then followed by external stationary gamma detectors [6]. The clearance curve is bicompartmental, one compartment being grey substance and the other compartment white substance. If the curves are followed for 10 minutes or more an average of white and grey flow may be obtained. It is also possible in such cases to make a bicompartmental analysis and obtain blood flow in white and grey substance separately. A more practical method is the initial slope analysis where the slope of the first one to two minutes of the clearance curve is used for flow calculation. This mainly represents flow in grey substance. The advantage of this is that it is much easier to maintain a steady state during functional activation, having alterations in blood pressure or pCO_2 for such a short measurement period. The original methodological studies were done with a single detector, but most studies in migraine have been done with 16, 35 or 254 detectors. Even with many detectors the spatial resolution of the method is not optimal because of its two dimensional nature. Each detector will pick up counts from a truncated cone of brain tissue in the whole depth of the hemisphere. Another limitation to this method is that only areas that receive tracer from the internal carotid artery can be studied. In most cases the primary visual cortex is thus not seen. Compton scatter is also an important factor which smooths out differences between regions. On the other hand the method has many advantages: a high count rate gives good measurement accuracy and allows measurements from many channels. Contamination with counts from extracerebral tissues is virtually non-existant, and the input function is as required, a true bolus delivery. So far, this method has been far more sensitive in disclosing functional activation and deactivation than any other method except PET. Movement of a hand or even a finger can be seen in virtually all individual patients, whereas methods utilising inhalation need samples from patients to see such changes.

Inhalation or intravenous bolus injection of [133] *Xenon and external stationary detection*

In the method outlined above a carotid puncture must be performed and hence the applicability of the method is limited to patients in whom a carotid arteriography is indicated. For this reason non-traumatic methods utilising inhalation or intravenous injection of [133] Xenon were developed [7,8]. There are many problems with these techniques. When the tracer is inhaled or injected intravenously, most of it is to be found in the respiratory air, since Xenon has a low affinity for blood. In order to get enough radioactivity into the brain a protracted inhalation over a minute or so is necessary, and thus the tracer arrives gradually into the brain. By computer methods correction can be made for this, but of course this always involves increased uncertainty about the input function. Also recirculation of [133] Xenon is considerable and must be corrected for. Extracranial tissues are labelled as well as brain and with external stationary detectors this cannot be sorted out, although certain correction procedures have been devised. The count rate is not nearly as high as with intra-arterial injection and therefore does not allow the use of large numbers of detectors. Very high amounts of radioactive Xenon are to be found in the nasal cavities and the pharynx which give a radiation artefact. Again correction procedures are possible for the airway artefact, but some error remains.

Inhalation of [133] *Xenon and single photon emission tomography*

When [133] Xenon inhalation or intravenous injection is used, tomographic detection can greatly reduce the problem of irradiation from extracerebral tissues [9,10]. It also provides a three dimensional view of regional cerebral blood flow and thus gives a much better spatial resolution than external stationary detectors, and it visualises deep structures as well as cortex. On the other hand this is certainly not an optimal method since there are still problems with the input

10

function, a somewhat unsatisfactory count rate and much Compton scatter. Overall, single photon emission tomography represents a vast improvement over [133]Xenon inhalation and stationary detectors, but cerebral cortex may still be studied much more accurately with intracarotid injection.

Positron emission tomography (PET)

This method utilises detection of very short-lived tracers emitting positrons. The technique is still in the developmental phase and technically very complicated. A team of physicists, engineers, radiopharmacists and doctors is necessary to run this equipment efficiently. The techniques give regional cerebral blood flow as well as regional cerebral oxygen consumption and oxygen extraction fraction. They may also be used for the determination of regional glucose metabolism and in the future a number of other applications will be available. Because of their complicated nature these methodologies have not yet been applied to the study of the acute migraine attack, but in the future they are likely to contribute significantly to our knowledge in this area.

Studies of regional cerebral blood flow during migraine attacks

Using intracarotid injection of [133]Xenon and 16 stationary detectors, Skinhøj and Paulson [11] were the first to describe decreased regional cerebral blood flow during prodromes of classic migraine. They also studied one patient during migraine headache where they felt that regional cerebral blood flow was probably increased. O'Brian et al [13] used [133]Xenon inhalation and two stationary detectors to study hemispheric blood flow which decreased about 10 per cent during prodromes in seven patients and increased eight per cent during headache in 10 patients. He did not use appropriate correction procedures later developed for this method. Skinhøj [13] presented intra-arterial [133]Xenon studies with 35 detectors in six patients, four of whom had classic migraine. These all had focally decreased cerebral blood flow during prodromes. Others were studied during headache and had an increased blood flow. No distinction was made between patients with classic and common migraine, and patients were not studied outside of attacks for comparison. Simard and Paulson [14] demonstrated almost complete abolition of normal CO_2 induced CBF increase during classic migraine prodromes in one patient. When restudied outside an attack, the patient had a normal response to carbon dioxide. Norris et al [15] followed a patient from the prodromal phase into the headache phase and after treatment. Cerebral blood was globally reduced during prodromes and rather high during headache, and it was unaltered after ergotamine had cured the headache. Mathew et al [16] found regional cerebral blood flow reduced in three patients studied during prodromes of classic migraine. They used a gamma camera and intra-arterial injection of [133]Xenon. They also found an increased cerebral blood flow

11

during the headache phase, but patients were not their own controls. Edmeads [17] presented a number of cases largely confirming previous studies, but they also pointed out that regional cerebral blood flow with their method (intra-arterial injection of ^{133}Xenon and 16 stationary detectors) was not necessarily reduced during visual prodromes. Marshall [18] used intra-arterial ^{133}Xenon injection and 15 detectors to study migraine equivalents, i.e. migrainous neurological symptoms without headache. Focal abnormalities were revealed at rest in two patients and a focal reduction of hyperventilatory response in three patients. The time relationship to the last attack was not stated. Sakai and Meyer [19] studied 43 patients with migraine using inhalation of ^{133}Xenon and eight stationary external detectors over each hemisphere. Correction for extracranial contamination and recirculation but not for airway artefact was performed. Three patients were studied during prodromes of classic migraine and had focally reduced blood flow. Twelve patients were studied during the headache phase of migraine, two with classic, and 10 with common migraine. Cerebral blood flow was increased approximately 30 per cent. The authors also found that increased blood flow was present up to 48 hours after the last migraine attack. When studied more than 48 hours after the last migraine attack migraineurs had normal cerebral blood flow. Autoregulation to reduce perfusion presssure by tilting was impaired. Analysis [19] revealed, however, that this was so only in four patients during attacks of classic migraine, whereas autoregulation was normal during common migraine attacks in two patients. It was normal in all migraine patients when free from attacks. With the same technique Sakai and Meyer later reported a markedly reduced response to breathing of 5% CO_2 in migraine patients during attacks [20]. Six to 20 hours post-headache the response to 5% CO_2 was normal, whereas the response was excessive when migraine patients were studied outside of an attack. CO_2 response tested by voluntary hyperventilation during migraine attacks was normal except in one patient studied during prodromes of classic migraine. A rather serious methodological criticism against these studies of both autoregulation and CO_2 response is the lack of arterial pCO_2 values. When comparing the response to small alterations in arterial pCO_2, end-expiratory values are not exact enough. It is also a problem that no clear distinction was made between classic and common migraine.

The only study utilising positron emission tomography (PET) dealt with a patient who suffered a stroke during a classic migraine attack [21]. The patient was studied 14 days after the attacks, at which time a CT-scan revealed a hypodense area in the left occipital region. In that area there was a reduced cerebral blood flow and a less reduced oxygen extraction, indicating luxury perfusion. More anteriorly, cerebral blood flow was increased with normal oxygen extraction and contralaterally in the right occipital cortex cerebral blood flow was decreased, but oxygen extraction increased, indicating a state of relative vasoconstriction. These extensive cerebral blood flow and oxygen extraction abnormalities indicated that there was something special about the case which distinguished it

12

from an ordinary stroke. Judge and Gauthiers [22] used 16 stationary detectors and inhalation of [133] Xenon in their study of 65 normal healthy volunteers and 17 patients studied within four days of a classic migraine attack, as well as 23 patients studied within two days of a common migraine attack. They found blood flow reduced in classic migraine and increased during common migraine. Bés et al [23] studied the reaction to a dopaminergic agent (Piribidil) in 10 normal volunteers and in 20 patients with migraine. The type of migraine was not stated. Migraineurs reacted much more strongly with nausea, vomiting and general malaise and could only tolerate less than half of the dose tolerated by normal controls. Similarly they suffered a marked reduction of mean arterial blood pressure and, interestingly, regional cerebral blood flow was increased by migraineurs but not in controls. A peripheral dopaminergic blocker, domperidone, did not reverse the effect of Piribidil in migraine patients, indicating hypersensitivity of central dopaminergic receptors in migraineurs. Staehlin-Jensen et al [24] studied two members of a family with hemiplegic migraine during attacks and found cerebral blood flow decreased whereas it was normal when outside of an attack. Gelmers [25] studied two patients, one had never suffered from migraine before, the other was known to suffer from common migraine. He used intracarotid injection of [133] Xenon and 35 external stationary detectors. During the study both patients developed headache and nausea but no sign of classic migraine. Simultaneously they both developed focal low flow areas in the posterior and temporal parts of the hemisphere. At follow-up both patients continued to suffer from common migraine attacks.

Our own studies of regional cerebral blood flow in migraine has fallen into three series. In an as yet unpublished series [26] we used [133] Xenon inhalation and tomography to study spontaneous attacks of common (N=11) and classic (N=11) migraine. None of these patients with common migraine had any focal blood flow abnormalities during the attack, these studies being compared to a study when the patients were free from migraine for at least a week. In particular there was no indication of focal oligaemia at any point in time and neither focal nor global blood flow was increased during the migraine attack. Focally reduced cerebral blood flow was observed in eight out of 11 patients with classic migraine attacks. This was so for the patients studied while still having prodromes, but also for patients in whom prodromes had recently disappeared and who were studied in the headache phase. Patients were followed with repeated measurements during the development of their attacks and did not develop reactive hyperaemia at any point in time. They were restudied after treatment and again when free from migraine for a week. There was no significant difference between blood flow immediately after treatment and when free from migraine for a week. Another series was done to reveal a hypothetical initial oligaemia just at the onset of a common migraine attack [27]. Since it is very difficult to know when such attacks begin, we studied patients with induceable migraine. Measurements were taken in the resting state, after provocation with

13

red wine and then they were repeated at 15 to 30 minute intervals until the patients had a fully developed common migraine attack. We obtained successful measurements in five patients using [133]Xenon inhalation and tomography and in three patients using [133]Xenon inhalation and 32 stationary detectors. At no point in time was oligaemia either focally or globally observed. Focal and global cerebral blood flow during the migraine attack was not different from rest. Taken together these two studies strongly indicate that common migraine attacks are not preceded by or associated with focal or global alterations of cerebral blood flow. We also studied regional cerebral blood flow with intracarotid injection of [133]Xenon and 254 external stationary detectors [28–30]. This procedure triggers an attack, and hence we were able to obtain measurements before and during the development of classic migraine attacks. In three patients in the first study we saw a small focal hyperaemia before the onset of attacks, but we are uncertain of its significance since it was not observed later. The typical finding was a reduced cerebral blood flow in the posterior part of the hemisphere. This spread anteriorly to a varying extent, sometimes to include the whole hemisphere; at other times it stopped at the occipital-parietal border or at the central sulcus. The rate of spread has been calculated to approximately 2mm/min [29]. The oligaemia did not respect territories of supply of major cerebral arteries, and this together with a gradual spread indicates that it is not caused by vasospasm. Also its modest magnitude indicates that vasospasm could not be the cause of the symptoms. In the same study various functional activation procedures such as speech, opening the eyes and listening were impaired in the oligaemic regions as was CO_2 reactivity, whereas autoregulation was normal [28–30]. The studies thus indicated an uncoupling between function, metabolism and cerebral blood flow. One patient revealed a similar kind of blood flow abnormality without having migraine either before, during or after the CBF study. He is the only one amongst the series of more than 250 patients studied with the same method who has developed such cerebral blood flow abnormalities without migraine symptoms. A further patient suffered from common migraine attacks, but had, during the study, symptoms indicating a classic migraine attack. Our study thus indicates that the described cerebral blood flow abnormalities are virtually pathognomonic for classic migraine, but that they may be induced in rare patients with common migraine or even without migraine by the intracarotid procedure. This is probably the explanation for the findings by Gelmers quoted above. It must be emphasised that focal reduction of cerebral blood flow has not been observed in conjunction with spontaneous attacks of common migraine.

A number of conclusions can be drawn from existing studies of regional cerebral blood flow during migraine attacks. First of all there is a uniformity of opinion that cerebral blood flow is focally or even globally reduced during prodromes of classic migraine. It is also likely that response to changes of arterial pCO_2 are abnormal during the prodromes of classic migraine, whereas autoregulation is not. Some of the older studies have described hyperaemia during the headache phase of classic migraine, whereas more recent studies found it normal. With regard to common migraine the largest and technically most satisfactory study has not demonstrated focal or global abnormalities in any phase of the attack. Several others have, however, measured increased CRF during the headache phase of common migraine. This problem must consequently be studied further, and there is also a great need for studies of the regulation of cerebral blood flow during common migraine attacks. On balance the cerebral blood flow studies do not at present lend much support to the vasospastic theory of migraine, since the newest and most extensive studies rather indicate a gradual spread of disturbed function located in the cortex.

Other evidence of vasoconstriction in migraine

Although the regional cerebral blood flow studies quoted above do not support the vasospastic theory of migraine, other evidence does. A number of strokes occur during migraine attacks and the deficits are often identical with the usual prodromes. Such individual cases are certainly impressive, but infarction in migraine is exceedingly rare. The vast majority of patients with classic migraine never experience permanent damage to the affected brain region. Strokes have also been described in association with common migraine attacks, and this is difficult to understand with our knowledge of normal cerebral blood flow in that condition. Many patients with cerebral vascular disease develop headache and nausea indistinguishable from a migraine attack. Common migraine as well as strokes occur in a large proportion of the population and by simple coincidence strokes must hit a fairly large number of migraineurs. It is therefore impossible to ascertain a causal relationship between migraine and stroke.

As mentioned previously, determination of arteriovenous oxygen differences during migraine attacks would be an effective way of demonstrating vasospasm. Unfortunately such measurements have not been done. Another way of studying possible cerebral ischaemia is by measurement of spinal fluid lactate and bicarbonate. Skinhøj [13] found increased lactic acid and decreased bicarbonate in spinal fluid during migraine attacks. The evaluation of these findings is complicated, since many factors other than vasoconstriction may affect spinal fluid lactic acid and bicarbonate. Furthermore, Skinhøj used a normal material gathered under somewhat different circumstances. It appears likely that at least some of Skinhøj's patients really had an increased lactic acid and decreased bicarbonate, but further studies are necessary to decide whether this reflects ischaemia or other factors.

If vasospasm is present in the brain during classic migraine attacks, it has to be at the arteriolar level for many of the reasons mentioned above. What could the mechanisms be? Traditionally circulating monoamines have been regarded as possible spasmogenic factors. Amongst monoamines 5-HT has notably been a

15

candidate. The level of 5-HT in blood falls during a migraine attack possibly reflecting release from thrombocytes with a transient increase in free 5-HT. We have shown, however, that 5-HT infused into the carotid artery does not alter regional cerebral blood flow in man [31]. We have demonstrated the same to be true for adrenaline/noradrenaline, angiotensin and isoprenaline [32,33]. Animal experiments were long at discrepancy with our findings, but as techniques for animal experimentation improved, and preparations were tested for intact cerebral autoregulation and blood brain barrier, they also failed to show significant vasoconstriction after intravascular infusion of monoamines [see 34]. This lack of effect of circulating monoamines on cerebral circulation agrees well with the demonstration of a tight physical as well as chemical blood brain barrier to monoamines [34]. If circulating monoamines are to play a role in the pathogenesis of migraine, an abnormality of the blood brain barrier must be assumed [35]. There are presently no studies to indicate impaired blood brain barrier in migraine patients. The other possibility is that vasoactive transmitters released from brain tissue might act on cerebral arterioles. This appears from a physiological point of view to be a much more likely mode of action. The neurological symptoms in classic migraine clearly indicate cortical dysfunction and many of the neurotransmitters are highly vasoactive. There is no physical blood brain barrier protecting the smooth muscle of the arterioles from brain interstitial fluid contents, and probably any spillover of transmitters into interstitial fluid has free access to the vascular smooth muscle.

Summary

In the first section of this paper, the physiology of cerebral blood flow regulation is discussed and methods for the measurement of regional cerebral blood flow and metabolism are critically reviewed. In view of the close ties between cerebral blood flow, metabolism and function, it is mandatory to consider the potential causes whenever a reduction of cerebral blood flow is observed: is it due to vasospasm, or is it secondary to a decreased neuronal function and, therefore, to reduced metabolic needs?

Older methods of measuring cerebral blood flow have important limitations, and results, produced by them, must be interpreted very cautiously. The more recent techniques, using inhalation or injection of [133]Xenon, have produced evidence to suggest that there may be a reduction of the cerebral blood flow during the prodromes of a classic migraine attack, whereas the flow during the headache phase would tend to be rather high. There is only one study where positron emission tomography has been used, and this in a single patient. In this patient, there were rather extensive cerebral blood flow and oxygen extraction abnormalities.

Our own group has used [133]Xenon and computerised tomographic measurements. Our data indicate that cerebral blood flow shows a gradually spreading reduction during the prodromes and into the headache phase of classic migraine attacks. We have not observed cerebral hyperaemia during the headache phase. Cerebral blood flow has been found normal in all our patients studied during attacks of common migraine. On balance, the available studies do not lend much support to the vasospastic theory of migraine.

Referring to the potential role of monoamines, such as 5-HT, it is unlikely that circulating monoamines could play a role as spasmogenic factors in the cerebral circulation, unless there is an abnormality in the blood-brain barrier. If such amines do play an important role, it is more likely that they are released from brain tissue since there is no barrier protecting the smooth muscle of the cerebral arterioles from the interstitial fluid contents.

References

1   Wolff HG. *Headache and Other Head Pain*. New York: Oxford University Press. 1963
2   Olesen J. Cerebral blood flow. Methods for measurement, regulation, effects and drugs and changes in disease. *Acta Neurol Scand 1974; 50:* suppl 57
3   Greenberg J, Hand P, Sylvestro A, Reivich M. Localized metabolic-flow couple during functional activity. *Acta Neurol Scand 1979; 60:* suppl 72: 12–13
4   Phelps ME, Huang SC, Hoffman EJ, Kuhl DE. Validation of tomographic measurement of cerebral blood volume with ^{11}C labelled carboxyhemoglobin. *J Nucl Med 1979; 20:* 328–334
5   Lenzi GL, Frackowiak RSJ, Jones T. Cerebral oxygen metabolism and blood flow in human cerebral ischemic infarction. *J Cereb Blood Flow Metab 1982; 29:* 321–335
6   Olesen J, Paulson OB, Lassen NA. Regional cerebral blood flow in man determined by the initial scope of the clearance of intra-arterially injected ^{133}Xe. *Stroke 1971; 2:* 635–646
7   O'Brist WD, Thompson HK, Wand HS, Wilkinson WE. Regional cerebral blood flow estimated by ^{133}Xe inhalation. *Stroke 1975; 6:* 245–256
8   Risberg J, Ali Z, Wilson EM et al. Regional cerebral blood flow by ^{133}Xe inhalation. *Stroke 1975; 6:* 142–148
9   Lassen NA, Henriksen L, Paulson OB. Regional cerebral blood flow in stroke by xenon-133 inhalation and emission tomography. *Stroke 1981; 12:* 284–288
10 Celcis P, Goldman T, Henriksen L, Lassen NA. A method for calculating regional cerebral blood flow from emission computed tomography of inert gas concentration; practical approach. *J Comput Assist Tomogr 1981; 5:* 641–645
11 Skinhøj E, Paulson OB. Regional blood flow in internal carotid distribution during migraine attack. *Br Med J 1969; 3:* 569–570
12 O'Brien MD. Cerebral-cortex-perfusion rates in migraine. *Lancet 1967; i:* 1036
13 Skinhøj E. Hemodynamic studies within the brain during migraine. *Arch Neurol 1973; 29:* 95–98
14 Simard D, Paulson OB. Cerebral vasomotor paralysis during migraine attack. *Arch Neurol 1973; 29:* 95–98
15 Norris JW, Hachinski VC, Cooper PW. Changes in cerebral blood flow during a migraine attack. *Br Med J 1975; 3:* 676–677
16 Mathew NT, Hrastnik F, Meyer JS. Regional cerebral blood flow in the diagnosis of vascular headache. *Headache 1976; 15:* 252–260
17 Edmeads J. Cerebral blood flow in migraine. *Headache 1977; 17:* 148–152
18 Marshall J. Cerebral blood flow in migraine. In Greene R, ed. *Concepts in Migraine Research*. New York: Raven Press. 1978: 131–139
19 Sakai F, Meyer JS. Regional cerebral hemodynamics during migraine and cluster headache measured by the ^{133}Xe inhalation method. *Headache 1978; 18:* 122–132

20   Sakai F, Meyer JS. Abnormal cerebrovascular reactivity in patients with migraine and cluster headache. *Headache 1979; 19:* 257–266

21   Bousser MG, Baron JC, Iba-Zizen MT et al. Migranous cerebral infarction: a tomographic study of cerebral blood flow and oxygen extraction fraction with the oxygen-15 inhalation technique. *Stroke 1980; 11:* 145–148

22   Juge O, Gautheir G. Mésures de debit sanguin cerebral regional (DSCR) par inhalation de xenon 133: applications cliniques. *Bull Schweiz Aka Med 1980; 36:* 101–115

23   Bès A, Guell A, Victor G et al. Effects of a dopaminergic agonist on CBF in migraine patients. In Heistad DD, Marcus ML, eds. *Cerebral Blood Flow: Effects of Nerves and Neurotransmitters.* New York: Elsevier Biomedical. 1982: 163–168

24   Stackelin Jensen T, Voldby B, Olivarius BF et al. Cerebral hemodynamics in familial hemiplegic migraine. *Cephalalgia 1981; 1:* 121–125

25   Gelmers HJ. Common migraine attacks preceded by focal hyperemia and parietal oligemia in the rCBF pattern. *Cephalalgia 1982; 2:* 29–32

26   Lauritzen M, Olesen J. Unpublished data

27   Olesen J, Tfelt-Hansen P, Henriksen L, Larsen B. The common migraine attack may not be initiated by cerebral ischemia. *Lancet 1981; ii:* 438–440

28   Olesen J, Larsen B, Lauritzen M. Focal hyperemia followed by spreading oligemia and impaired activation of rCBF in classic migraine. *Ann Neurol 1981; 9:* 344–352

29   Lauritzen M, Skyhøj Olsen T, Lassen NA, Paulson OB. The changes of regional cerebral blood flow during the course of classical migraine attacks. *Ann Neurol:* in press

30   Lauritzen M, Skyhøj Olsen T, Lassen NA, Paulson OB. The regulation of regional cerebral blood flow during and between migraine attacks. *Ann Neurol:* in press

31   Olesen J. Effect of serotonin on regional cerebral blood flow (rCBF) in man. *Cephalalgia 1981; 1:* 7–10

32   Olesen J. The effect of intracarotid epinephrine, norepinephrine, and angiotensin on the regional cerebral blood flow in man. *Neurology 1972; 22:* 978–987

33   Olesen J, Hougard K, Hertz M. Isoproterenol and propranolol: ability to cross the blood-brain barrier and effects on cerebral circulation in man. *Stroke 1978; 9:* 344–349

34   Bès A, Géraud G, eds. *Cerebral Circulation and Neurotransmitters.* Excerpta Medica: Amsterdam. 1980

35   Harper AM, MacKenzie ET, McCulloch J, Pikard JD. Migraine and the blood-brain barrier. *Lancet 1977; i:* 1034–1036

2

ANTIVASOCONSTRICTOR EFFECTS OF DRUGS USED IN MIGRAINE THERAPY

J M Van Nueten

Support for the involvement of vascular disturbances in migraine comes from the observation that patients with peripheral vascular disorders can also display symptoms seen in migraine patients during an attack (e.g. headache, nausea) [1]. Conversely, it has been shown that migraine patients frequently suffer from peripheral vascular diseases such as Raynaud's phenomenon, suggesting a common underlying deficiency [2]. A typical migraine attack is preceded by an aura, during which cerebral blood flow probably is reduced [3,4]. During the attacks vasospasms may occur, especially in the presence of a deficient blood brain barrier [4–6]. If the vasospasms are located at the arteriolar level, the extreme precapillary constriction will lead to a significant decrease in local blood flow, resulting in insufficient tissue perfusion, tissue ischaemia and dysfunction [1,7,8].

Vasospasms can be due either to an abnormal responsiveness of the vascular smooth muscle cells or to abnormally high levels of endogenous vasoconstrictor substances [9]. They are caused by contractions of vascular smooth muscle cells resulting from an increase in cytoplasmic Ca^{2+}-concentration. Furthermore, in some conditions hypoxia has been shown to induce a decrease in tissue blood flow [10], most likely because of vasoconstriction subsequent to an increased Ca^{2+}-influx in the smooth muscle cell of the vascular wall [8]. In cerebral vascular tissue in particular, increases of the influx of extracellular calcium ions (Ca^{2+}) induced by vasoactive substances, are reinforced by hypoxia [8,11,12].

Despite a variety of other theoretical explanations for migraine, including the attractive hypoxia hypothesis [13,14], it still appears that a number of vasoactive substances (e.g. prostaglandins, catecholamines and, in particular, 5-hydroxytryptamine) may play a major role [13–17]. Thus, it is likely that during the migraine attack, vasoactive substances are released or activated [6,18,19]. For example, it is well known that in hypoxia, blood platelets release 5-hydroxytryptamine and synthesise prostaglandin-like material (e.g.

thromboxane A_2). Vasoconstriction induced by platelet products is a Ca^{2+}-dependent phenomenon [12,20]. Release of vasoactive substances from platelets has been proposed as a possible mechanism in the aetiology of migraine [21—24]. Particularly in the case of 5-hydroxytryptamine the vasoconstrictor effect of one endogenous mediator may be amplified by the simultaneous presence of minute amounts of other vasoactive substances [8,25—27]. In this context, it is interesting, that serum taken from patients undergoing a migraine crisis amplifies the vasoconstrictor response to norepinephrine in extracranial arteries [18,28].

To avoid pathological situations at the microcirculatory level the balance between vasoconstrictor and vasodilator substances must be maintained [29,30]. A given vasoactive substance may induce opposite vascular responses depending on the initial vascular tone [19,31,32]. Attenuation of the vasodilator component of a vasoactive substance, or induction of vasoconstriction may be related to the therapeutic effect observed with some drugs during the headache phase of the migraine attack [33—35].

Migraine is a multifactorial disease [36] which reflects the fact that cerebrovascular tissue is exposed to a number of endogenously released vasoactive substances and to hypoxic conditions. Likewise, the therapeutic effect of antimigraine drugs could be due to several factors. This chapter summarises their effect on cerebral vascular smooth muscle.

Calcium (Ca^{2+})

Vascular smooth muscle contracts when it is exposed to potassium (K^+) in the presence of Ca^{2+}. This effect of K^+ is due to cell membrane depolarisation

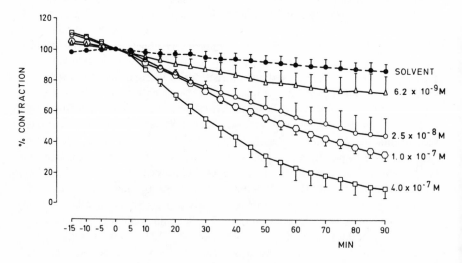

Figure 1. Effect of flunarizine (M) on K^+-induced contractions of canine basilar arteries (means ± SEM; n=5)

20

resulting in an increased entry of extracellular Ca^{2+} [20,37,38]. In cerebral arteries flunarizine, which is used for the prevention of migraine attacks [17, 39–40] inhibits the contractile responses of canine basilar (Figure 1) and internal carotid arteries to K^+. This is because flunarizine causes dose-dependent inhibition of Ca^{2+}-entry [12,42]. In comparative studies on different canine vascular preparations, flunarizine was particularly potent on brain arteries [42,43]. Similar findings were reported for nimodipine, another Ca^{2+}-entry blocker with potential antimigraine properties [44–46].

Inhibition of Ca^{2+}-induced vascular contraction has also been reported with drugs used in migraine therapy such as cyproheptadine, domperidone, amitryptiline and, to a lesser extent, pizotifen (Table I).

TABLE I. Inhibition of contractions of rat caudal arteries in response to 5-hydroxytryptamine (5-HT), norepinephrine (Nor) and Ca^{2+} ED_{50} values (M)

Anti-migraine drugs	5-HT	Nor	Ca^{2+}
pizotifen (1) (5)	1.6×10^{-9} (5)	7.5×10^{-7}	3.3×10^{-7}
cyproheptadine (1) (5)	2.7×10^{-9} (5)	7.0×10^{-7}	1.1×10^{-8}
methysergide (1) (2) (5)	3.6×19^{-9} (5)	Θ (6)	Θ
chlorpromazine	4.5×10^{-9}	7.9×10^{-9}	2.9×10^{-7}
amitriptyline	1.6×10^{-8}	1.0×10^{-6}	NT (7)
domperidone (2) (3)	3.5×10^{-7}	7.5×10^{-7}	5.5×10^{-6}
flunarizine	3.6×10^{-7} (5)	6.7×10^{-7}	1.1×10^{-8}
metoclopramide (3)	8.2×10^{-7} (5)	Θ	Θ
propranolol (4)	2.3×10^{-6} (5)	Θ	Θ

(1)   partial agonist
(2)   inhibits 5-HT induced relaxation (canine coronary artery)
(3)   dopamine-antagonist
(4)   β-adrenergic antagonist
(5)   serotonergic antagonism was reported in the literature [15,16,59,61]
(6) Θ: inactive
(7)   NT: not tested

Catecholamines

Norepinephrine is a normal neurotransmitter in the blood vessel wall. It is released when the sympathetic nerves are excited and usually causes vasoconstriction mediated by alpha-adrenoceptors. Sympathetic innervation is particularly rich in the cerebrovascular area [47].

The contractile response of the isolated rabbit ear artery to stimulation of the sympathetic nerves is inhibited by α-adrenergic blocking agents (e.g. phentolamine), clonidine, cyproheptadine, pizotifen) [27], but also by cinnarizine and

21

flunarizine (Van Nueten, unpublished observations). It is well established that flunarizine inhibits contractions of systemic blood vessels and also decreases vascular reactivity to catecholamines after systemic administration to rats and dogs [48,49]. Inhibition of norepinephrine-induced vascular contractions is also observed with ergotamine, domperidone and amitriptyline (Table I). In feline cerebral arteries α-adrenergic blocking agents inhibit contractions induced by catecholamines (Figure 2) [50]. In peripheral vascular tissue ergotamine and

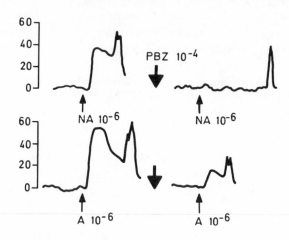

Figure 2. Contractions induced by norepinephrine (NA) and epinephrine (A) on isolated middle cerebral arteries of the cat were inhibited by phenoxybenzamine (PBZ); concentrations in molar values. (From Nielson and Owman [50], with permission)

dihydroergotamine also inhibit alpha-adrenergic responses [51]; the latter findings are confirmed in vivo [52]. The therapeutic effect of the dopamine-antagonist domperidone [53], was suggested to be due to its inhibitory action on dopamine super-reactivity of migraineurs [54,55]. One cannot exclude that this effect may be reinforced by the vascular effects of the compound.

5-hydroxytryptamine (5-HT)

Complex effects of 5-hydroxytryptamine

Although its exact role in the chain of events contributing to migraine is still unclear 5-hydroxytryptamine is very likely involved in the migraine attack [14,31,51,57–59]. This monoamine has been implicated in the pathogenesis of pain-inducing cerebrovascular reactions [60,61]. A rich and well defined population of 5-HT-receptors and of serotonergic nerves is present in the cerebral vascular wall [31,61,62].

The effects of 5-hydroxytryptamine on the blood vessel wall are complex;

22

they include venular constriction; contraction of most arterial and venous smooth muscle; arteriolar dilatation, in particular in the splanchnic and cerebral circulation; and inhibition of peripheral adrenergic neurotransmission [63]. Thus, in a given vascular bed, the net effect of the monoamine is determined by the balance between its vasoconstrictor and vasodilator actions [6,9,31,64–67]. 5-hydroxytryptamine can induce either a decrease or an increase of cerebral blood flow in vivo (Figure 3) depending upon the vascular area [56,68]. Physiological concentrations of 5-HT, when injected intracisternally in dogs, caused long-lasting cerebral spasms, suggestive of the importance of 5-HT in the aetiology of such spasms [69].

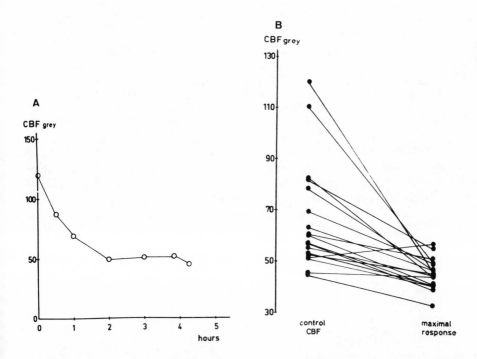

Figure 3. Reaction of the canine cerebral blood flow in grey matter (ml/100g/min) during a continuous infusion of 5-hydroxytryptamine (0.8μg/kg/min). A. Representative example. B. Comparison between control values and corresponding values at maximal 5-HT effect. Method: Crypton[85] elimination method. (From Ekström-Jodal et al [68], with permission)

Vasoconstrictor effects of 5-hydroxytryptamine

Isolated cranial arteries are particularly sensitive to the vasoconstrictor effect of 5-hydroxytryptamine (Figure 4) [16,33,66,70]. Quite a number of drugs used for migraine therapy, although they have widely different pharmacological

23

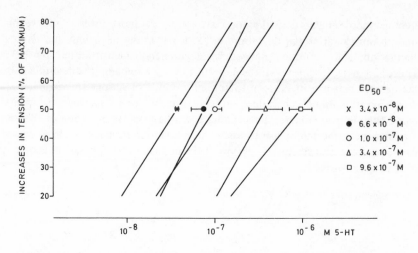

Figure 4. Mean contractile responses of canine blood vessels to 5-HT. X: basilar artery (100%=1.40±0.16g); •: internal carotid artery (100%=3.10±0.71g); o: coronary artery (100%=3.48±0.81g); △: gastrosplenic artery (100%=7.23±1.89g); □: gastrosplenic vein (100%=2.54±0.65g). Calculated regression lines. (From Van Nueten [66] with permission)

properties, inhibit 5-HT induced contractions of cerebral and peripheral vascular tissues (Table I). This inhibition observed on temporal arteries from migraine patients (Figure 5) is comparable to that observed on vessels from 'non-migraine' patients, suggesting a similar population of 5-HT receptors [61]. Compounds

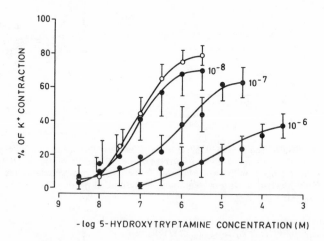

Figure 5. Contractile response to 5-hydroxytryptamine and effect of increasing concentrations of methysergide ($10^{-8}-10^{-6}$ M; -20 min) on human temporal arteries from migraine patients. Experiments were done in the presence of 10^{-6} M cocaine and 10^{-7} M propranolol. (From Skärby et al [61], with permission)

24

inhibiting 5-HT-induced vascular contractions include specific 5-HT-antago-nists, dopamine-antagonists, Ca^{2+}-entry blocking drugs, and β-adrenergic blocking agents (Table I), indicating a common link in the mechanism of action of these compounds. As far as 5-HT antagonists are concerned, a therapeutic action in migraine was observed with pizotifen, cyproheptadine and methys-ergide. Preliminary clinical observations, with the specific serotonergic 5-HT$_2$ antagonist ketanserin have failed to produce convincing antimigraine proper-ties and may, therefore, suggest no or minor involvement of 5-HT$_2$ receptors in the migraine attack (Amery, personal communication).

Vasodilator effects of 5-hydroxytryptamine

It is possible that the vasodilator responses to 5-hydroxytryptamine contribute to pain during migraine attacks. Therefore, partial serotonergic agonists may be useful in inhibiting this vasodilator component. Such partial agonism (intrinsic vasoconstrictor combined with inhibitory effects) is particularly evident for

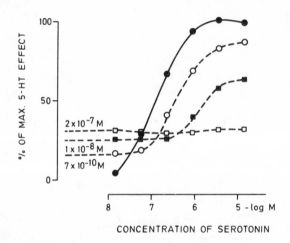

CONCENTRATION OF SEROTONIN

Figure 6. Dose-response curves for 5-hydroxytryptamine on human temporal artery strips obtained during autopsy 15 hours after death; 5-HT alone (solid line) or in the presence of increasing concentrations of ergotamine added 60 min previously (dashed line). (From Müller-Schweinitzer and Weidmann [33], with permission)

ergotamine (Figure 6), dihydroergotamine and methysergide, and to a lesser extent for pizotifen and cyproheptadine [27,33,66,70].

Prevention of 5-HT-induced vasodilatation can also be obtained with dopamine-antagonists such as domperidone at concentrations devoid of any vasoconstrictor activity (Van Nueten, unpublished observations).

25

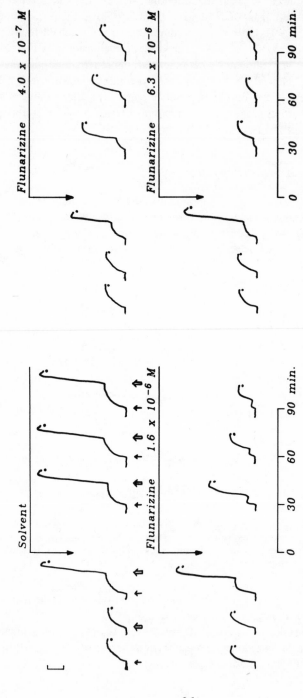

Figure 7. Isometric tension recordings in four segments of the same canine basilar artery, demonstrating the amplifying effect of 5-hydroxytryptamine (3.4×10^{-9} M, ($\uparrow$)) on the contractile responses to 2.8×10^{-7} M prostaglandin $F_{2\alpha}$ ($\Uparrow$) and the inhibition of the amplifying effect of flunarizine

26

Amplifying effects of 5-hydroxytryptamine

Both in isolated blood vessels and in the intact animal, 5-hydroxytryptamine potentiates (amplifies) the contractile responses to a variety of vasoconstrictor agonists [26,67,71–74]. Its amplifying effect, by exaggerating the constrictor effects of other neurohumoral mediators, may contribute to abnormal vascular responses. In canine basilar arteries, flunarizine prevents the amplifying effect of 5-hydroxytryptamine on vascular contractions induced by prostaglandin $F_{2\alpha}$ (Figure 7). Inhibition of such amplifying effect may be of particular importance in the intact organism since the concentrations of 5-hydroxytryptamine which cause amplification [74,75] correspond to the concentrations of the monoamine found in human plasma [76].

Since the vasodilator component of 5-hydroxytryptamine may trigger the migraine attack, increasing the sensitivity of cerebral blood vessels to circulating vasoconstrictor substances may be beneficial. Such potentiation is observed with minute concentrations of clonidine, methysergide, pizotifen, cyproheptadine or ergotamine [16,25,27].

Hypoxia

The responsiveness of the blood vessel wall to vasoconstrictor substances is modulated by local conditions to which the vascular smooth muscle cells are exposed [77]. For example, acute hypoxia causes marked further increase in tension in canine blood vessels when these vessels are first exposed to a vaso-constrictor substance [11]; these hypoxic contractions are inhibited by fluna-rizine [8,12,20]. This is also the case in canine cerebral blood vessels (Figure 8). These findings may help to explain why flunarizine has a prophylactic effect in migraine [13].

Blood constituents

When blood platelets aggregate they release vasoactive substances such as throm-boxane A_2 and prostaglandins E_2 and $F_{2\alpha}$ [12,24,78,79]. Activated platelets induce a marked contraction of canine basilar arteries, which can be prevented by flunarizine in a concentration-dependent way (Figure 9). The inhibition by flunarizine has a gradual onset and a prolonged duration. In a similar study on the rat caudal artery, biochemical measurements of the various mediators involved, as well as pharmacological analyses showed that 5-hydroxytryptamine and prostaglandins – in particular thromboxane A_2 – are the principal mediators responsible for platelet-mediated vasoconstriction. The primary site of action of flunarizine is at the level of the Ca^{2+}-entry in the vascular smooth muscle cells [80]. The finding that flunarizine is effective on platelet-mediated vaso-constriction, is in agreement with the inhibition by flunarizine of vascular

27

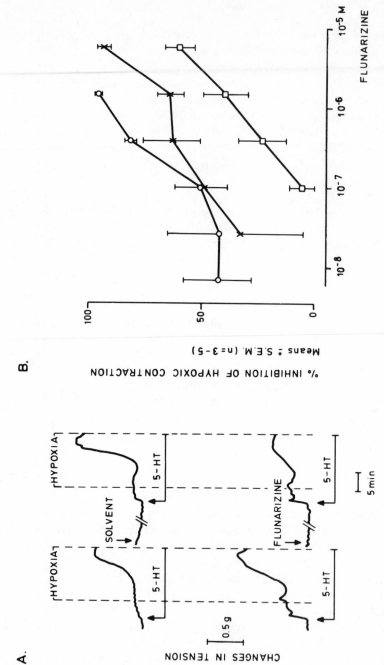

Figure 8. A. Isometric tension recordings in two basilar artery segments from the same dog, showing the effect of solvent (0.1% ethanol) and flunarizine (10^{-7} M, 90min contact time) on the contractile response to hypoxia in the presence of 5-hydroxytryptamine (3.6×10^{-9} M; 5-HT). B. Inhibitory effect of flunarizine on hypoxia-induced contractions of canine basilar (o), middle cerebral (x) and internal carotid (□) arteries in the presence of 5-HT. The data are shown as means ± SEM expressed as per cent inhibition of the contraction induced by hypoxia before the addition of the drug and corrected for control values. The incubation period for flunarizine or its solvent was 90 minutes. (From Van Nueten et al [8], with permission)

28

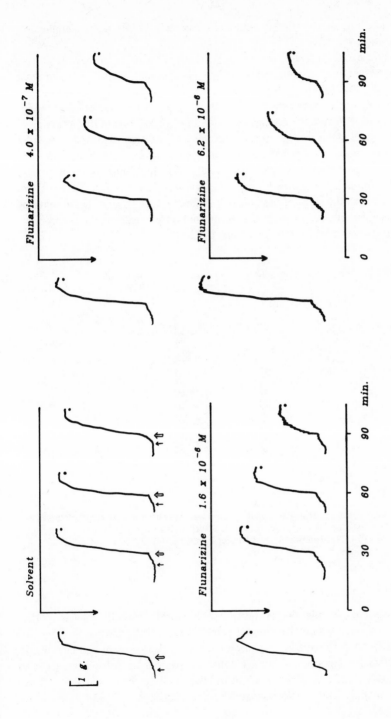

Figure 9. Isometric tension recordings in four segments of the same canine basilar artery, demonstrating the contractile response to rat platelets (2.5 x 10^{11}/L) stimulated with thrombin (0.002 NIHu/L). Flunarizine inhibits these contractions in a concentration-dependent way

29

contractions induced by the exogenous substances 5-hydroxytryptamine and prostaglandin $F_{2\alpha}$ [81].

Intense vasoconstriction of cerebral arteries may be a major factor contributing to the development of cerebral ischaemia in patients with cerebrovascular diseases [82–84]. Cerebral arterial spasms can be induced by fresh and clotted autologous blood, by serum and by fibrinogen degradation products [28,82–86]. The role of cerebrovascular spasms due to blood components in the aetiology of migraine is still unclear, but it is intriguing to note that sera obtained from migraine patients in the pre-attack and post-onset stage amplify the vasoconstrictor action of vasoactive substances (e.g. 5-HT, histamine, norepinephrine) on isolated human and bovine extracranial arteries [28]. This amplifying effect is thus related to the stage of the migraine attack (Figure 10). Similar amplifying effects were also observed with human serum and fibrinogen degradation products which may trigger cerebral arterial spasms [82,87].

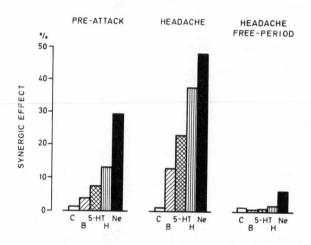

Figure 10. Sera obtained from five female patients during the migraine crisis enhanced the contractile response of human extracranial artery strips to bradykinin (B), 5-hydroxytryptamine (5-HT), histamine (H) and norepinephrine (NE). (From Nattero et al [28], with permission)

Conclusions

The pathogenesis of migraine is multifactorial; cerebrovascular malfunction is only one of the factors involved in migraine. Thus, cerebral vasospasms may play a role in triggering the headache phase of migraine. Vasospasms can be induced by the excessive amounts of endogenous vasoconstrictor substances, such as released from blood platelets, or found in blood and cerebrospinal fluid. Moreover, during migraine attacks vasoactive substances may be activated by the concomitant presence in minute amounts, of substances with amplifying properties. Hypoxic conditions may considerably enhance vasoconstrictor responses to endogenous vasoactive substances. The influence of a given vasoactive substance on the cerebral vascular bed will depend upon its initial vascular tone, the presence of other substances (with amplifying or inhibitory properties), the dependency of the contractile response of the vascular smooth muscle cells upon Ca^{2+}, and on local hypoxia. An important role for the action of these substances in the pathogenesis of migraine is suggested by the fact that a number of heterogeneous drugs used in the therapy of the disease have strong antivasoconstrictor properties.

Summary

Cerebral vascular malfunction is one of the factors thought to be involved in migraine, a multifactorial disease. For example, cerebral vasospasms are induced by the presence of high quantities of endogenous vasoactive substances. They may also be activated by the concomitant presence in minute amounts of substances with amplifying properties. In particular the imbalance between vasoconstrictor and vasodilator substances or effects may be involved in episodes of migraine. A number of drugs used in the therapy of migraine inhibit vasoconstriction induced by calcium, norepinephrine and 5-hydroxytryptamine as well, and this may suggest a role for these substances in the pathogenesis of migraine. The long-lasting antivasoconstrictor effect of the Ca^{2+}-entry blocker flunarizine may help to explain, at least in part, its therapeutic effect in the prophylaxis of migraine. The recently reported therapeutic effects of domperidone, possibly due to its antagonism of dopamine hypersensitivity, may similarly be reinforced by the vascular effects of the compound.

Acknowledgments

The author wishes to thank Drs P M Vanhoutte and J Schuurkes for valuable discussion. The valuable contributions of W De Ridder, J Van Mierlo, L Leijssen and C Verellen in preparing the manuscript are greatly acknowledged.

References

1   Olesen J. The role of vasoconstriction in the pathogenesis of migraine. *This volume.* 1984
2   Miller D, Waters DD, Warnica W et al. Is variant angina the coronary manifestation of a generalized vasospastic disorder? *N Engl J Med 1981; 304:* 763–766
3   Skinhøj E, Paulson OB. Regional blood flow in internal carotid distribution during migraine attack. *Br Med J 1969; 3:* 569–570
4   Olesen J, Larsen B, Lauritzen M. Focal hyperemia followed by spreading oligemia and impaired activation of rCBF in classic migraine. *Ann Neurol 1981; 9:* 344–352
5   Check WA. Chronic vasoconstriction may have role in migraine headaches. *Arch Intern Med 1980; 140:* 19

6   Harper AM, MacKenzie ET. Effects of 5-hydroxytryptamine on pial arteriolar calibre in anaesthetized cats. *J Physiol 1977; 271:* 735–746

7   Gerold M, Haeusler G. α_2-Adrenoceptors in rat resistance vessels. *Arch Pharmacol 1983; 322:* 29–33

8   Van Nueten JM, De Ridder W, Van Beek J. Hypoxia and spasms in the cerebral vasculature. *J Cerebr Blood Flow Metab 1982; 2:* S29–S31

9   Vanhoutte PM. Heterogeneity of vascular smooth muscle. In Kaley G, Altura BM, eds. *Microcirculation.* Baltimore: University Park Press. 1978: 181

10   Sparks HV, Gorman MW. Ischemic vasodilation or ischemic vasoconstriction. In Vanhoutte PM, Leusen I, eds. *Vasodilatation.* New York: Raven Press. 1981: 193

11   Vanhoutte PM. Effects of anoxia and glucose depletion on isolated veins of the dog. *Am J Physiol 1976; 230:* 1261–1268

12   Van Nueten JM, De Clerck F. Protection against hypoxia-induced decrease in tissue blood flow. In Clifford Rose F, Amery WK, eds. *Cerebral Hypoxia in the Pathogenesis of Migraine.* London: Pitman. 1982: 176

13   Amery WK, Wauquier A, Van Nueten JM et al. The anti-migrainous pharmacology of flunarizine (R 14 950), a calcium antagonist. *Drugs Exptl Clin Res 1981; VII 1:* 1–10

14   Amery WK. Brain hypoxia: the turning-point in the genesis of the migraine attack? *Cephalalgia 1982; 2:* 83–109

15   Edvinsson L, Hardebo JE, Owman C. Pharmacological analysis of 5-hydroxytryptamine receptors in isolated intracranial and extracranial vessels of cat and man. *Circul Res 1978; 42:* 143–151

16   Hardebo JE, Edvinsson L, Owman CH, Svendgaard N-Aa. Potentiation and antagonism of serotonin effects on intracranial and extracranial vessels. *Neurology 1978; 28:* 64–70

17   Clifford Rose F. Possible role for flunarizine in the prophylaxis of migraine. In Clifford Rose F, Amery WK, eds. *Cerebral Hypoxia in the Pathogenesis of Migraine.* London: Pitman. 1982: 185

18   Nattero G, Bisbocci D, Brandi G et al. Haemodynamic and humoral aspects in premenstrual headache. *Headache, New Vistas.* Florence: Biomedical Press. 1977: 111

19   White PR, Hagen AA. Cerebrovascular actions of prostaglandins. *Pharmac Ther 1982; 18:* 313–331

20   Van Nueten JM. Selectivity of calcium entry blockers. In Godfraind T, Albertini A, Paoletti R, eds. *Calcium Modulators.* Amsterdam: Elsevier Biomedical Press. 1982: 199

21   Gawel M, Burkitt M, Rose FC. The platelet release reaction during migraine attacks. *Headache 1979; 19:* 323–327

22   Hannington E. Migraine: a blood disorder? *Lancet 1978; ii:* 501–502

23   Medina JL, Fareed J, Diamond S. Lithium carbonate therapy for cluster headache. Changes in number of platelets, and serotonin and histamine levels. *Arch Neurol 1980; 37:* 559–563

24   Wachowicz B. Platelet activation: its possible role in the migraine mechanism. *Adv Neurol 1982; 33:* 243–246

25   Speight TM, Avery GS. Pizotifen (BC-105): a review of its pharmacological properties and its therapeutic efficacy in vascular headaches. *Drugs 1972; 3:* 159–203

26   Bevan JA, Duckles SP, Lee TJ-F. Histamine potentiation of nerve- and drug-induced responses of a rabbit cerebral artery. *Circ Res 1975; 36:* 647–653

27   Fozard JR. Comparative effects of four migraine prophylactic drugs on an isolated extracranial artery. *Europ J Pharmacol 1976; 36:* 127–139

28   Nattero J, Franzone J, Croce F et al. Animal and human arteries 'in vitro' response to serum of migraineurs. *Int J Clin Pharmacol Ther Toxicol 1980; 18:* 367–370

29   Van Nueten JM, Vanhoutte PM. Improvement of tissue perfusion with inhibitors of calcium ion influx. *Biochem Pharmacol 1980; 29:* 479–481

30   Vanhoutte PM. Effects of calcium entry blockers on tissue hypoxia. *J Cer Blood Flow Metab 1982; 2:* S42–S44

31   Edvinsson L, Hardebo JE. Demonstration of 5-hydroxytryptamine receptors through inhibition by methergoline in cat pial arteries in vitro. *Br J Pharmac 1978; 64:* 281–283

32   Lamar JC, Hardebo JE. Interaction of a potential antimigraine drug (Org GC 94) with the vasomotor action of serotonin. *Eur J Pharmacol 1979; 60:* 263–275

33   Müller-Schweinitzer E, Weidmann H. Regional differences in the responsiveness of isolated arteries from cattle, dog and man. *Agents and Actions 1977; 7/3:* 383–389

34   Saxena PR, de Vlaam-Schluter GM. Role of some biogenic substances in migraine and relevant mechanism in antimigraine action of ergotamine. Studies in an experimental model for migraine. *Headache 1974; 13:* 142–163

35   Graham JR, Wolff HG. Mechanism of migraine headache and action of ergotamine tartrate. *Arch Neurol Psychiatry 1938; 39:* 737–763

36   Berde B, Fanchamps A. Bedeutung humoraler Mediatoren fur Pathogenese und Behandlung der Migrane. *Munch Med Wochenschr 1975; 117(38):* 1489–1496

37   Bolton TB. Mechanisms of action of transmitters and other substances on smooth muscle. *Physiol Rev 1979; 59:* 606–718

38   Casteels R. Electro- and pharmacomechanical coupling in vascular smooth muscle. *Chest 1980; 78:* 150–156

39   Amery WK. Flunarizine, a calcium channel blocker: a new prophylactic drug in migraine. *Headache 1983; 23:* 70–74

40   Diamond S, Schenbaum H. Flunarizine, a calcium channel blocker, in the prophylactic treatment of migraine. *Headache 1983; 23:* 39–42

41   Louis P, Spierings ELH. Comparison of flunarizine (Sibelium®) and pizotifen (Sandomigran®) in migraine treatment: a double-blind study. *Cephalalgia 1982; 2:* 197–203

42   Van Nueten JM, Vanhoutte PM. Calcium entry blockers and vascular smooth muscle heterogeneity. *Fed Proc 1981; 40:* 2862–2865

43   Van Nueten JM, Vanhoutte PM. Selectivity of calcium antagonism and serotonin antagonism with respect to venous and arterial tissues. *Angiology 1981; 32:* 476–484

44   Toward R, Kazda S. The cellular mechanism of action of nimodipine (Bay e 9736), a new calcium antagonist. *Br J Pharmacol 1979; 67:* p409–p410

45   Gelmers HJ. Nimodipine, a new calcium antagonist, in the prophylactic treatment of migraine. *Headache 1983; 23:* 106–109

46   Andersson K-E, Edvinsson L, MacKenzie ET et al. Influence of extracellular calcium and calcium antagonists on contractions induced by potassium and prostaglandin $F_{2\alpha}$ in isolated cerebral and mesenteric arteries of the cat. *Br J Pharmac 1983; 79:* 135–140

47   Saxena PR. Agonists and antagonists of vascular receptors. *Adv Neurol 1982; 33:* 309–314

48   Godfraind T, Dieu D. The inhibition by flunarizine of the norepinephrine-evoked contraction and calcium influx in rat aorta and mesenteric arteries. *J Pharmacol Exp Ther 1981; 217:* 510–515

49   Van Nueten JM. Vasodilatation or inhibition of peripheral vasoconstriction? In Vanhoutte PM, Leusen I, eds. *Mechanisms of Vasodilation. Satellite Symposium 27th International Congress Physiological Science.* Basel: Karger. 1978: 137

50   Nielsen KC, Owman C. Contractile response and amine receptor mechanisms in isolated middle cerebral artery of the cat. *Brain Res 1971; 27:* 33–42

51   Fozard JR. The animal pharmacology of drugs used in the treatment of migraine. *J Pharm Pharmac 1975; 27:* 297–321

52   Pacha W, Salzmann R. Inhibition of the re-uptake of neuronally liberated noradrenaline and α-receptor blocking action of some ergot alkaloids. *Br Pharmacol Soc 1970:* 439P–440P

53   Amery WK, Waelkens J. Prevention of the last chance: an alternative pharmacological treatment of migraine. *Headache 1983; 23:* 37–38

54   Boccuni M, Fanciullacci M, Michelacci S, Sicuteri F. Impairment of postural reflex in migraine: possible role of dopamine receptors. In Corsine GU, Gessa GL, eds. *Apomorphine and Other Dopaminomimetics.* New York: Raven Press. 1981: 267

55   Bès A, Géraud G, Güell A, Arné-Bès MC. Hypersensibilité dopaminergique dans la migraine: un test diagnostique? *Nouv Presse Med 1982; 11:* 1475–1478

56   Deshmukh VD, Harper AM. The effect of serotonin on cerebral and extracerebral blood flow with possible implications in migraine. *Acta Neurol Scandinav 1973; 49:* 649–658

57 Sicuteri F. Vasoneuroactive substances and their implication in vascular pain. *Res Clin Stud Headache 1967; 1:* 6–45

58 Anthony M, Lance JW. The role of serotonin in migraine. In Pearse J, ed. *Modern Topics in Migraine.* London: William Heinemann Ltd. 1975: 107

59 Fozard JR. Basic mechanisms of antimigraine drugs. *Adv Neurol 1982; 33:* 295–307

60 Anthony M, Hinterberger H, Lance JW. The possible relationship of serotonin to the migraine syndrome. *Res Clin Stud Headache 1969; 2:* 29–59

61 Skärby T, Tfelt-Hansen P, Gjerris F et al. Characterization of 5-hydroxytryptamine receptors in human temporal arteries: comparison between migraine sufferers and nonsufferers. *Ann Neurol 1982; 12:* 272–277

62 Griffith SG, Lincoln J, Burnstock G. Serotonin as a neurotransmitter in cerebral arteries. *Brain Res 1982; 247:* 388–392

63 Shepherd JT, Vanhoutte PM, eds. *The Human Cardiovascular System, Facts and Concepts.* New York: Raven Press. 1979: 1

64 Saxena PR, van Houwelingen P, Bonta IL. The effects of mianserin hydrochloride on the vascular responses evoked by 5-hydroxytryptamine and related vasoactive substances. *Eur J Pharmacol 1971; 13:* 295–305

65 Toda N, Fujita Y. Responsiveness of isolated cerebral and peripheral arteries to serotonin, norepinephrine and transmural electrical stimulation. *Circ Res 1973; 33:* 98–104

66 Van Nueten JM. 5-hydroxytryptamine and precapillary vessels. *Fed Proc 1983; 42:* 223–227

67 Van Nueten JM, Janssen PAJ, Van Beek J et al. Vascular effects of ketanserin (R 41 468), a novel antagonist of 5-HT$_2$ serotonergic receptors. *J Pharmacol Exp Ther 1981; 218:* 217–230

68 Ekström-Jodal B, von Essen C, Häggendal E, Roos B-E. Effects of 5-hydroxytryptamine on the cerebral blood flow in the dog. *Acta Neurol Scandinav 1974; 50:* 27–38

69 Allen GS, Gold LHA, Chou SN et al. Cerebral arterial spasm. Part 3: In vivo intracisternal production of spasm by serotonin and blood and its reversal by phenoxybenzamine. *J Neurosurg 1974; 40:* 451–458

70 Van Neuten JM, Janssen PAJ, Vanhoutte PM. Pharmacological properties of serotonergic responses in vascular, bronchial and gastrointestinal smooth muscle. *Proceedings 4th International Symposium on Vascular Neuroeffector Mechanisms, Kyoto, Japan.* 1983: in press

71 Hurwitz R, Campbell RW, Gordon P, Haddy FJ. Interaction of serotonin with vasoconstrictor agents in the vascular bed of the denervated dog forelimb. *J Pharmacol Exp Ther 1961; 133:* 57–62

72 de la Lande IS, Cannell VA, Waterson JG. The interaction of serotonin and noradrenalin on the perfused artery. *Br J Pharm Pharmacol 1966; 28:* 255–272

73 Fozard JR. Drug interactions on an isolated artery. In Cumings JN, ed. *Background to Migraine.* London: William Heinemann. 1973: 150

74 Van Nueten JM, Janssen PAJ, De Ridder W, Vanhoutte PM. Interaction between 5-hydroxytryptamine and other vasoconstrictor substances in the isolated femoral artery of the rabbit; effect of ketanserin (R 41 468). *Eur J Pharmacol 1982; 77:* 281–287

75 Van Nueten JM. Serotonergic amplification mechanisms in vascular tissues. In De Clerck F, Vanhoutte PM, eds. *5-Hydroxytruptamine in Peripheral Reactions.* New York: Raven Press. 1982: 77

76 Crawford N. Plasma-free serotonin (5-hydroxytryptamine). *Clin Chim Acta 1963; 8:* 39–45

77 Vanhoutte PM. Effects of calcium entry blockers on tissue hypoxia. *J Cereb Blood Flow Metabol 1982; 2:* S42–S44

78 De Clerck F, David JL. Pharmacological control of platelet and red blood cell function in the microcirculation. *J Cardiovasc Pharmacol 1981; 3:* 1388–1412

79 De Clerck F, Van Nueten JM. Platelet-mediated vascular contractions: inhibition of the serotonergic component by ketanserin. *Thromb Res 1982; 27:* 713–727

80   De Clerck F, Van Nueten JM. Platelet-mediated vascular contractions. Inhibition by flunarizine, a calcium-entry blocker. *Biochem Pharmacol 1983; 32:* 765–771

81   Godfraind T, Miller RC. Actions of prostaglandin $F_{2\alpha}$ and noradrenaline on calcium exchange and contraction in rat mesenteric arteries and their sensitivity to calcium entry blockers. *Br J Pharmac 1982; 75:* 229–236

82   Forster C, Whalley ET. Vascular smooth muscle response to fibrinogen degradation products and 5-hydroxytryptamine: possible role in cerebral vasospasm in man. *Br J Clin Pharmac 1980; 10:* 231–236

83   Boisvert DPJ, Weir BKA, Overton TR et al. Cerebrovascular responses to subarchnoid blood and serotonin in the monkey. *J Neurosurg 1979; 50:* 441–448

84   Boullin DJ, Du Boulay GH, Rogers AT. Aetiology of cerebral arterial spasm following subarachnoid haemorrhage: evidence against a major involvement of 5-hydroxytryptamine in the production of acute spasm. *Br J Clin Pharmac 1978; 6:* 203–215

85   Watts C. Reserpine and cerebral vasospasm. *Stroke 1977; 8:* 112–114

86   Starling LM, Boullin DJ, Grahame-Smith DG et al. Responses of isolated human basilar arteries to 5-hydroxytryptamine, noradrenaline, serum, platelets, and erythrocytes. *J Neurol Neurosurgery Psychiatry 1975; 38:* 650–656

3

THE ROLE OF ARTERIOVENOUS SHUNTING IN MIGRAINE

E L H Spierings

Heyck's migraine shunt theory

Arteriovenous shunting as a factor in the pathogenesis of the migraine attack was postulated by Heyck in the 1950s [1]. In the English edition of his book [2], which appeared one year before his death in 1982, Heyck states that the notion evolved from his doubts concerning the correctness of Wolff's assumption that the migraine headache is caused by *general* vasodilatation [3]. Heyck's doubts originated from his observation that during the migraine attack the very large majority of patients look pale and show laxity of facial tissue tone, which, to put it in his own words, "definitely points to a condition of bloodlessness in the tissue". The fact that "pronounced migraine attacks are (also) accompanied by an increased filling, tension and pulsation of the major arterial branches" while "the major veins also stand out", made him conclude that during attacks of migraine "there is an increased blood flow in the major afferent and efferent vessels while at the same time the tissue (capillary) supply is deficient".

To corroborate his hypothesis, Heyck punctured in seven patients with distinct hemicranial migraine the external jugular vein and a peripheral artery to determine the regional arteriovenous oxygen content difference. Approximately 80 per cent of the blood flowing in the external jugular vein is derived from the non-cerebral tissues of the head [4], and it is the cranial non-cerebral circulation that is, as shown by Wolff [3], particularly involved in the pathogenesis of the migraine headache.

The results that Heyck obtained in his experiments are presented in Figure 1. They show that the arteriovenous oxygen content difference is significantly lower on the side of the headache when compared to the other side of the head. Furthermore, they demonstrate that, when administration of dihydroergotamine led to subsidence of the headache, this beneficial effect was associated with an increase and 'normalisation' of the arteriovenous oxygen content difference.

36

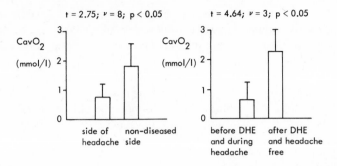

Figure 1. Arteriovenous oxygen content difference ($CavO_2$) over the cranial circulation. The venous samples were obtained from the external jugular vein. In the lefthand diagram the sides of the head are compared in cases of unilateral headache. In the righthand diagram the side of the head affected by the pain is studied before and after administration of dihydroergotamine (DHE) and subsidence of the headache. The data are obtained from Heyck [2, 3], are converted into SI units and are statistically analysed using the Student's t-test for unpaired and paired samples, respectively. (Reproduced from Spierings [5])

Heyck argues that the low arteriovenous oxygen content difference on the side of the headache *cannot* be due to general vasodilatation because of the pallor and the flaccid skin turgor that patients show during attacks of migraine and because the regional skin temperature is low, as has been observed by Lance and Anthony [6] using infra red thermography. Heyck sees only one explanation which could clear out 'the apparent contradictions in the behaviour of the large vessels compared to the state of tissue blood supply, namely, the assumption that AV shunts are formed in the vascular periphery allowing the blood to pass over directly from the arterial to the venous circulation". This is schematically illustrated in Figure 2.

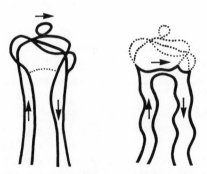

Figure 2. Heyck hypothesised that arteriovenous anastomoses or shunts are intimately involved in the vascular changes underlying the migraine attack, and that, while of minor importance under normal conditions (left), the arteriovenous anastomoses open widely at the onset of the attack (right). (Reproduced from Prusiński [7])

37

Also with regard to the pathogenesis of the aura symptoms of classical migraine, Heyck postulated the involvement of arteriovenous anastomoses, as their opening may, through capillary steal, lead to tissue ischaemia and the aura symptoms are thought to be due to cerebral ischaemia. To find support for this claim Heyck measured the arteriovenous oxygen content difference over the *cerebral* circulation, sampling blood from the internal jugular vein, in two patients who exhibited symptoms of confusion and disorientation during their migraine headache. In both cases he found the arteriovenous oxygen content difference to be considerably low when compared to normal, which again indicated to him an increased shunting of blood.

Pallor, skin colour and blood flow changes

It is hard to conceive that Harold Wolff, an astute clinician who studied many patients during attacks of migraine and who himself was a migraineur, had never noticed that when patients change colour in relation to the attack they usually turn pale and hardly ever become red. Still, this fact has never prevented him from postulating that the migraine headache is caused by general vasodilatation, and I agree with him for two reasons. First of all, because the migraine pain is mostly located in the temporal or frontotemporal regions of the head and rarely affects the face. This is probably due to the fact that the frontal branch of the superficial temporal artery is preferentially involved in the process of migrainous vasodilatation. Secondly, because even if the migraine pain is located in the face, and it then usually affects the orbital or maxillary regions, it may be caused by dilatation of deeply located vessels, like the choroidal plexus or the maxillary artery, thereby not being able to bring about a change in skin colour.

A different behaviour in relation to the migraine attack of the superficial vasculature of the face, or at least of that of the forehead, from that of the side of the head is also suggested by the results of the studies summarised in Table I. The studies focused on the haemodynamic changes that take place during the migraine attack in the cranial non-cerebral circulation. Their results suggest that these changes consist of a decreased flow to the forehead and of an increased flow to the lateral side of the head, which is a pattern of changes also true for cluster headache [12].

However, even if Heyck is right as far as the paleness and the vasodilatation is concerned, it is still questionable whether his assumption that pallor of the skin indicates decreased capillary flow and is compatible with increased arteriovenous shunting is correct. As has been shown in a study, skin colour is chiefly determined by the state of filling of the subpapillary venous plexuses [13]. Arteriovenous anastomoses, if present, probably also drain into these veins which would make their opening result in increased filling of the plexuses and, therefore, associated with reddening rather than with whitening of the skin.

38

TABLE I. Results of the studies on the behaviour of the cranial non-cerebral circulation during attacks of migraine

Authors	Technique	Area or structures studied	Findings (interpretation)	Laterality related to headache
Tunis and Wolff [8,9]	Pulse wave registration	Superficial temporal artery	⬈ amplitude of pulsations (⬈ flow)	Not stated
Elkind et al [10]	^{24}Na clearance	Frontotemporal skin	⬈ clearance (⬈ cutaneous blood flow)	Ipsilateral
Lance and Anthony [6]	Thermography	Forehead	8/13 (62%) skin temperature: ipsilateral < contralateral (⬊ flow)	ipsilateral
Sakai and Meyer [11]	^{133}Xe inhalation	Lateral side of the skull	⬈ extracerebral flow index (⬈ blood volume and/or flow)	Not stated

Arteriovenous anastomoses or shunts

Sucquet [14], in a study published in 1862, was the first to provide indirect evidence for the presence of arteriovenous anastomoses in man. In regard to the head, he located the arteriovenous anastomoses in the lips, nose, forehead, cheeks and ears. However, Berlinerblau [15] and Hoyer [16], who applied the same resin injection technique as Sucquet, were unable to confirm his observation. Still, more recent studies on the presence of arteriovenous anastomoses in the human head have not only confirmed Sucquet's findings [17–21], but also extended them to the deep pial plexus of the brain [22] and to the dura mater [23, 24].

Despite an extremely thorough search through the literature, I found no indication pointing to the presence of arteriovenous anastomoses at the site of the head mostly affected by migraine, i.e. the frontotemporal and temporal regions. One could also suppose that the opening of arteriovenous anastomoses at that location occurs at the level of the dura mater where arteriovenous anastomoses have been demonstrated to be present in abundance by Rowbotham and Little [23]. However, then the swelling up of blood vessels of both arterial and venous nature of the temple, as is seen in severe cases of migraine, would go unexplained because the dura mater is vascularised predominantly by the middle meningeal artery which is a branch of the maxillary artery.

Arteriovenous oxygen content difference

I have also not been able to find any indication in the literature with regard to the significance of the arteriovenous oxygen content difference in relation to the shunting of blood through arteriovenous anastomoses. This lack of information is probably due to the fact that, until the advent of the radioactive microsphere techique [25–26] more than a decade ago, it has been virtually impossible to accurately study arteriovenous anastomotic blood flow.

In the radioactive microsphere technique small plastic spheres are used that are labelled with a radioactive tracer and that are introduced directly into the arterial circulation. Provided that microspheres and blood mix homogeneously, the microspheres will be then distributed throughout the tissues in proportion to the local blood flow and within the tissues over the capillaries and the arterio-venous anastomoses, if the latter are present. Due to the fact that their walls contain a thick multilayered and often sphincter-like musculature with a dense innervation, the diameter of the arteriovenous anastomoses varies but is in general larger than 20μm [27], making them wider than the capillaries which measure from 5–10μm [28]. Therefore, when microspheres of approximately 15μm diameter are used it is possible to distinguish capillary flow from flow through arteriovenous anastomoses because the microspheres entering the capillaries will become trapped in them while those entering the arteriovenous anastomoses will pass through them. The microspheres which pass through the arteriovenous anastomoses and appear in the venous circulation, will ultimately become trapped in the lungs, therefore not re-entering the arterial system in any appreciable number [29–31]. This is schematically illustrated in Figure 3.

In order to find out whether the mode of action of antimigraine drugs is compatible with Heyck's migraine shunt theory, we employed the 15μm radioactive microsphere technique to study the effect of these drugs on the distribution of carotid blood flow over the capillaries and the arteriovenous anastomoses [32–35, 37]. In the experiments, which were performed in cats, the microspheres were directly injected into the carotid artery through a cannula which was placed retrogradely into the lingual artery. It has to be remembered here that in the cat the internal carotid artery is a vestigial structure, reduced to a fibrotic string, and that the brain receives blood not only from the vertebral but also from the external carotid artery. The contribution to the circulation of the brain by the external carotid arteries, however, amounts to only approximately 15 per cent of total carotid blood flow as we have been able to determine in our experiments (Figure 4). In the experiments we measured the carotid blood flow by means of an electromagnetic sine wave flow probe placed around the artery.

Apart from the carotid blood flow and the distribution of carotid blood flow over the capillaries and the arteriovenous anastomoses we determined in the same experiments the arteriovenous oxygen content difference over the cranial

40

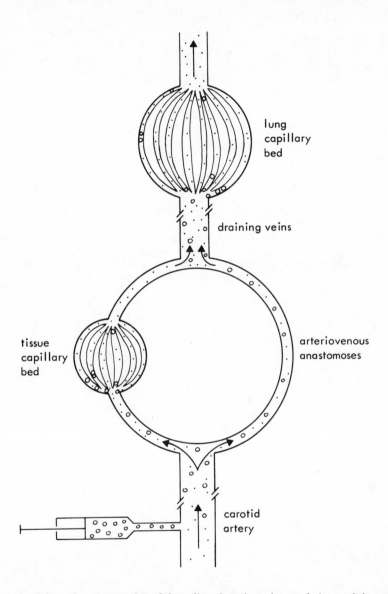

Figure 3. Schematic representation of the radioactive microsphere technique as it is applied to the study of the distribution of carotid blood flow over the capillaries and the arterio-venous anastomoses. The dots represent the red blood cells and the open circles the 15μm isotope-labelled plastic microspheres. (Reproduced from Spierings and Saxena [32])

circulation. Like Heyck, we drew the venous samples from the external jugular vein but through a cannula which was inserted into the transverse (facial) vein in the direction of the external jugular vein. Forty experiments were performed in this way and the data obtained from the base-line measurements were used to

41

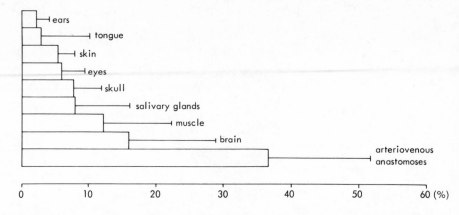

Figure 4. Distribution of carotid blood flow in the cat as determined by direct injection of 15μm microspheres into the carotid artery. Carotid blood flow averaged 21.2 ± 12.7 (SD) ml/min (n = 40). The data are expressed as means ± SD. (Reproduced from Spierings [5])

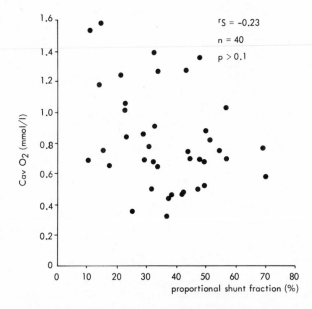

Figure 5. Scatter diagram in which the arteriovenous oxygen content difference ($CavO_2$) over the cranial circulation with the venous sample drawn from the external jugular vein, is plotted against the proportion of carotid blood flow shunted through the arteriovenous anastomoses as determined by the 15μm microsphere technique. The Spearman rank test was used to calculate the correlation coefficient r_S. (Reproduced from Spierings [5])

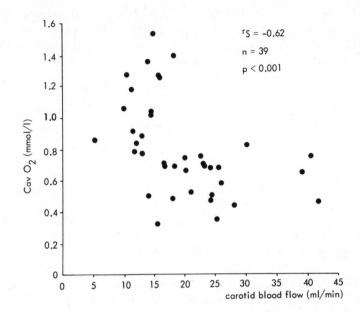

Figure 6. Scatter diagram in which the arteriovenous oxygen content difference ($CavO_2$) over the cranial circulation with the venous sample drawn from the external jugular vein, is plotted against carotid blood flow. One pair of data (80.7ml/min, 1.58mmol/L) has been omitted because of the excessively high carotid blood flow value. The Spearman rank test was used to calculate the correlation coefficient r_S. (Reproduced from Spierings [5])

analyse for correlations with the arteriovenous oxygen content difference. The analysis revealed an absence of correlation ($r_S = -0.23$) between the arteriovenous oxygen content difference and the proportion or fraction of carotid blood flow shunted through the arteriovenous anastomoses (Figure 5). In contrast, the arteriovenous oxygen content difference showed a significant (negative) correlation ($r_S = -0.62$) with carotid blood flow (Figure 6). Multiplication of the carotid blood flow by the shunt fraction in order to obtain the absolute amount of blood shunted through the arteriovenous anastomoses decreased the correlation coefficient to -0.51.

Correlation data and Heyck's observations

If the above presented correlation data obtained in experiments in cats are also true for man, they imply that Heyck's observations on the changes in arteriovenous oxygen content difference reflect changes in arterial blood flow rather than changes in the distribution of flow over the capillaries and the arteriovenous anastomoses. In this way his finding that the arteriovenous oxygen content

43

difference is lower on the side of the headache when compared to the non-affected side of the head (lefthand diagram in Figure 1) indicates increased arterial blood flow on the side of the pain. If arteriovenous anastomoses are present at the location of the headache, the increased arterial blood flow will be associated with increased flow through the arteriovenous anastomoses, but only as a secondary reaction. Such an increase in arteriovenous anastomotic blood flow is different from the one that would result from opening of arterio-venous anastomoses because it is *not* associated with a decrease in capillary perfusion, the latter being an essential part of Heyck's theory.

The above reasoning can also be applied to the observed increase in arterio-venous oxygen content difference resulting from the administration of dihydro-ergotamine (righthand diagram in Figure 1). Again, if the correlations found in the experiments in cats are also true for man, the increase in arteriovenous oxygen content difference following administration of the drug is a reflection of a decrease in arterial blood flow. This conclusion has to be drawn, although in the same experiments from which the correlation data are derived, we observed an effect of dihydroergotamine on the distribution of carotid blood flow compatible with a constrictor action of the drug on the arteriovenous anastomoses (Figure 7). However, again this effect correlated only very poorly with the effect of the drug on the arteriovenous oxygen content difference (Figure 8), which, as shown by Heyck in migraine patients, consists of an increase. In the

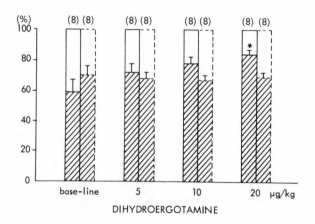

Figure 7. Effect of dihydroergotamine, 5, 10 and 20μg/kg i.v., on the distribution of carotid blood flow over the capillaries *(striped bars)* and the arteriovenous anastomoses *(open bars)*. The distribution was determined by the 15μm microsphere technique. The data are expressed as means ± SEM. Both the control group *(dashed-lined bars)* and the experimental group *(solid-lined bars)* consist of eight animals. A significant difference (p ≤ 0.05) between the means of the two groups is indicated by an asterisk and is calculated according to the two-tailed Wilcoxon rank sum test. (Reproduced from Spierings [36])

44

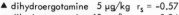

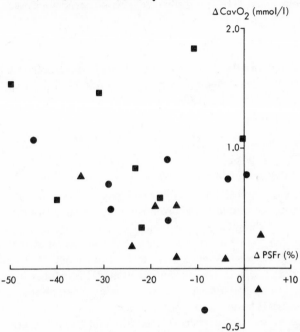

Figure 8. Scatter diagram in which the effect of dihydroergotamine, 5, 10 and 20μg/kg i.v., on the distribution of carotid blood flow, as presented in Figure 7, is plotted against that on the arteriovenous oxygen content difference ($CavO_2$), as presented in Figure 9. The Spearman rank sum test was used to calculate the correlation coefficients r_S. (Reproduced from Spierings [36])

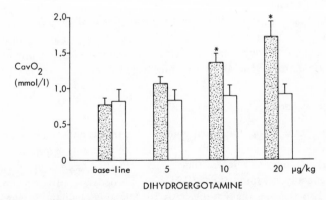

Figure 9. Effect of dihydroergotamine, 5, 10 and 20μg/kg i.v., on the arteriovenous oxygen content difference ($CavO_2$) over the cranial circulation. The venous samples were obtained from the external jugular vein. The data are expressed as means ± SEM. Both the control group *(open bars)* and the experimental group *(speckled bars)* consist of eight animals. A significant difference ($p < 0.05$) between the means of the two groups is indicated by an asterisk and is calculated according to the two-tailed Wilcoxon rank sum test. (Reproduced from Spierings and Saxena [37])

above described experiments we were able to confirm this observation by Heyck and in addition demonstrated that the effect of dihydroergotamine on the arteriovenous oxygen content difference is dose-dependent, as shown in Figure 9.

Migraine aura and arteriovenous shunting

As mentioned above, Heyck also incriminated the arteriovenous anastomoses in the pathogenesis of the transient neurological symptoms that precede or, occasionally, occur simultaneously with the headache in cases of classical migraine. In doing so he assumed that:

1. opening of arteriovenous anastomoses leads, through capillary steal, to tissue ischaemia, and

2. the symptoms of the migraine aura are caused by cerebral ischaemia.

The observation that the arteriovenous oxygen content difference over the cerebral circulation was low when compared to normal in two patients who were confused and disoriented during their migraine headache Heyck presented as support for the 'aura part' of his theory. However, as far as the significance of the low arteriovenous oxygen content difference is concerned, certainly we can repeat what was said in the previous section. Namely, that if the correlations as observed in cats are also true for man, the low arteriovenous oxygen content difference reflects an increase in arterial blood flow rather than a redistribution of flow due to opening of arteriovenous anastomoses and resulting in a decrease in capillary perfusion.

It is also becoming increasingly likely that the aura symptoms of classical migraine are *not* caused by cerebral ischaemia, as suggested by Wolff [3], but that they are the result of a primary neuronal process. Of this process Milner [38] has suggested that it consists of a spreading depression heralded by neuronal excitation, which is a kind of neuronal event that *cannot* be triggered by cerebral ischaemia [39]. The result of the cerebral blood flow studies performed during the last couple of years using the Xenon-clearance technique provide support for such a 'neuronal view' on the pathogenesis of the aura symptoms [40, 41].

Concluding remarks

Heyck's hypothesis on the involvement of arteriovenous anastomoses in the pathogenesis of the migraine headache and of the aura symptoms that may precede it, presents an interesting concept and a fascinating alternative to Wolff's generally accepted theory [3]. On the occasion of the symposium on Cerebral Hypoxia in the Pathogenesis of Migraine, held in Brighton in the autumn of 1981, I critically compared both theories as far as they deal with the migraine aura [36]. My conclusion then was that there is actually no evidence that could support Heyck's assumption that opening of arteriovenous anastomoses

46

is the basic process underlying the aura symptoms, and I still maintain this opinion.

Furthermore, as I have shown in this paper, the grounds on which the 'headache part' of Heyck's theory rests, including both clinical observations and experimental data, are not very solid. For example, it is questionable whether pallor of the skin is compatible with increased shunting of blood through arteriovenous anastomoses; also there is no evidence available in the literature that arteriovenous anastomoses are present in the frontotemporal and temporal regions of the head where the migraine pain is mostly felt; and finally the significance of the changes in arteriovenous oxygen content difference in relation to arteriovenous shunting has never been considered great [42] and is further diminished by our above presented observations in cats.

The fact that, as we have demonstrated, a major anti-migraine drug like ergotamine acts on the microcirculation in a way that suggests closure of arteriovenous anastomoses [32, 33], which has also been observed by Stolzenburg in histological studies back in the 1930s [43], does not, as I think, diminish the significance of my statements. The reason for this is that our experiments were not performed in man but in cat and that the effect of the drug was not correlated with its anti-migraine action. Therefore, the results of our experiments justify in my opinion only the following statement: They provide a mode of action for ergotamine on which its potent anti-migraine effect possibly depends, provided that opening of arteriovenous anastomoses plays the by Heyck suggested role in the pathogenesis of the migraine attack. However, it remains to be seen whether Heyck's fiction will ever turn into fact.

Summary

As an alternative to Wolff's theory, Heyck proposed the involvement of arteriovenous anastomoses in the pathogenesis of the migraine attack. However, there is no evidence that arteriovenous shunts are present at the site of the head mostly affected by the migraine pain, i.e. the frontotemporal and temporal regions. In addition, it is questionable whether changes in arteriovenous oxygen content difference, as provided by Heyck in support of his theory, are a reliable expression of changes in the proportion of blood flow shunting through the arteriovenous anastomoses. Using the radioactive microsphere technique, we found a negative correlation between the arteriovenous oxygen content difference and the proportion of carotid blood flow shunted through the arteriovenous anastomoses. Even the fact that we showed that ergotamine closes arteriovenous anastomoses in the cranial circulation of the cat, does not prove Heyck's theory. In order to be useful as an argument in favour of Heyck's theory, the action of ergotamine on the arteriovenous shunting has to be demonstrated in man and be shown to correlate with its potent antimigraine effect.

47

Acknowledgment

I would like to thank my wife, Malina, for valuable assistance in the preparation of this manuscript.

References

1 Heyck H. *Der Kopfschmerz*. Stuttgart: Georg Thieme Verlag. 1958
2 Heyck H. *Headache and Facial Pain*. Stuttgart: Georg Thieme Verlag. 1981
3 Dalessio DJ. *Wolff's Headache and Other Head Pain*. New York: Oxford University Press. 1980
4 Shenkin HA, Harmel MH, Kety SS. Dynamic anatomy of the cerebral circulation. *Arch Neurol Psychiatry 1948; 60:* 240–252
5 Spierings ELH. *The Pathophysiology of the Migraine Attack*. Alphen aan den Rijn/ Brussels: Stafleu's Wetenschappelijke Uitgeversmaatschappij. 1980
6 Lance JW, Anthony M. Thermographic studies in vascular headache. *Med J Aust 1971; 1:* 240–243
7 Prusiński A. *Bóle głowy, ich przyczyny i leczenie*. Warsaw: Państwowy Zakład Wydawnictw Lekarskich. 1973
8 Tunis MM, Wolff HG. Analysis of cranial artery pulse waves in patients with vascular headache of the migraine type. *Am J Med Sci 1952; 224:* 565–568
9 Tunis MM, Wolff HG. Studies on headache: Long-term observations of the reactivity of the cranial arteries in subjects with vascular headache of the migraine type. *Arch Neurol Psychiatry 1953; 70:* 551–557
10 Elkind AH, Friedman AP, Grossman J. Cutaneous blood flow in vascular headache of the migraine type. *Neurology 1964; 14:* 24–30
11 Sakai F, Meyer JS. Regional cerebral hemodynamics during migraine and cluster headaches measured by the ^{133}Xe inhalation method. *Headache 1978; 18:* 122–132
12 Spierings ELH. Craniovascular accompaniments of the vascular headache of the migraine type. *Headache 1979; 19:* 397–399
13 Wetzel NC, Zotterman Y. On differences in the vascular colouration of various regions of the normal skin. *Heart 1926; 13:* 357–367
14 Sucquet JP. *D'une circulation dérivative dans les membres et dans la tête chez l'homme*. Paris: A Delahaya. 1862
15 Berlinerblau F. Ueber den directen Uebergang von Arterien in Venen. *Arch Anat Physiol (Lpz) 1875:* 177–188
16 Hoyer H. Ueber unmittelbare Einmündung kleinster Arterien in Gefässäste venösen Charakters. *Arch Mikr Anat 1877; 13:* 603–644
17 Märk W. Ueber arterio-venöse Anastomosen, Gefässperren und Gefässe mit epitheloiden Zellen beim Menschen. *Z Mikr Anat Forsch 1941; 50:* 392–445
18 Patzelt V. Ueber arterio-venöse Anastomosen in der Nase, Oberlippe und Zunge des Menschen. *Z Mikr Anat Forsch 1943; 54:* 207–218
19 Prichard MML, Daniel PM. Arterio-venous anastomoses in the human external ear. *Am J Anat 1956; 90:* 309–317
20 Temesrékási D. Mikroskopischer Bau und Funktion der Schwellgewebes der Nasenmuschel des Menschen. *A Mikr Anat Forsch 1969; 80:* 219–229
21 Cauna N. The fine structure of the arteriovenous anastomosis and its nerve supply in the human nasal respiratory mucosa. *Anat Res 1970; 168:* 9–22
22 Rowbotham FG, Little E. A new concept of the circulation and the circulations of the brain. *Br J Surg 1965; 52:* 539–542
23 Rowbotham GF, Little E. New concepts on the aetiology and vascularisation of meningiomata; the mechanisms of migraine; the chemical processes of the cerebro-spinal fluid; and the formation of collections of blood or fluid in the subdural space. *Br J Surg 1965; 52:* 21–24

24   Kerber CW, Newton TH. The macro and microvasculature of the dura mater. *Neuroradiology 1973; 6:* 175—179

25   Hales JRS. Radioactive microsphere techniques for studies of the circulation. *Clin Exp Pharmacol Physiol 1974; Suppl 1:* 31—46

26   Heymann MA, Payne BD, Hoffman JIE et al. Blood flow measurements with radionuclide-labelled particles. *Prog Cardiovasc Dis 1977; 20:* 55—79

27   Grant RT, Bland EF. Observations on arteriovenous anastomoses in human skin and in the bird's foot with special reference to the reaction to cold. *Heart 1932; 15:* 385—411

28   Berne RM, Levy NM. *Cardiovascular Physiology.* St Louis: CV Mosby Co. 1972

29   Kaihara S, Van Heerden PD, Migita T et al. Measurement of distribution of cardiac output. *J Appl Physiol 1968; 25:* 696—700

30   Warren DJ, Ledingham JGG. Measurement of cardiac output distribution using microspheres. Some practical and theoretical considerations. *Cardiovasc Res 1974; 8:* 570—581

31   Fan FC, Schuessler GB, Chen RYZ et al. Determinations of blood flow and shunting of 9- and 15-μm spheres in regional beds. *Am J Physiol 1979; 237:* H25—H33

32   Spierings ELH, Saxena PR. The action of ergotamine on the distribution of carotid blood flow — the migraine shunt theory revisited. *Headache 1980; 20:* 143—145

33   Spierings ELH, Saxena PR. Effect of ergotamine on cranial arteriovenous shunting in experiments with constant flow perfusion. *Eur J Pharmacol 1979; 56:* 31—37

34   Spierings ELH, Saxena PR. Effect of isometheptene on the distribution and shunting of 15μm microspheres throughout the cephalic circulation of the cat. *Headache 1980; 20:* 103—106

35   Spierings ELH, Saxena PR. Antimigraine drugs and cranial arteriovenous shunting in the cat. *Neurology 1980; 30:* 696—701

36   Spierings ELH. Arterial vasoconstriction versus arteriovenous shunting in the migraine aura. In Rose FC, Amery WK, eds. *Cerebral Hypoxia in the Pathogenesis of Migraine.* London: Pitman. 1982: 12—21

37   Spierings ELH, Saxena PR. Pharmacology of arteriovenous anastomoses. In Critchley M, Friedman A, Gorini S et al, eds. *Headache: Physiopathological and Clinical Concepts.* New York: Raven Press. 1982: 291—294

38   Milner PM. Note on a possible correspondence between the scotomas of migraine and spreading depression of Leão. *EEG Clin Neurophysiol 1958; 10:* 705

39   Leão AAP. Further observations on the spreading depression of activity in the cerebral cortex. *J Neurophysiol 1947; 10:* 409—419

40   Olesen J, Larsen B, Lauritzen M. Focal hyperemia followed by spreading oligemia and impaired activation of rCBF in classic migraine. *Ann Neurol 1981; 9:* 344—352

41   Lauritzen M, Skyhøj Olsen T, Lassen NA et al. Changes in regional cerebral blood flow during the course of classic migraine attacks. *Ann Neurol 1983; 13:* 633—641

42   Marshall J. Cerebral blood flow in migraine. In Greene R, ed. *Current Concepts in Migraine Research.* New York: Raven Press. 1978; 131—139

43   Stolzenburg HJ. Experimentelle Untersuchungen über das Verhalten der arteriovenösen Anastomosen. *Z Mikr Anat Forsch 1937; 41:* 348—358

4

THE EFFECTS OF ANTIMIGRAINE DRUGS ON ARTERIOVENOUS ANASTOMOSES*

P R Saxena

Introduction

The idea that antimigraine drugs may affect the calibre of arteriovenous (A-V) anastomoses (AVAs) originates from the astute observations of the late Professor Hartwig Heyck [1,2]. He pointed out that the occurrence of a vasodilation in the branches of the carotid artery, proposed as the main cause of migraine headache [3,4], is paradoxical to the presence of facial pallor and tissue laxity in the vast majority of patients. Instead, Heyck [1,2] and, later, Rowbotham and Little [5] proposed that the main feature of migraine attacks, whatever be the original trigger factor(s), is an opening of AVAs which would shunt blood away from the capillary (nutrient) bed directly into the veins. Although Heyck [1,2] supported this view by demonstrating that during migraine headaches the oxygen content of external jugular venous blood significantly increases, it is also pertinent to evaluate this hypothesis by examining the pharmacological effects of antimigraine drugs on AVAs. In this presentation I will summarise such studies, most of which have been performed in my laboratory. At the outset it is, however, essential to provide background information about the methodological and physiological aspects of AVAs so that the readers can better evaluate the results presented.

RADIOACTIVE MICROSPHERE METHOD FOR THE STUDY OF AVAs

The AVAs, which form smooth muscle-containing precapillary communications between the arterial and venous sides of the circulation in many areas of the body [6,7], have been studied by several methods. These include histological preparations [8,9], a direct observation under microscope in a living animal

---

* Dedicated to Professor Dr Hartwig Heyck, who died on October 1, 1982

[10], the use of diffusible and non-diffusible tracers [11,12] and the appearance of particles of known size, such as the glass beads, in the venous blood [13,14]. The last method, however, produced equivocal results due to sedimentation and non-uniformity in the size of the particles and the problems in counting. The availability of plastic microspheres, labelled with radioactive tracers, in several uniform sizes has overcome these difficulties and many investigators have started employing such spheres for a *quantitative* estimation of A-V shunting [see 15–17].

General principle of the microsphere method

When radioactive microspheres of a proper size are injected into an arterial blood stream, they mix with the blood homogeneously and are distributed to the various tissues in proportion to the blood flow. Although a *complete* entrapment of the spheres in the peripheral circulation on their first passage is stated as a major requirement of the method [16,18], such a strict requirement, besides being unattainable for tissues (skin, ears) where a significant number of large AVAs (<60μm diameter) exist [6–10,19,20], applies only to the measurement of *total* (capillary plus non-capillary) tissue blood flow. Microspheres of practically all sizes that have been used do *shunt* to the venous side [13,15,16].

Significance of microsphere shunting

The significance of A-V shunting of microspheres can be evaluated if one knows the relative diameters of the vessels connecting the arterial and venous sides of the circulation (capillaries, preferential thoroughfare channels and AVAs) and of the vessels where microspheres of different sizes get impacted. The diameter of capillaries, examined in many tissues and in many species, is less than 10μm [21–24]. The preferential thoroughfare channels, often defined as the distal (endothelial) portion of the metarterioles [25], in the tissues where they are present (e.g. the mesentery, tongue, skeletal muscles) have a diameter between 8–18μm [21]. The diameter of AVAs varies considerably (5μm to over 100μm) but is generally greater than 25μm (6,7,19,21]. The exact diameter of the vessels where microspheres get impacted has also been measured. In the cheek pouch of the anaesthetised hamster, Dickhoner et al [26] found that microspheres of 9, 15 and 24μm diameter (D_m) impact in vessels having mean diameters (D_v) of 11.5, 27.7 and 42.3 respectively. A comparison of the above values suggests that microspheres with a diameter of 10μm and above appear in the venous side mainly via relatively wide AVAs. Thus, the proportion of microspheres appearing in the venous blood draining an organ, or detected in tissues which serve as a sieve for a region (lungs and liver) can be used as an *index* of *non-capillary* (non-nutrient) blood flow shunted via AVAs. On the other hand, the microspheres trapped in tissues will, in practice, provide blood flow values

51

somewhere between *capillary* (nutrient) and *total* flows. The extent of the contribution of non-capillary blood flow to tissue blood flow, as well as to the venous drainage shall depend on the relative diameters of AVAs in the particular tissues and the sphere size used.

Sites from where the microspheres shunt

Several studies have shown that microspheres of 15μm and larger do not appear in venous blood draining the brain [15,18,27], heart [16,27,28], kidneys [27, 29], gastrointestinal tract [27,30] and the skeletal muscles and bones applied by the femoral artery [31]. Microspheres do, however, shunt across the canine femoral circulation [15,31] and this has been localised in the skin and paws [31]. The most A-V shunting has been found in the carotid circulation of several species; the fraction of 15μm spheres injected into the common carotid artery was 34 to 52 per cent in cats [32–35], 41 per cent in dogs [36] and about 80 per cent in pigs [29]. In more recent experiments [37] we have determined the distribution of microspheres of four different sizes, 10, 15, 25, 35μm diameter, in the common carotid arterial bed of the pig (Table I). It should be

TABLE I. Per cent (mean ± SEM) of common carotid blood distributed to head tissues in seven pigs

| | Microsphere size (μm) | | | |
	10	15	25	35
Lungs (AVAs)	84.1±2.3	83.6±2.3	81.6±1.8[ab]	68.2±2.3[abc]
Brain	1.1±0.6	1.2±0.6	1.2±0.6	1.2±0.6
Ears	0.6±0.2	0.5±0.1	0.5±0.1	1.7±0.2[abc]
Skin	0.8±0.2	0.7±0.2	2.7±0.5[ab]	14.4±2.7[abc]
Skeletal muscles	4.2±0.8	4.3±0.8	3.9±0.7	4.2±0.7
Tongue	1.3±0.2	1.4±0.3	1.6±0.3[ab]	1.6±0.3[ab]
Bones	3.6±0.9	3.8±1.0	3.9±1.0	3.8±1.0
Eyes	0.9±0.1	1.2±0.2[a]	1.4±0.2[ab]	1.4±0.3[ab]
Salivary glands	2.0±0.7	2.1±0.7	1.9±0.7	1.9±0.7

a, b and c denote comparisons (p<0.05) with values obtained with microspheres of 10, 15 and 25μm diameters, respectively (paired t-test). Data from Saxena and Verdouw [37]

noted that there is an inverse relationship between the sphere size and the AVA-flow. Furthermore, since blood flow distributed to the tongue, eye and, in particular, to the skin and ears were higher with spheres of larger size than with smaller ones, it seems that in the pig the AVAs are located in these tissues. However, they may also be present in the nasal mucosa [38], rete mirabile [39] and dura mater [5].

52

SOME PHYSIOLOGICAL ASPECTS OF AVAs

Innervation of AVAs

There is ample histological evidence that AVAs have a dense peripheral innervation comprising mainly afferent (sensory), cholinergic and adrenergic fibres [7,40–42]. In addition, a non-adrenergic non-cholinergic innervation has been described [43] which may be purinergic in nature [44]. The exact role that these nerves play in the regulation of blood flow through AVAs is as yet not clearly understood. Though acetylcholine causes a widening of the calibre of AVAs [7], both sympathetic nerve stimulation [38,45,46] and noradrenaline [31,45,47,48] decrease and phentolamine [31,47,48] increases AVA-flow. The beta-adrenergic agonist isoprenaline either does not modify [31,47] or only slightly increases [48] AVA-flow in dogs, chicken and sheep. However, in the human digital AVAs there seems to be a distinct beta-drenergic vasodilator mechanism that may be humorally activated but has no functional role in modulating sympathetic vasoconstriction [12]. The AVAs normally remain under a tonic adrenergic vasoconstrictor influence [31,47,48] which diminishes during heat-induced vasodilation [48]. Apart from this passive vasodilation, the AVAs also seem to possess an active neurogenic vasodilatory mechanism. After adrenergic blockade, stimulation of foot nerves in chicken and ducks causes vasodilation [47,49] which cannot be attenuated by blockers of cholinergic, beta-adrenergic or histaminergic receptors [49]. Since the non-adrenergic non-cholinergic vesicles found in association with AVAs resemble purinergic vesicles [44] and since ATP is quite potent in increasing AVA-flow in the chicken foot [47], the non-adrenergic non-cholinergic vasodilation may be operating via ATP (or an allied substance) released from the purinergic nerves.

5-Hydroxytryptamine (5-HT)

Constriction of AVAs by 5-HT

Apart from the neurohumoral agents described above, AVAs can be constricted by 5-HT. In a preliminary study, it was shown that the amine decreased the number of glass spheres appearing in the fluid perfusing the isolated rabbit ear [50]. Subsequently, Saxena et al [51] found that intravenous administration of 5-HT in the rabbits decreases the proportion of microspheres found in the lungs (after left atrial injection), which apart from a small bronchial arterial component [52], mainly represents peripheral A-V shunting. Furthermore, the drug also reduces microsphere shunting in the common carotid arterial bed of cats [29, 32]. Lastly, intracarotid infusion of 5-HT in the pig decreases the AVA-fraction of carotid blood flow but increases its fraction distributed to the extracerebral tissues (Figure 1), mainly the skin and ears [29].

53

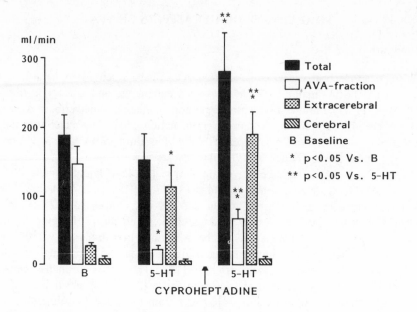

Figure 1. Modification by cyproheptadine ($1mg/kg^{-1}$/i.v.) on the effects of intracarotid infusions of 5-HT ($2\mu g/kg^{-1}/min^{-1}$) on the distribution of carotid artery blood flow into AVA, extracerebral and cerebral fractions in the pig. Data from Saxena and Verdouw [29]

Types of receptors for 5-HT

Cyproheptadine, which blocks D-receptors for 5-HT [53] – or the 5-HT$_2$-receptors according to the present-day terminology [54,55] – completely reverses the effect of 5-HT on the total carotid blood flow. However, the vasoconstrictor response of AVAs is only partially attenuated and the vasodilatory response is enhanced (Figure 1). These results show that 5-HT causes vasoconstriction of the large arteries via D (5-HT$_2$)-receptors which are only partly involved in the constriction of AVAs caused by 5-HT. A major part of the vasoconstriction in these non-nutrient vessels and the vasodilation in the extracerebral tissues are mediated by 'atypical' 5-HT receptors [29] that may perhaps be of the 5-HT$_1$ type [56]. In our recent studies (Verdouw and Saxena, unpublished) we have confirmed the above view. Both methysergide and ketanserin [57] behave like cyproheptadine in the carotid region against 5-HT. The constriction of AVAs via 'atypical' 5-HT receptors also explains why drugs of the methysergide type, quite potent in antagonising the contraction of isolated arterial segments [58], do not effectively attenuate the 5-HT-induced enhancement in the carotid vascular resistance observed in vivo [59,60]. The in vitro studies, though quite elegant for receptor characterisation, are limited, due to technical feasibility, only to the large arteries where the D-type receptors are present. In the *in vivo* studies, one deals mainly with the AVAs and arterioles where the 'atypical' receptors are located [29].

Possible role of 5-HT in circulation

The vascular pharmacology of 5-HT-contractions of large arteries [61,62], AVAs [29,30] and some veins [59], and a dilatation of arterioles [29,61], points to a possible role of 5-HT in the local regulation of blood flow (Figure 2). Despite a

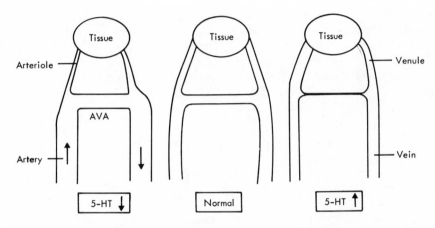

Figure 2. Schematic representation of the hypothesised role of 5-HT in the fractionation of carotid arterial blood into nutrient (arterioles and capillaries) and non-nutrient (AVA) parts. The arrows in the arteries and vein show the direction of blood flow, whereas those next to '5-HT' denote a decrease and increase in the concentration of the amine in blood

rather low plasma 5-HT concentration the cranial circulation, where the vessels are quite sensitive to 5-HT [63] and where AVAs are in abundance [29,32–37], may be selectively affected. When the plasma concentration of this amine becomes elevated, the tissues may receive enough blood despite a constriction of large arteries because the AVAs may then close. In case the concentration of 5-HT falls, as it does during migraine attacks [64], large arteries and AVAs may dilate while the arterioles constrict. This would allow AVA-flow to increase at the expense of tissue (nutrient) blood flow – a situation that seems to be present in migraine [1,2]. It is pertinent to point out that administration of 5-HT may alleviate [65], while that of reserpine can induce [66] migraine attacks.

ANTIMIGRAINE DRUGS AND AVAs

If the AVAs open up during migraine attacks it is reasonable to expect that at least some antimigraine drugs may constrict these non-nutrient vessels. Indeed, even before the 'shunt' hypothesis was considered in the pathophysiology of migraine [1,2], Stolzenburg in 1937 [67] had suggested that ergotamine may close AVAs. The studies performed in our laboratory confirm and extend this suggestion to a number of other drugs.

Ergot alkaloids

Ergotamine

Johnston and Saxena [68] studied the effect of ergotamine ($5-20\mu g/kg^{-1}$) on regional tissue blood flow and on the shunting of microspheres ($15\mu m$) in and oxygen saturation of the external jugular venous blood in the cat. They reported that while ergotamine does not change tissue blood flow to a number of structures, including the brain, gastrointestinal tract, spleen, skin, skeletal muscles, it reduces the number of microspheres reaching the lungs (i.e. AVA-flow plus bronchial artery flow). The drug also decreases the jugular AVA-flow and,

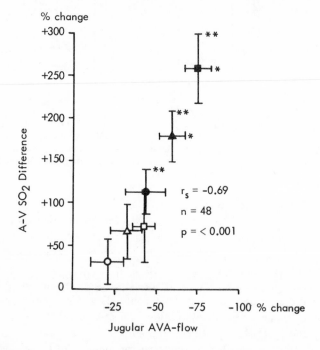

Figure 3. Effect of 5 (●), 10 (▲), and 20 (■) $\mu g/kg^{-1}$/i.v. of ergotamine, or the corresponding volume of saline (open symbols) on A-V (jugular) oxygen saturation (SO_2) difference and jugular AVA-flow in cats. *: significantly (p<0.05, Mann-Whitney U-test) different from the changes caused by saline in AVA-flow; **: significantly (p<0.05, Mann-Whitney U-test) different from the changes caused by saline in A-V SO_2 difference; r_s: Spearman rank correlation coefficient. Data from Johnston and Saxena [68]

perhaps thereby, increases the A-V oxygen saturation difference of the jugular venous blood [68]. These two effects show a reasonable correlation with each other (Figure 3). The reduction of microsphere shunting in the jugular venous blood by ergotamine was also confirmed in the pig by Schamhardt et al [69].

The effect of ergotamine on the complete distribution of the common carotid arterial blood has also been studied by us [32–34,36]. In the cat we reported that about 40 per cent of carotid blood is shunted via the AVAs which, as discussed above, are mainly located in the skin, ears, eyes, nasal mucosa, tongue, dura mater and rete mirabile. Only about five to 10 per cent of carotid blood enters the brain and the rest (about 40 per cent) is distributed to the various extracerebral structures of the head. As shown in Figure 4, ergotamine reduces

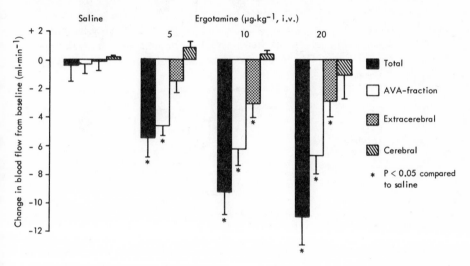

Figure 4. Effect of saline and ergotamine on total carotid blood flow and its distribution in AVA, extracerebral and cerebral fractions in cats. Data from Saxena [32]

the total carotid blood flow mainly due to a reduction of AVA-flow. The cerebral component of the carotid blood, as was also reported with total cerebral blood flow [68,70], remains unchanged while the extracerebral component is only moderately reduced by the drug. Similar findings have been reported in the dog [36]. The redistribution of carotid blood does not appear to be a consequence of a reduction of total carotid blood flow by ergotamine because the drug is equally effective in experiments where the common carotid artery was perfused with a constant blood volume [33].

An attempt has been made to analyse the receptors involved in the constriction of AVAs by ergotamine by comparing its effects in normal dogs and in dogs pretreated with phentolamine and pizotifen, which block alpha-adrenergic and D-type of 5-HT receptors, respectively [36]. In the saline-treated group, ergotamine

57

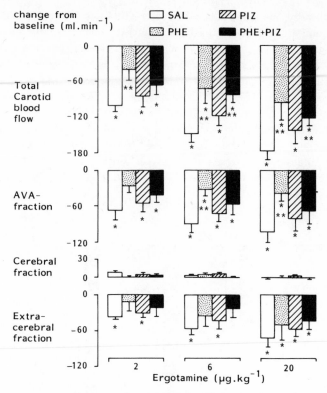

Figure 5. Effect of ergotamine on total carotid blood flow and its AVA, cerebral, and extra-cerebral fractions in dogs pretreated with either saline (SAL), phentolamine, $0.5mg/kg^{-1}$ (PHE), pizotifen, $0.5mg/kg^{-1}$ (PIZ), or a combination of the two antagonist drugs (PHE+PIZ). *: significantly ($p < 0.05$, paired t-test) different from the baseline values; **: significantly ($p < 0.05$, Mann-Whitney U-test) different from the changes in the saline-treated group. Reproduced from Saxena et al [36]

decreases total carotid flow. The decrease in AVA-fraction is significantly more than that in the extracerebral fraction, but no change is observed in the amount of carotid blood delivered to the brain (Figure 5). Pizotifen does not modify the effects of ergotamine while phentolamine, either alone or in combination with pizotifen, only slightly reduces its effects on total carotid and AVA-flows. This moderate attenuation of the responses to ergotamine may be secondary to a reduction of total carotid blood flow by phentolamine, particularly because neither the percentage distribution nor the vascular resistance changes due to ergotamine are modified by phentolamine [36]. Thus, the constriction of AVAs and arterioles in the carotid region by ergotamine mainly occur by a 'direct' vascular action and not by a mediation of alpha-adrenergic receptors or D-type 5-HT receptors. This view is consistent with our earlier findings [71] that even considerably high and, perhaps, non-specific concentrations of alpha-adrenolytics (phentolamine, 5mg/kg^{-1} and dibenzyline, 10mg/kg^{-1}) are able to reduce the vasoconstriction in the total carotid vascular bed induced only by low (1 and 2μg/kg^{-1}), but not by high (>4μg/kg^{-1}), doses of ergotamine.

In conclusion, it has been clearly shown that ergotamine preferentially decreases AVA-flow and increases A-V (jugular) O_2 saturation (or content) difference. This is in conformity with our earlier results [60,71] showing that this drug has a more selective vasoconstrictor action in the carotid and femoral vascular beds (Figure 6), the two regions where there is abundant A-V shunting

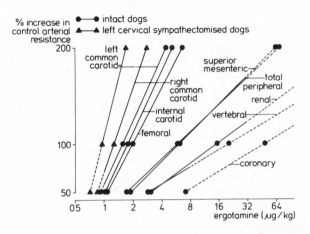

Figure 6. Regression lines for the vasoconstrictor effect of ergotamine in different canine vascular regions. The interrupted part of the lines represent the calculated dose-range not actually employed in the experiments). Reproduced from Saxena and de Vlaam-Schluter [71]

[29,31–36]. Recently in a Doppler ultrasound investigation in migraine patients [72], it has been reported that ergotamine (2–6mg orally) causes an exclusive increase of resistance in the external carotid area without appreciable changes in the internal carotid area. In humans, the internal carotid artery almost exclusively supplies the brain, where there is neither a significant number of AVAs [15, 18,27] nor any reduction of blood flow by ergotamine [68,70].

Dihydroergotamine

Dihydroergotamine is another drug which is sometimes used to treat acute attacks of migraine. As shown in Figure 7, this agent, like ergotamine, decreases carotid blood flow, fractional shunting and enhances the A-V (jugular) oxygen content difference [34]. No studies have so far been conducted regarding the receptors involved in its effects on AVAs but the situation could be the same as with ergotamine.

59

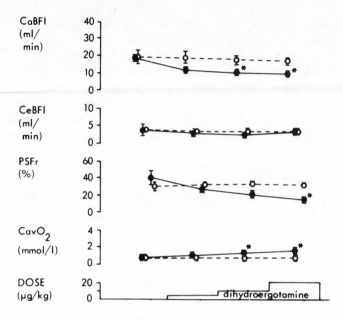

Figure 7. Effect of dihydroergotamine (5, 10 and $20\mu g/kg^{-1}$, i.v.) on total carotid blood flow (CaBFL) and its cerebral (CeBFL)- and AVA (PSFr)-fractions, and on the A-V (jugular) content difference ($CavO_2$) in cats. *: significant ($p < 0.05$; Mann-Whitney U-test) difference between ergotamine (•) and saline (o) treated animals. Reproduced from Spierings and Saxena [34]

Anti-5-HT drugs

Methysergide

The potent anti-5-HT (D-receptors) effects of methysergide and its value in the prophylactic treatment of migraine are well established. While some investigators believe that these two properties of methysergide are causally related [73], others have suggested that a 5-HT-like effect may be involved in its therapeutic action [74,75]. This is particularly due to the reasons that:

1 Methysergide is not very effective in antagonising the 5-HT induced carotid vasoconstriction [60,76];

2 The blood levels of 5-HT decrease, rather than increase, during migraine headaches [64]; and,

3 Methysergide, unlike some other anti-5-HT agents [57], also possesses pro-5-HT effects [55,74,75,77] and elicits a selective carotid vasoconstrictor response in both monkeys and dogs in doses above $10\mu g/kg^{-1}$ [74,76].

In rabbits, Forsyth and Saxena [78] reported that, like 5-HT (the effect of which is partially antagonised), $0.5mg/kg^{-1}$ dose of methysergide decreases

60

microsphere content of lungs (AVA-flow plus bronchial artery flow). We have recently obtained more direct evidence that methysergide $(50-350\mu g/kg^{-1})$ reduces AVA-fraction (non-nutrient) of carotid blood flow, but either does not change (cerebral-fraction) or even slightly increases (extracerebral-fraction) the nutrient part of carotid flow (Table II). However, it must be pointed out that

TABLE II. The effect of cumulative doses of methysergide on common carotid blood flow and its fractionation in seven pigs. Values are in ml/min^{-1} (mean ± SEM)

| | Methysergide ($\mu g/kg^{-1}$; i.v.) | | | |
	0	50	150	350
Total carotid	214±37	201±37*	191±36*	178±34*
AVA	188±33	168±34*	154±34*	132±32*
Extracerebral	24±4	29±3	31±3	41±5*
Cerebral	2±1	3±1	5±2	5±2

*: significantly different (p<0.05) from baseline values (paired t-test). Data from Verdouw and Saxena (unpublished)

the drug did not have a clear effect on A-V shunting in cats when used in doses of $25-100\mu g/kg^{-1}$ [34]. In comparison with ergotamine and dihydroergotamine, methysergide, unlike other drugs of this type, seems to have a relatively weak vasoconstrictor effect on the AVAs in the carotid circulation. One of the reasons for a weak effect on AVAs could be that methysergide has an additional pre-junctional inhibitory effect on sympathetic neurotransmission [79], which may result in AVA-dilation. Under conditions of low sympathetic activity [79], but not otherwise [74,79], methysergide causes vasoconstriction in the femoral vascular bed where there is also sufficient AVA-flow [31]. It is possible that the post-synaptic 5-HT receptors on the AVAs [29] and on the dog saphenous vein [77] and the presynaptic receptors on the sympathetic nerves [79] are similar because they are not blocked by cyproheptadine and methysergide and they are stimulated by methysergide.

Cyproheptadine

Though only a limited number of studies have been performed with cyproheptadine, it does not seem to constrict AVAs [29]. As stated earlier, the drug neither causes carotid vasoconstriction, nor does it effectively block the increase in *total* carotid resistance by 5-HT [29,60]. On the different vascular segments in the carotid region, the responses to 5-HT are either blocked (large arteries) or partially attenuated (AVAs) or even enhanced (arterioles) by cyproheptadine [29].

Pizotifen

In dose levels of up to $50\mu g/kg^{-1}$, pizotifen has no direct effect on the internal or external carotid circulation of either the monkey [76] or the dog (Saxena, unpublished). The drug possesses only a slight anti-5-HT effect in the carotid circulation [76]. Thus, like cyproheptadine, pizotifen is unlikely to constrict AVAs, though a direct proof has not yet been sought.

Drugs affecting adrenergic transmission

Isometheptene

Isometheptene, an aliphatic amine, has been used either alone or in combination with acetaminophen and dichloralphenazone (Midrin®) for both acute and interval treatment of migraine [80,81]. In intravenous doses of $0.25-1.0$mg/ kg^{-1}, the drug causes a moderate hypertension and tachycardia [35]. The carotid blood flow, particularly its AVA-fraction, is decreased while the A-V (jugular) oxygen content difference increases in cats (Figure 8). Though the

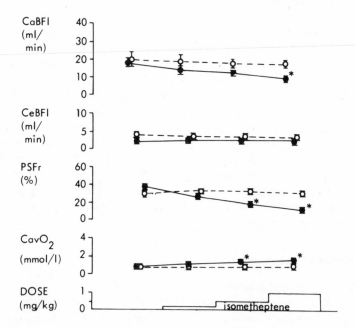

Figure 8. Effect of isometheptene ($0.25, 0.5$ and 1.0mg/kg^{-1}, i.v.) on total carotid blood flow (CaBFL) and its cerebral (CeBFL)- and AVA (PSFr)-fractions, and on the A-V (jugular) oxygen content difference (CavO$_2$) in cats. *: significant ($p<0.05$; Mann-Whitney U-test) difference between isometheptene (●) and saline (○) treated animals. Reproduced from Spierings and Saxena [35]

attenuation by alpha-adrenolytic drugs of the isometheptene-induced constriction of AVAs has not yet been demonstrated, such an effect of the drug is in keeping with its known indirect sympathomimetic properties [82].

Clonidine

Clonidine was introduced in the prophylactic treatment of migraine on the basis of animal experiments showing that repeated daily administration of the drug reduced the reactivity of the vessels to both vasoconstrictor and vasodilator drugs [83]. However, it must be remembered that clonidine also acts on vascular post-synaptic alpha$_2$-adrenoceptors [84] and, thus, may constrict AVAs, particularly in a lower dose-range. This property has so far only been explored in the carotid circulation of *young* Yorkshire pigs where the sympathetic nervous system is not well developed (Verdouw and Saxena, unpublished). Nevertheless, acute intracarotid bolus injection of clonidine (1 and 5μg/kg^{-1}) in these animals causes a short-lasting alpha-adrenoceptor mediated reduction in AVA-flow. But, even if this drug is more effective in constricting AVAs in other species, the dose-range used will be critical as clonidine is well known for reducing sympathetic nervous activity by a central action [85]. A reduction of sympathetic nervous system tone dilates AVAs [31, 47,48].

Beta-adrenoceptor antagonists

Propranolol and some other beta-adrenoceptor antagonists, particularly those without a partial agonistic action, are effective in the treatment of migraine [86–88]. The mechanism of the antimigraine action of beta-adrenoceptor antagonists is not known [88] and no direct studies are available regarding their effect on the fractionation of arterial blood into AVA- and capillary-fractions. But, Cohen and Coffmann [12] have reported a humoral vasodilatory mechanism in the AVAs of human digital circulation. Beta-adrenoceptor antagonists can potentially block such a mechanism. However, there is no indication so far if a beta-adrenergic vasodilatory mechanism also operates in the regulation of cranial AVAs in migraine.

Other drugs

Apart from the above drugs, there are several other agents (e.g. analgesics, indomethacin, metoclopramide, calcium channel blockers etc) which are also employed in the treatment of migraine. No convincing studies are yet available, either on their direct effect or on the effects of biogenic substances (which they can antagonise (e.g. prostaglandins, dopamine) on AVAs.

Summary and conclusions

There is ample histological evidence that AVAs normally exist in many tissues and in many different species. The use of radioactive microspheres in experimental animals can be employed to localise large AVAs. In the head such AVAs are mainly present in the facial skin, nasal mucosa, eyes, tongue, and in the dura mater. They are not present in sufficient numbers in the brain tissue itself but, due to a strategical position of the cranial AVAs, they can modify cerebral blood flow indirectly. The AVAs are innervated with cholinergic, purinergic and adrenergic nerves. The cholinergic and purinergic nerves seem to dilate AVAs while the adrenergic nerves can cause both a 'passive' dilation and an 'active' constriction.

Amongst the humoral agents involved in migraine, 5-HT has a profound effect on AVAs. The amine-induced redistribution of common carotid arterial blood towards the capillaries occurs at the expense of AVA-flow. The AVA constriction is mainly mediated by 'atypical' 5-HT receptors, but the D-receptors may also be involved to some extent.

A number of antimigraine drugs have been examined for their possible effects on the fractionation of arterial blood into nutrient (capillary) and non-nutrient (AVA) fractions. The ergot alkaloids, ergotamine and dihydroergotamine, powerfully and selectively reduce common carotid artery blood flow, particularly its AVA-fraction, and increase A-V (jugular) oxygen content difference. The vasoconstrictor effect of ergotamine on AVAs is independent of the reduction of carotid blood flow, and it does not seem to be mediated by either alpha-adrenergic or D-type of 5-HT receptors. Amongst the anti-5-HT drugs effective in migraine, it is only methysergide that causes a selective carotid vasoconstriction and some reduction of AVA-flow, probably by stimulating the 'atypical' 5-HT receptors. However, the effect of methysergide is much less potent than that of ergotamine and dihydroergotamine. Cyproheptadine and pizotifen do not contract AVAs.

The antimigraine drugs which stimulate alpha-adrenergic receptors (isometheptene and clonidine) can also decrease AVA-flow. Isometheptene seems more effective than clonidine; the latter drug causes central inhibition of sympathetic tone which may dilate AVAs. The effects of other antimigraine drugs on AVAs have not yet been studied. But, the presence of a beta-adrenoceptor mediated humoral vasodilatory mechanism in digital AVAs in man suggests that the beta-adrenoceptor antagonists may be able to reduce AVA-flow in some situations.

In conclusion, the data presented here show that AVAs form an important part of microcirculation in many. areas of the body. The calibre of AVAs can be regulated by neural and humoral mechanisms and some of the antimigraine drugs, particularly the ergot alkaloids, are potent constrictors of non-nutrient channels. This effect may play an important role in their therapeutic action.

Acknowledgments

I wish to thank my co-authors and technical assistants who contributed in the investigations cited in this publication. Thanks are also due to the journals *Headache* (Figures 5 and 8), *Cephalalgia* (Figure 6) and *Neurology* (Figure 7) for permission to reproduce figures from our previous publications.

References

1   Heyck H. *Der Kopfschmerz, Differentialdiagnostik und Therapie für die Praxis.* Stuttgart: Thieme. 1958: 301
2   Heyck H. Pathogenesis of migraine. *Res Clin Stud Headache 1969; 2:* 1–28
3   Graham JR, Wolff HG. Mechanism of migraine headache and action of ergotamine tartrate. *Arch Neurol Psychiat 1938; 39:* 737–763
4   Dalessio DJ. *Wolff's Headache and Other Head Pain. Fourth Edition.* New York: Oxford University Press. 1980
5   Rowbotham GF, Little E. New concepts on the aetiology and vascularization of meningiomata: the mechanism of migraine, the chemical process of cerebrospinal fluid, and the formation of collections of blood or fluid in the subdural space. *Br J Surg 1965; 52:* 21–24
6   Clark ER, Clark EL. Observations on living arteriovenous anastomoses as seen in transparent chambers introduced into the rabbit's ear. *Am J Anat 1934; 54:* 229–286
7   Sherman JL. Normal arteriovenous anastomoses. *Medicine 1963; 92:* 247–267
8   Goodall AM. Arterio-venous anastomoses in the skin of the head and ears of the calf. *J Anat 1955; 89:* 100–105
9   Molyneux GS. Observations on the structure, distribution and significance of arteriovenous anastomoses in sheep skin. In Lyne AG, Short BF, eds. *Biology of Skin and Skin and Hair Growth.* Sydney: Angus and Robertson. 1965: 591–602
10   Grant RT, Bland EF. Observations on arterio-venous anastomoses in human skin and in bird's feet with special reference to reaction to cold. *Heart 1931; 15:* 385–411
11   Brakke AM. *Arteriovenous Shunts in Peripheral Circulation. Thesis, Catholic University of Nijmegen.* Rotterdam: Bronder-Offset n.v. 1971
12   Cohen RA, Coffmann JD. Beta-adrenergic vasodilator mechanism in the finger. *Circ Res 1981; 49:* 1196–1202
13   Prinzmetal M, Ornitz EM Jr et al. Arteriovenous anastomoses in liver, spleen and lungs. *Am J Physiol 1948; 152:* 48–52
14   Delaney JP, Grim E. Canine gastric blood flow and distribution. *Am J Physiol 1964; 207:* 1195–1202
15   Hales JRS. Radioactive microsphere techniques for studies of the circulation. *Clin Exp Pharmacol Physiol 1974; suppl 1:* 31–36
16   Heymann MA, Payne BD, Hoffman JIE, Rudolph AM. Blood flow measurements with radionuclide labelled particles. *Progr Cardiovasc Dis 1977; 20:* 55–79
17   Saxena PR, Schamhardt HC, Forsyth RP et al. Computer programs for the radioactive microsphere technique. Determination of regional blood flows and other haemodynamic variable in different experimental circumstances. *Comp Progr Biomed 1980; 12:* 63–84
18   Marcus ML, Heistad DD, Ehrhardt JC et al. Total and regional cerebral blood flow measurements with $7-10\mu$, 15μ, 25μ and 50μ diameter microspheres. *J Appl Physiol 1976; 40:* 501–507
19   Daniel PM, Prichard MML. Arteriovenous anastomoses in the external ear. *Q J Exp Physiol 1956; 41:* 107–123
20   Greenfield ADM. The circulation through the skin. In Hamilton WF, Dow P, eds. *Handbook of Physiology, Section 2, Vol II.* Washington: American Physiological Society. 1963: 1325–2351

21 Burton AC. Relation of structure to function of the tissues of the wall of blood vessels. *Physiol Rev 1944; 34:* 619–642

22 Baez S. Skeletal muscle and gastrointestinal microvascular morphology. In Kaley G, Altura BM, eds. *Microcirculation, Vol I.* Baltimore: University Park Press. 1977: 69–94

23 Laursen H, Diemer NH. Capillary size, density and ultrastructure in brain of rats with urase-induced hyperammonaemia. *Acta Neurol Scand 1980; 62:* 103–115

24 Potter RF, Groom AC. Capillary diameter and geometry in cardiac and skeletal muscle studied by means of corrosion casts. *Microvasc Res 1983; 25:* 68–84

25 Chambers R, Sweifach BW. The topography and function of the mesenteric capillary microcirculation. *Am J Anat 1944; 75:* 173–205

26 Dickhoner WH, Bradley BR, Harrel GS. Diameter of arterial microvessels trapping 8–10μm, 15μm and 25μm microspheres as determined by vital microscopy of hamster cheek pouch. *Invest Radiol 1978; 13:* 313–317

27 Fan FC, Schuessler GB, Chen RYZ et al. Determination of blood flow and shunting of 9- and 15-μm spheres in regional beds. *Am J Physiol 1979; 237:* H25–H33

28 Utley J, Carlson EL, Hoffman JIE et al. Total and regional myocardial blood flow measured with 25μ, 15μ, 9μ and filtered 1–10μ diameter microspheres and antipyrine in dogs and sheep. *Circ Res 1974; 34:* 391–405

29 Saxena PR, Verdouw PD. Redistribution by 5-hydroxytryptamine of carotid arterial blood at the expense of arteriovenous blood flow. *J Physiol (Lond) 1982; 332:* 501–520

30 Maxwell LC, Shepherd AP, Riedel GL et al. Effect of microsphere size on apparent intramural distribution of intestinal blood flow. *Am J Physiol 1981; 241:* H408–H414

31 Spence RJ, Rhodes BA, Wagner HN. Regulation of arteriovenous anastomic and capillary blood flow in dog leg. *Am J Physiol 1972; 222:* 326–332

32 Saxena PR. Arteriovenous shunting and migraine. *Res Clin Stud Headache 1978; 6:* 89–102

33 Spierings ELH, Saxena PR. Effect of ergotamine on cranial arteriovenous shunting in experiments with constant flow perfusion. *Eur J Pharmacol 1979; 56:* 31–37

34 Spierings ELH, Saxena PR. Antimigraine drugs and cranial arteriovenous shunting in the cat. *Neurology 1980; 30:* 696–701

35 Spierings ELH, Saxena PR. Effect of isometheptene on the distribution and shunting of 15μm microsphere throughout the cephalic circulation of the cat. *Headache 1980; 20:* 103–106

36 Saxena PR, Koedam NA, Heiligers J et al. Ergotamine-induced constriction of cranial arteriovenous anastomoses in dogs pretreated with phentolamine and pizotifen. *Cephalalgia 1983; 3:* 71–81

37 Saxena PR, Verdouw PD. Tissue blood flow and arteriovenous shunting in pigs measured with microsphere of four different sizes. *Am J Physiol:* submitted

38 Änggård A. Capillary and shunt blood flow in the nasal mucosa of the cat. *Acta Otolaryng 1974; 78:* 418–422

39 Gillilan LA, Markesberry WR. Arteriovenous shunts in the blood supply to the brain of some common laboratory animals – with special reference to the rete mirabile conjugatum in the cat. *J Comp Neurol 1963; 121:* 305–311

40 Hurley HJ Jr, Mescon H. Cholinergic innervation of the digital arteriovenous anastomoses of human skin. A histochemical localization of cholinesterase. *J Appl Physiol 1956; 9:* 82–84

41 Iljima T, Tagawa T. Adrenergic and cholinergic innervation of arteriovenous anastomosis in the rabbit ear. *Anat Rec 1976; 185:* 373–379

42 Waris T, Kyosola K, Partanen S. The adrenergic innervation of arteriovenous anastomoses in the subcutaneous fascia of rat skin. *Scand J Plast Reconstr Surg 1980. 14;* 215–220

43 Molyneux GS, Harmon B. Innervation of arteriovenous anastomoses in the web of the foot of the domestic duck, *Anas platyrhynchos:* structural evidence for the presence of non-adrenergic non-cholinergic nerves. *Am J Anat 1982; 135:* 119–128

44   Burnstock G. Cholinergic and purinergic regulation of blood vessels. In Bohr DF, Somlyo AP, Sparks HV, eds. *Handbook of Physiology. Sec. 2: The Cardiovascular System, Vol II.* Bethesda: The American Physiology Society. 1980: 567–612

45   Folkow B, Sivertsson R. Aspects of the difference in vascular 'reactivity' between cutaneous resistance vessels and A-V anastomoses. *Angiologica 1964; 1:* 338–345

46   Baker CH, Davis DL, Sutton ET. Neural control of nutritional and non-nutritional circuits in the dog hind paw. *Am J Physiol 1978; 234:* H384–H391

47   Hillman PE, Scott NR, Van Tienhoven A. Vasomotion in chicken foot: dual innervation of arteriovenous anastomoses. *Am J Physiol 1982; 242:* R582–R590

48   Hales JRS, Foldes A, Fawcett AA, King RB. The role of adrenergic mechanisms in thermoregulatory control of blood flow through capillaries and arteriovenous anastomoses in the sheep hind limb. *Pflugers Arch 1982; 395:* 93–98

49   McGregor DD. Noncholinergic vasodilator innervation in the feet of ducks and chickens. *Am J Physiol 1979; 237:* H112–H117

50   Rondell PA, Palmer LE, Bohr DR. Influence of pharmacologic agents on capillary – AVA flow distribution in the perfused rabbit ears. *Fed Proc 1957; 16:* 109

51   Saxena PR, Forsyth RP, Johnston BM et al. Regional and systemic haemodynamic changes evoked by 5-hydroxytryptamine in awake and anaesthetized rabbits. *Eur J Pharmacol 1978; 50:* 61–68

52   Modell HI, Beck K, Butler J. Functional aspects of canine bronchial-pulmonary vascular communications. *J Appl Physiol Res Environ Exerc Physiol 1981; 50:* 1045–1051

53   Gaddum JH, Picarelli Z. Two kinds of tryptamine receptors. *Br J Pharmacol 1957; 12:* 323–328

54   Peroutka SJ, Snyder SH. Multiple serotonin receptors: differential binding of [^{3}H] 5-hydroxytryptamine, [^{3}H]lysergic acid diethylamide and [^{3}H]spiroperidol. *Mol Pharmacol 1981; 16:* 687–699

55   Humphrey PPA. Introductory remarks: some comments on pharmacological characterization of 5-hydroxytryptamine receptors. In *Proceedings of Fourth International Symposium on Vascular Neuroeffector Mechanisms, Tokyo.* In press

56   Kalkman HO, Boddeke HWGM, Doods HN et al. Hypotensive activity of serotonin receptor agonists in rats is related to their affinity for 5-HT$_1$ receptors. *Eur J Pharmacol 1983; 91:* 155–156

57   Van Nueten JM, Janssen PAJ, Van Beek J et al. Vascular effects of ketanserin (R41468), a novel antagonist of 5-HT$_2$ serotonergic receptors. *J Pharmacol Exp Ther 1981; 218:* 217–230

58   Rivinsson L, Handebo JE, Owman C. Pharmacological analysis of 5-hydroxytryptamine receptors in isolated intracranial and extracranial vessels of cat and man. *Circ Res 1978; 42:* 143–151

59   Saxena PR, Van Houwelingen P, Bonta IL. The effects of mianserin hydrochloride on the vascular responses evoked by 5-hydroxytryptamine and related vasoactive substances. *Eur J Pharmacol 1971; 13:* 295–305

60   Saxena PR. The effects of antimigraine drugs on the vascular responses by 5-hydroxytryptamine and related biogenic substances on the external carotid bed of dogs: possible pharmacological implications to their antimigraine action. *Headache 1972; 12:* 44–54

61   Haddy FJ, Gorden P, Emanuel DA. Influence of tone upon responses of small and large vessels to serotonin. *Circ Res 1959; 7:* 123–130

62   Heistad DD, Marcus ML, Sandberg S et al. Effect of sympathetic nerve stimulation on cerebral blood flow and on large cerebral arteries of dogs. *Circ Res 1976; 41:* 342–350

63   Toda N, Fujita F. Responsiveness of isolated cerebral and peripheral arteries to serotonin, and transmural electrical stimulation. *Circ Res 1973; 33:* 98–104

64   Anthony M, Hinterberger H, Lance JW. The possible relationship pf serotonin to the migraine syndrome. *Res Clin Stud Headache 1969; 2:* 29–59

65   Kimball RW, Friedman AP, Vallejo E. Effect of serotonin in migraine patients. *Neurology 1960; 10:* 107–111

66   Tandon RN, Sur BK, Nath K. Effect of reserpine injections in migrainous and normal control subjects, with estimations of urinary 5-hydroxyindole acetic acid. *Neurology 1969; 19:* 1073–1079

67   Stolzenburg HJ. Experimentelle Untersuchungen uber das Verhalten der arteriovenosen Anastomosen. *Z Mikr Anat Forsch 1937; 41:* 348–358

68   Johnston BM, Saxena PR. The effect of ergotamine on tissue blood flow and the arteriovenous shunting or radioactive microspheres in the head. *Br J Pharmacol 1978; 63:* 541–549

69   Schamhardt HC, Verdouw PD, van der Hoek TM et al. Regional myocardial perfusion and wall thickness and arteriovenous shunting after ergotamine administration to pigs with a fixed coronary stenosis. *J Cardiovasc Pharmacol 1979; 1:* 673–686

70   Hatchinski V, Norris JW, Edmeads J et al. Ergotamine and cerebral blood flow. *Stroke 1978:* 594–597

71   Saxena PR, de Vlaam-Schluter GM. Role of some biogenic substances in migraine and relevant mechanism in antimigraine action of ergotamine – studies in an experimental model for migraine. *Headache 1974; 13:* 142–163

72   Puzich R, Girke W, Heidrich H et al. Dopplersonographische Untersuchungen der extrakraniellen Hirngefäse bei Migräne-Patienten nach Gabe von Ergotamintartrat. *Dtsch Med Wschr 1983; 108:* 457–461

73   Fozard JR. Basic mechanisms of antimigraine drugs. *Adv Neurol 1982; 33:* 295–307

74   Saxena PR. Selective vasoconstriction in carotid vascular bed by methysergide: possible relevance to its antimigraine effect. *Eur J Pharmacol 1974; 27:* 99–105

75   Raskin NH. Pharmacology of migraine. *Ann Rev Pharmacol Toxicol 1981; 21:* 463–478

76   Spira PJ, Mylecharane EJ, Lance JW. The effects of humoral agents and antimigraine drugs on the cranial circulation of the monkey. *Res Clin Stud Headache 1976; 4:* 37–75

77   Apperley E, Feniuk W, Humphrey PPA et al. Evidence for two types of excitatory receptors for 5-hydroxytryptamine in dog isolated vasculature. *Br J Pharmacol 1980; 68:* 215–224

78   Forsyth RP, Saxena PR. The influence of methysergide on 5-hydroxytryptamine-induced changes in regional distribution of blood flow. *J Pharm Pharmacol 1978; 30:* 503–507

79   Feniuk W, Humphrey PPA, Watts AD. Modification of the vasomotor actions of methysergide in the femoral arterial bed of the anaesthetized dog by changes in sympathetic nerve activity. *J Autonom Pharmacol 1981; 1:* 127–132

80   Yuill GM, Swinburn WR, Liversedge LA. A double-blind crossover trial of isomethepene mucate compound and ergotamine in migraine. *Br J Clin Prac 1972; 26:* 76–79

81   Diamond S. Treatment of migraine with isometheptene, acetominophen, and dichloralphenazone combination: a double-blind crossover trial. *Headache 1976; 15:* 282–287

82   Bowman WC, Rand MJ. *Textbook of Pharmacology. 2nd Edition.* Oxford: Blackwell Scientific Publications. 1980

83   Zaimis E, Hannington E. A possible pharmacological approach to migraine. *Lancet 1969; 2:* 299–300

84   Timmermans PBMM, van Zwieten RA. The postsynaptic $alpha_2$-adrenoceptor. *J Autonom Pharmacol 1981; 1:* 171–183

85   Schmitt H, Schmitt H. Interactions between 2-(2,6-dichlorophenylamine) 2-imidazoline hydrochloride (ST 155, CATAPRESSAN) and alpha-adrenergic blocking drugs. *Eur J Pharmacol 1970; 9:* 7–13

86   Widroe T-E, Vigander T. Propranolol in the treatment of migraine. *Br Med J 1974; 2:* 699–701

87   Standnes B. The prophylactic effect of timolol versus propranolol and placebo in common migraine; beta-blockers in migraine. *Cephalalgia 1982; 2:* 165–170

88   Weerasuriya K, Patel L, Turner P. Beta-adrenoceptor blockade and migraine. *Cephalalgia 1982; 2:* 33–45

5

PLATELETS AND MIGRAINE

J L David, F De Clerck

Introduction

Increased risks of cerebral ischaemia have been reported in migrainous patients [1–3]. In both cerebral ischaemic and migraine attacks, platelets exhibit abnormal behaviour [4,5].

Moreover, migraine periods parallel changes in plasma 5-HT [6], a vasoactive amine stored in platelets and released in response to a number of stimuli together with some other constituents which may play a role in the pathogenesis of migraine [7].

These observations have led many investigators to measure platelet contents, aggregation and release during the various periods of migraine and in several types of this disease.

The purpose of this paper is to review briefly platelet modifications which have been observed in a number of migrainous patients and which may be relevant to the pathophysiology of migraine.

Uptake of 5-hydroxytryptamine

The main part of 5-hydroxytryptamine (5-HT) in the blood is stored in specific platelet granules, named dense bodies [8].

The uptake of 5-HT by the platelet is an energy-consuming process which occurs in the plasma membrane [9,10].

In vitro, it takes place against a concentration gradient and reaches a saturation level, provided that the 5-HT concentration does not exceed the threshold above which diffusion will dominate [11]. The active uptake depends on the NA^+/K^+ gradient across the plasma membrane which is generated by the activity of an ATPase. ADP inhibits the uptake, possibly by changing NA^+/K^+ gradient [12]. Receptors involved in the active transport of 5-HT across the plasma membrane seem to differ from the receptor by which 5-HT induces platelet shape change and aggregation [13].

In headache-free migrainous patients, the uptake of 5-HT by platelets as well as the endogenous content of this amine was found to be increased [14]. However, in a more recent study, the uptake was found lowered in some patients [15] but ranged from normal to totally abnormal [16].

The discrepancies between the reported results may be due in part to the differences in technical procedures [11], the temperature of the medium being a determinant factor. Km and Vmax were normal at $37°C$ during headache-free period; however, the mean increase in Km at $37°C$ from $25°C$ was more marked in migraineurs than in control, suggesting a permanent membrane abnormality [17].

In the attack period in one group of patients studied there was a significant correlation between time elapsed since the latest migraine attack and the Vmax of uptake [18], but in another group of patients, the 5-HT uptake was not reduced during the first three days after an attack [19].

In patients with a common migraine attack, platelets in suspension in their own plasma exhibited a reduced 5-HT uptake with low values for both Km and Vmax [20,21]. It is noteworthy that the uptake was normalised after resuspension of the platelets in control plasma or after isolation on a dextran gradient. These findings suggest that the uptake may be inhibited by one or several plasma factors during an attack, at least in some migrainous patients.

Release of 5-hydroxytryptamine

The release reaction occurs when platelets are stimulated at a critical level by a number of agents, including ADP, epinephrine, thrombin and collagen [22]. Released ADP and 5-HT can recruit more platelets to become activated [23]. Furthermore, sub-threshold concentrations of an agonist can be amplified by another. For instance, 5-HT strongly amplifies the release induced by several agents such as ADP or collagen [24].

It is well documented that the platelet 5-HT content significantly decreases before the onset of the migraine attack; at the same time the plasma level of this amine rises and then falls during the headache, while excretion of 5-HIAA increases [25]. After a migraine attack, platelet 5-HT content was rapidly restored to its preheadache level. However, the threshold for the release induced ex vivo by epinephrine or norepinephrine remained significantly high for at least three days, corresponding to a clinical refractory period [19].

In attack-free intervals, platelets from migrainous patients showed no difference in endogenous release of 5-HT when compared to platelets from control subjects [14].

Plasma taken from migrainous patients during an attack released significantly more labelled 5-HT from platelets of both normal and migrainous subjects.

70

This plasma releasing activity was also present, but at lower levels in attack-free intervals [26]. However, in another study, results from cross-incubations with assay of endogenous 5-HT showed that the plasma releasing activity was solely acting on platelets of migraineurs and did not affect platelets of healthy subjects [27].

Intraplatelet taurine

Taurine, a sulphur containing beta-aminoacid, is uniquely concentrated by the platelets [28]. It was reported that platelet levels of taurine were significantly greater during the headache phase of migraine than in the post-headache phase [29]. Taurine is proposed to have smooth muscle-relaxing properties; therefore, a higher platelet concentration of this neuromodulator during headache could leave less available taurine to interact with smooth muscle cell, this indirectly promoting constriction.

Intraplatelet adenine nucleotides

Platelets of migrainous patients contain significantly more ADP and total adenine nucleotides at all times than normal platelets [30,31]. The implications of these findings are not clear but it must be kept in mind that the release of 5-HT and ATP-ADP are intricately connected [23]. Moreover, there is evidence that ADP inhibits the uptake of 5-HT possibly by changing the Na^+/K^+ gradient [12].

Platelet and vascular prostaglandin products

Platelet stimulation makes arachidonic acid available for generation of thromboxane A_2 (TXA_2), a powerful aggregating and vasoconstricting substance. On the contrary, in the vessel wall arachidonic acid is the precursor of prostacyclin (PGI_2) which inhibits platelet aggregation and induces vasodilation [32].

The question is to know whether migraine platelets can generate more TXA_2 and/or less sensitive to the inhibitory effect of PGI_2.

Preliminary results have shown no significant differences in the total formation of platelet prostaglandins and of TXB_2, the stable end-product of TXA_2 [33].

Intraplatelet monoamineoxidase (MAO)

Human platelets contain the B form of MAO [34] which oxidises phenylethylamine, tyramine and tryptamine, the latter two also being a substrate of the A form. 5-HT, a substrate of the A form, is poorly influenced by platelet MAO. Platelet MAO activity has been found significantly decreased during migraine attacks when compared with its activity outside of an attack [35]. The transitory decrease of MAO during a migraine attack may be induced by a circulating plasma inhibitory factor [36].

Conflicting results which have been reported during the headache-free period may be due to differences in the technical procedures used; alternatively they may reflect the heterogeneity of the migraineurs, a small part of them probably having a permanent deficit [37,38].

Moreover, variations of platelet MAO during the menstrual cycle cloud the interpretation of the results obtained in migraineurs.

The permanently depressed platelet MAO activity appeared to be a consequence of smaller number of MAO molecules and not of a loss of their efficiency [39].

Additionally, there is no link between the platelet size and migraine nor between specific MAO activity and the platelet size in control subjects, migrainous patients or patients with cluster headache [40]. Thus, lower mean MAO activity reported in these patients could not be attributed to a preponderance of older, smaller and less reactive circulating platelets. It should be stressed that low values of MAO are not confined to migraineurs only [37].

The possible role of the reduction of platelet MAO in the pathogenesis of migraine is still subject to speculation. The absence of any relationship between the decrease in platelet MAO and the predisposition of dietary migraine triggered by monoamines seems to be established [21]. As previously suggested, a reduction in activity of MAO platelets and perhaps in the other tissues may represent a compensatory response with relevance to the therapeutic effect of MAO inhibitors in intractable migraine attacks.

Platelet phenolsulfotransferase (PST)

This enzyme, which plays a role in the catabolism of phenols, is present in the platelets in its two forms P and M. The form P acts on exogenous phenols and presumably on a range of unknown phenols. The form M acts on monoamine phenols such as noradrenaline and tyramine [41].

Patients with dietary migraine have a relative deficiency of the P form of PST compared with non-dietary migraine patients or controls [42,43]. The form M is also somewhat reduced in dietary migraine but less significantly. These findings suggest that dietary phenols may trigger dietary migraines due to a platelet abnormality. However, taking into account the degree of overlap in values between dietary migraineurs and controls, low intraplatelet concentration of this enzyme seems to be only one of the predisposing factors among many others in the development of a migraine attack.

Platelet aggregation and coagulation ex vivo

Platelet aggregation can be induced ex vivo in citrated plasma and is easily measured by the turbidometric technique [44]. As for the release reaction, various agents can induce aggregation at a rate and an extent depending on their nature and their concentration [45]; 5-HT induces a weak aggregation but strongly amplifies the response to other inducers [24,46].

In one study, the initial rate of the aggregation response to 5-HT was increased in migrainous patients between attacks but was lower during the headache phase [47].

In another study, the threshold of ADP required to induce the platelet release reaction was lower but without a significant increase of the initial rate of aggregation [48]. Furthermore, disaggregation was less marked than in controls. The hyperactivity of platelets was not related to the severity of the headache nor to the occurrence of migrainous neurological symptoms.

Aggregation induced by ADP, epinephrine, thrombin and 5-HT was found to be increased during the prodromes but decreased during the headache phase [49]. It is striking that the variations of platelet aggregability parallel the increase in plasma 5-HT level during the prodromes and its reduction during the headache phase [6].

However, in patients with classic migraine, hyperaggregation was only induced by 5-HT but not by ADP or epinephrine [50]. A significantly increased extension of aggregation induced by 5-HT was reported in some patients with severe prodromal symptoms in comparison with their age- and sex-matched controls [19].

Signs of hypercoagulability have been detected in patients with complicated migraine during complicated or uncomplicated attacks. Plasma coagulability was consistently more increased when the headache was associated with a focal cerebral dysfunction [51,52]. In patients with uncomplicated migraine, plasma coagulability dropped during the later phase of the attack, probably due to the release of endogenous heparin. In the same study, platelet aggregability to ADP, measured by a screen filtration system was increased during a complicated migraine attack, but fell in the same patients when the attack was uncomplicated. Therefore prolonged focal cerebral dysfunction might reflect a thromboembolic phenomenon.

On the whole, most of the reported results suggest that in migrainous patients platelet aggregability is increased between the attacks and that release operates more easily. It is likely that a selection of patients and technical differences account for some of the inconsistency between the data from the literature.

Platelet activation in vivo

Among the products of release, beta-thromboglobulin (BTG) and platelet factor 4 (pf4) are two platelet specific proteins which are stored in the alpha-granules. An increase of their plasma level reflects an in vivo release upon stimulation of the platelets or results from their destruction in the circulation [53].

It must be emphasised that the results of RIA of BTG and pf4 are dependent upon their plasma half-life which are respectively 100 minutes and 10 minutes [54]. Unfortunately, platelet activation may occur during blood sampling and the subsequent steps before their assay by RIA in plasma. This artefact which is to be feared when platelets are hypersensitive must be prevented by careful technical procedures [55].

In one study, there was no significant difference in plasma BTG concentrations between controls and migraine patients during headache-free periods. During headache attacks, plasma BTG was significantly increased in only 50 per cent of patients, but without any relation to the intensity or the severity of the headache [56].

More recently, it has been shown that the levels of plasma BTG and pf4 were increased in some patients during the headache-free period [57]. During the attack, the two platelet proteins increased further, especially in patients having relatively high levels already during headache-free periods. In these patients, intraplatelet 5-HT dropped during the attacks but remained within the normal range during the headache-free periods, even when platelet protein levels were increased in plasma. The lack of information about the correlation between release of 5-HT and platelet proteins in vivo does not allow of a valid conclusion being drawn concerning this observation.

The values of plasma concentration of BTG were significantly higher in classic migrainous patients than in control subjects [58]. Moreover, BTG levels in patients suffering from classic migraine in headache-free periods were similar to those occurring in classic migraine attacks and in common migraine attacks. These results indicate that in classic migrainous patients, platelet activation in vivo occurs very frequently during headache-free periods; the authors suggest that focal symptoms which characterise classic migraine attacks are not related to platelet release. However, as previously mentioned, high plasma levels of BTG and mainly pf4 must be interpreted with caution in view of the high reference values which do not exclude artefactual release ex vivo [55].

The index of Wu and Hoak [59] enables one to evaluate circulating platelet aggregates. Briefly, the lower the index, the more platelet aggregates are present in the blood sample immediately diluted in a formol-EDTA solution.

Circulating platelet aggregates have been found in several cases of acute cerebral insufficiency [4]. In migrainous patients, the index was significantly lower during the headache-free interval [49,19]. The circulating aggregates could play a role in producing a prodromal symptom of migraine.

Similar to the interpretation of plasma BTG — pf4 levels, the possibility that aggregation occurs during blood sampling must be kept in mind [55].

Platelet membrane modification

Functional abnormalities of platelets during both headache and headache-free periods point to a permanent alteration of the platelet membrane structure [60].

Therefore, its lipid composition has been analysed in two groups of migrainous patients with frequent (more than five per cent) and infrequent (less than five per cent) severe headaches. This study has shown that infrequent migraineurs had a significantly lower content of saturated fatty acids and a higher content of long-chain (22°C) polyunsaturated fatty acids. The saturation index of several phospholipids, the level of phosphatidylcholine and the ratio phosphatidylcholine/phosphatidylethanolamine were found to be increased; these changes would suggest that the platelet membrane would be more fluid in infrequent migraineurs than those of frequent migraineurs.

The hypersensitivity to ADP and to epinephrine of platelets with a less fluid membrane [61] may account for the hyperaggregability reported in migraineurs.

On the contrary, the membranes of platelets of migraine-suffering and control individuals were found to have a similar composition in terms of cholesterol level and cholesterol/phospholipid ratios, suggesting that the hyperreactivity in this pathology is mediated by other differences between platelets [62].

Influence of oral contraceptives

In patients without a migraine history before starting oral contraception, oral contraceptives were able to produce changes in platelet behaviour similar to those found in non-treated migraine patients [63]. For instance, the aggregation induced by 5-HT was no different in a group of patients who had started suffering from migraine attacks after oral contraception was started (group 1) to another group of patients whose attacks had become more frequent and severe after they started such medication (group 2). However, platelet reactivity to 5-HT significantly decreased after stopping oral contraception in patients in group 1, but remained high in the patients in group 2.

In this study, platelet reactivity to ADP, epinephrine and norepinephrine was not modified.

Previously, it has been shown that taking a combined oral contraceptive pill with a relatively larger oestrogenic activity increases (at day 21) and reduces (at day 28) the receptors for 5-HT and norepinephrine on the platelets. The aggregation induced by both amines and the active uptake of 5-HT, being a true functional association [64].

Influence of plasma constituents

Increased levels in plasma factor(s) such as free fatty acids [65] and noradrenaline [66] have been considered as possible causes for the release of 5-HT from platelets which occurs at the onset of a migraine attack.

Several authors have suggested that stress, dietary factors or fasting may precipitate an attack by releasing catecholamines which directly stimulate the platelets [67] or increase the plasma concentration of fatty acids which can also induce aggregation and release [68].

The presence in plasma of an unknown 5-HT-releasing factor in migraine patients has been demonstrated on several occasions [26,27].

These results have led to speculation about the situation in which plasma levels of free-fatty acids, especially arachidonic acid, would be increased and could induce platelet aggregation and release [32].

Moreover, some unidentified plasma factor(s) seem to inhibit uptake of 5-HT during the attacks [20,69].

Although the role of tyramine as a triggering factor of a migraine attack is still debated, it is worth keeping in mind that platelets from headache-free migrainous patients were more sensitive to the tyramine-releasing effect than platelets from control subjects [14].

According to a recent report, platelet 5-HT uptake was restored by a dietary tryptophan restriction as migrainous symptomatology improved [70].

Migraine in thrombocytopenia

The striking association between the appearance of typical migraine episodes and periods of severe thrombocytopenia in a patient without any previous history of migraine and the coincidence of both remissions has been confirmed in several cases of idiopathic thrombocytopenia or systemic lupus erythematosus [71]. In such patients, control of thrombocytopenia by corticoids or splenectomy was accompanied by a dramatic improvement of the migraine. As remarked by the authors, more fundamental data corroborate these clinical observations:

platelets from patients with idiopathic thrombocytopenia clump more often than those in normal subjects;

plasma from patients with idiopathic thrombocytopenia releases much more 5-HT from normal platelets than does plasma from normal individuals [72];

plasma from some migrainous patients can produce an abnormal release of 5-HT from normal platelets [42];

IgG levels are reported to be increased in migraine patients [73].

These findings have led to the following hypothesis: platelets sensitised by circulating antiplatelet antibodies (IgG) might repeatedly and abruptly induce a release of 5-HT into the arterial bloodstream. Sudden and brief increases of levels of free 5-HT would be compatible with the levels usually reported just before the onset of migraine. Then, the rapid metabolism of the released 5-HT and the destruction of sensitised platelets by the spleen might further reduce the availability of 5-HT. This situation would be compatible with low 5-HT level during the headache phase. Therefore, some types of migraine may have an immunological pathogenesis related to sudden changes in 5-HT metabolism.

Moreover, an inverse relationship between the free plasma- and intraplatelet-5-HT has been reported both in patients with idiopathic thrombocytopenia and in the majority of patients with systemic lupus erythematosus [74].

Migraine and thrombocythaemia

Cerebral ischaemia is a potential complication of thrombocythaemia. Some rare cases of this proliferative disorder are striking by the severity of headaches [75] or by the incidence of symptoms suggestive of a migrainous event [76].

Migraine and mitral valve prolapse

Mitral valve prolapse occurs in about six per cent of young women. The increased rate of cerebral ischaemic events in these patients is well documented. A high incidence of migraine syndrome was also observed. A role of platelets in the pathophysiologic mechanism of these associations is strongly suggested [77].

Conclusions

Several experimental and clinical data suggest firstly, that at least in a number of migraine patients, platelets are permanently modified and secondly, that probably not one single plasma factor would on its own be able to enhance platelet reactivity to a critical level or trigger the observed platelet reactions.

The formation of circulating aggregates and the release of vasoactive substances such as 5-HT and/or thromboxane A_2 could initiate a chain reaction resulting in headache rather than being an epiphenomenon devoid of any physiological impact.

Summary

Platelet modifications have been reported in migraine patients. Permanent abnormalities in membrane lipid composition, at least in the more severe cases, may be correlated to some aspects of the platelet dysfunction. During headache-free periods, hyperaggregability and anomalies in 5-HT uptake are among the more common features ex vivo. Furthermore, circulating aggregates were detected in vivo during the same period. In attacks, the platelet 5-HT content is lowered, probably due to the occurrence of the release reaction and inhibition of 5-HT re-uptake; both modifications being likely to be triggered by plasma factor (S). A possible role of immunoglobulins has been convincingly demonstrated in patients suffering from migraine and immune thrombocytopenia. Variations in platelet enzyme activities, depending upon the type and stage of migraine led to speculations rather than certainties about the role of MAO and PST.

Although platelets are likely to be involved in the pathophysiology of migraine, the available data are often in conflict because of methodological differences and the heterogeneity of the migraine patients.

References

1 Amery WK. Brain hypoxia: the turning point in the genesis of the migraine attack? *Cephalalgia 1982; 2:* 83–109
2 Guest IA, Woolf AL. Fatal infarction of brain in migraine. *Br Med J 1964; 1:* 225
3 Leviton A, Malvea B, Graham JR. Vascular diseases, mortality and migraine in the parents of migraine patients. *Neurology 1974; 24:* 669–672
4 Dougherty Jr JH, Levy DE, Weksler BB. Platelet activation in acute cerebral ischaemia (serial measurements of platelet function in cerebrovascular disease). *Lancet 1977; i:* 821–824
5 Kalendovsky Z, Austin J, Steele P. Increased platelet aggregability in young patients with stroke. *Arch Neurol 1975; 32:* 13–20
6 Lance JW, Anthony M, Hinterberger H. The control of cranial arteries by humeral mechanisms and its relation to the migraine syndrome. *Headache 1967; 7:* 93–102
7 Hanington E. Migraine: a blood disorder. *Lancet 1978; ii:* 501–503
8 Da Prada M, Richards JG, Kettler R. Amine storage organelles in platelets. In Gordon JL, ed. *Platelets in Biology and Pathology.* Amsterdam, New York, Oxford: Elsevier-North Holland Biomedical Press. 1981: 107–145
9 Pletscher A. Metabolism, transfer and storage of 5-hydroxytryptamine in blood platelets. *Br J Pharmacol Chemother 1968; 32:* 1–16
10 Sneddon JM. Blood platelets as a model for monoamine containing neurones. *Prog Neurobiol 1973; 1:* 151–198
11 Malmgren R. Methodological aspects of studies on the 5-HT uptake mechanism in normal platelets. *Acta Pharmacol Toxicol 1981; 49:* 277–284
12 Drummond AH, Gordon JL. Specific binding sites for 5-hydroxytryp blood platelets. *Biochem J 1975; 150:* 129–132
13 Schachter M, Grahame-Smith DG. 5-hydroxytryptamine and the platelet: specific binding and active uptake. In De Clerck F, Van Houtte P, eds. *5-hydroxytryptamine in Peripheral Reactions.* New York: Raven Press. 1982:49–59
14 Dalsgaard-Nielsen T, Genefke IK. Serotonin release and uptake in platelets from healthy persons and migrainous patients in attack-free intervals. *Headache 1974; 14:* 26–32
15 Malmgren R et al. Acetylsalicylic asthma and migraine – a defect in serotonin (5-HT) uptake in platelets. *Thromb Res 1978; 13:* 1137–1139
16 Malmgren R, Olsson P, Tornling G, Unge G. The 5-hydroxytryptamine take-up mechanism in normal platelets and platelets from migraine and asthmatic patients. *Thromb Res 1980; 18:* 733–741
17 Oxman T, Hitzemann R, Smith R. In *The Migraine Trust. 4th Int Symp.* 1982: 26–27
18 Coppen A, Swade C, Wood K, Carroll JD. Platelet 5-hydroxytryptamine accumulation and migraine. *Lancet 1979; ii:* 914
19 Hanington E, Jones RJ, Amess JAL, Wachowicz B. Migraine: a platelet disorder. *Lancet 1981; ii:* 720–723
20 Launay JM, Pradalier A, Dreux C, Dry J. Platelet serotonin uptake and migraine. *Cephalalgia 1982; 2:* 57–59
21 Sandler M. Transitory platelet monoamine oxidase deficit in migraine: some reflections. *Headache 1977; 17:* 153–158
22 De Clerck F, David JL. Pharmacological control of platelet and red blood cell function in the microcirculation. *J Cardiovasc Pharmacol 1981; 3:* 1388–1412
23 Holmsen H. Platelet secretion (release reaction) – mechanism and pharmacology. *Adv Pharmacol Ther 1979; 4:* 97–109
24 De Clerck F, Herman AG. 5-hydroxytryptamine and platelet aggregation. *Fed Prod 1983; 42:* 228–232

25   Salmon S, Bonciani M, Fanciullacci M et al. A putative 5-HT central feedback in migraine and cluster headache attacks. *Adv Neurol 1982; 33:* 265
26   Dvilansky A, Rishpon S, Nathan I. Release of platelet 5-hydroxytryptamine by plasma taken from patients during and between migraine attacks. *Pain 1976; 2:* 315
27   Mück-Seler D, Deanovic Z, Dupelj M. Platelet serotonin (5-HT) and 5-HT releasing factor in plasma of migrainous patients. *Headache 1979; 19:* 14–17
28   Al-Ubaidi FF, Lascelles PT. Uptake and metabolism of ^{14}C-*arachidonic acid by platelets in patients with migraine. The Migraine Trust. 4th Int Symp. Abstract book.* London. 1982: 23–25
29   Dhopesh VP, Baskin SI. Change in platelet taurine and migraine. *Headache 1982; 22:* 165–166
30   Rydzewski W, Wachowicz B. Adenine nucletides in and between migraine attacks. In Samuelsson B, Paoletti R, eds. *Advances in Prostaglandin and Thromboxane Research.* New York: Raven Press. 1976: 737–746
31   Hanington E, Jones RJ, Amess JAL. Platelet nucleotides in migraine. *Lancet 1982; ii:* 437
32   Moncada S, Vane JR. Arachidonic acid metabolites and the interactions between platelets and blood-vessel wall. *N Engl J Med 1979; 300:* 1142–1147
33   Ahtee L, Boullin DJ, Paasonen MK. Transport of taurine by normal human blood platelets. *Br J Pharmacol 1974; 52:* 245–251
34   Donnelly CH, Murphy DL. Substrate-and inhibitor-related characteristics of human platelet monoamine oxidase. *Biochem Pharmacol 1977; 26:* 853–858
35   Glover V et al. Transitory decrease in platelet monoamine-oxidase activity during migraine attacks. *Lancet 1977; i:* 391–393
36   Sandler M. Cerebrovascular changes in migraine: secondary manifestations of a circulating humoral agent? *J Neurol Transmission 1978; Suppl 14:* 51–59
37   Glover V, Peatfield R, Zammit-Pace R et al. Platelet monoamine oxidase activity and headache. *J Neurol Neurosurg Psychiatr 1981; 44:* 786–790
38   Thomas DV. Platelet monoamine oxidase in migraine. *Adv Neurol 1982; 33:* 279
39   Summers KM, Brown GK, Craig IW et al. Platelet monoamine oxidase: specific activity and turnover number in migraine. *Clin Chim Acta 1982; 121:* 139–146
40   Peatfield RC, Gawel MJ, Guthrie DL et al. Platelet size: no correlation with migraine or monoamine oxidase activity. *J Neurol Neurosurg Psychiatr 1982; 45:* 826–829
41   Sandler M, Usdin E. In Sandler M, Usdin E, eds. *Phenolsulfotransferase in Mental Health Research.* London: MacMillan. 1981
42   Glover V, Littlewood J, Sandler M et al. Biochemical predisposition to dietary migraine: the role of phenosulphotransferase. *Headache 1983; 23:* 53–58
43   Littlewood J et al. Platelet phenolsulphotransferase deficiency in dietary migraine. *Lancet 1982; i:* 983–986
44   Belmaker RH, Murphy DL, Wyatt RL, Loriaux DL. Human platelet monoamine oxidase changes during the menstrual cycle. *Arch Gen Psychiatr 1974; 31:* 553
45   Vargaftif BB, Chignard M, Benveniste J. Present concepts on the mechanisms of platelet aggregation. *Biochem Pharmacol 1981; 30:* 263–271
46   Hilton BP, Cumings JN. An assessment of platelet aggregation induced by 5-hydroxytryptamine. *J Clin Pathol 1971; 24:* 250–258
47   Hilton BP, Cumings JN. 5-hydroxytryptamine levels and platelet aggregation responses in subjects with acute migraine headache. *J Neurol Neurosurg Psychiat 1972; 35:* 505
48   Couch JR, Hassanein RS. Platelet aggregability in migraine. *Neurology 1977; 27:* 843
49   Deshmukh SV, Meyer J Stirling. Cyclic changes in platelets dynamics and the pathogenesis and prophylaxis of migraine. *Headache 1977; 17:* 101–108
50   Jones RJ,Forsythe AM, Amess JAL. Platelet aggregation in migraine patients during the headache-free interval. *Adv Neurol 1982; 33:* 275–278
51   Kalendovsky Z, Austin J, Steele P. Increased platelet aggregability in young patients with stroke. *Arch Neurol 1975; 32:* 13–20
52   Kalendovsky Z, Austin JH. Changes in blood clotting systems during migraine attacks. *Headache 1977; 16:* 293–312
53   Kaplan KL, Owen J. Plasma levels of a beta-thromboglobulin and platelet factor-4 as indices of platelet activation in vivo. *Blood 1981; 57:* 199 –202

79

54 Dawes J, Smith RC, Pepper DS. The release, distribution and clearance of human beta-thromboglobulin and platelet-factor 4. *Thromb Res 1978; 12:* 851–861

55 David JL, De Clerck F. Detection of platelet activation in vivo: significance and limitations of the available tests. In De Clerck F, Van Houtte PM, eds. *5-hydroxytryptamine in Peripheral Reactions.* New York: Raven Press 1982: 61

56 Gawel M, Burkitt M, Clifford Rose F. The platelet release reaction during migraine attacks. *Headache 1979; 19:* 323–327

57 D'Andrea G, Toldo M, Cortelazzo S, Milone FF. Platelet activity in migraine. *Headache 1982; 22:* 207–212

58 D'Andrea G, Cananzi A, Toldo S et al. Platelet behaviour in classic migraine: responsiveness to small doses of aspirin. *Thromb Haemostas 1983; 49:* 153

59 Wu KK, Hoak JC. A new method for quantitative detection of platelet aggregates in patients with arterial insufficiency. *Lancet 1974; ii:* 924–926

60 Oxman TE, Hitzemann RJ, Smith R. Platelet membrane lipid composition and the frequency of migraine. *Headache 1982; 22:* 261–267

61 Shattil SJ, Cooper RA. Role of membrane lipid composition, organisation and fluidity in human platelet function. *Prog Hemost Thromb 1978; 4:* 59–86

62 Bottomley JM, Hanington E, Jones RJ, Chapman D. Platelet lipid composition in human migraine. *Headache 1982; 22:* 256–260

63 Hanington E, Jones RJ, Amess JAL. Platelet aggregation in response to 5-HT in migraine patients taking oral contraceptives. *Lancet 1982; i:* 967–968

64 Peters JR, Elliott JM, Grahame-Smith DG. Effect of oral contraceptives on platelet noradrenaline and 5-hydroxytryptamine receptors and aggregation. *Lancet 1979; ii:* 933–936

65 Hsu LKG, Crisp AH, Kalucy RS et al. Early morning migraine nocturnal plasma levels of catecholamines, tryptophan, glucose and free fatty acids and sleep encephalographs. *Lancet 1977; i:* 447–451

66 Hockaday JM, Williamson DH, Whitty CWM. Blood glucose levels and fatty acid metabolism in migraine relating to fasting. *Lancet 1971; i:* 1153–1156

67 O'Brien JR. Some effects of adrenaline and anti-adrenaline compounds on platelets in vitro and in vivo. *Nature (London) 1963; 200:* 763–764

68 Hornstra G. *Dietary Fats and Arterial Thrombosis.* Thesis. RUL Maastricht: The Netherlands

69 Praladier A, Launay JM. 5-hydroxytryptamine uptake by platelets from migrainous patients. *Lancet 1982; i:* 862

70 Unge G, Malmgren R, Theorell H, Olsson P. Effects of dietary protein-tryptophan restriction upon 5-HT uptake in platelets and clinical symptoms in migraine with skin manifestations. In *The Migraine Trust. 4th Int Symp 1982;* 14–15

71 Damasio H, Beck D. Migraine, thrombocytopenia and serotonin metabolism. *Lancet 1978; i:* 240–242

72 Hirschman RJ, Shulman NR. The use of platelet serotonin release as a sensitive method for detecting antiplatelet antibodies and a plasma anti-platelet factor in patients with idiopathic thrombocytopenic purpora. *Br J Haematol 1973; 24:* 793–802

73 Lord GDA, Duckworth JW. Immunoglobulin and complement studies in migraine. *Headache 1977; 17:* 163–168

74 Parbtani A, Cameron JS. Platelets, serotonin, migraine and immune complex disease. *Lancet 1978; ii:* 679

75 Hanington E. Migraine as a blood disorder: preliminary studies. *Adv Neurol 1982; 33:* 253–256

76 Bousser MG, Conard J, Lecrubier C, Bousser J. Migraine ou accidents ischémiques transitoires au cours d'une thrombotytémie essentielle. Action de la ticlopidine. *Ann Méd Interne 1980; 131:* 87–90

77 Litman GI, Friedman HM. Migraine and the mitral prolapse syndrome. *Am Heart J 1978; 96:* 610–614

6

EFFECTS OF ANTIMIGRAINE DRUGS
ON PLATELET BEHAVIOUR

F De Clerck, J L David

Introduction

Recently, abnormalities in platelet behaviour have been proposed as a major factor or even as a primary cause in the pathogenesis of migraine attacks [1–4]. Briefly, depending upon the stage of the disease when tested, platelets of migraineurs are hyperreactive in their response to aggregating agents such as ADP, thrombin, epinephrine, 5-hydroxytryptamine (5-HT), platelet activator in patient's plasma, in their proneness to undergo the release reaction in vitro as well as in vivo, and show a reduced MAO activity as well as uptake capacity for 5-HT [5–17]; these changes may lead to excessive release/production of vasoactive products such as 5-HT, PGE_2, $PGF_{2\alpha}$ and thromboxane A_2 (TXA_2) which may produce cerebral vasoconstriction and ischaemia supposed to occur during the prodromal phase of migraine [8,10–12,17,18].

Based upon rationale, treatment with several 'anti-platelet' drugs has been applied in migraine, with varying success [1,19–21]. The aim of the present study is to review the effects of some drugs currently used in the treatment of this disease (ergotamine, pizotifen, methysergide, clonidine, propranolol, flunarizine, nimodipine, domperidone, aspirin) on several aspects of platelet behaviour according to their mechanism of action using an earlier proposed classification of anti-platelet drugs into inhibitors of induction, transmission and extrusion [22–24].

Definition of the various stages of platelet activation

According to Holmsen [22] the response of platelets to various agonists occurs in three consecutive stages: induction, transmission and execution. *Induction* represents the interaction of a given agonist with its receptor on the platelet membrane. *Transmission* represents an energy-requiring process, subsequent to membrane receptor occupancy, involving the release of a transmitter or second messenger from the membrane to affect cellular target structures; this second messenger probably is Ca^{2+} mobilised from a membrane-bound and a vesicular pool into the cytoplasm, its removal again from the cytoplasm being regulated by cAMP-dependent processes. *Execution* then represents a uniform sequence of consecutive, morphological and biochemical reactions described [25,26] as shape change, reversible aggregation and, depending upon the nature and concentration of the inducer(s), the release of intragranular material and the production of arachidonic acid metabolites producing irreversible aggregation (extrusion phase) [24].

Convincing evidence suggests that a rise of free Ca^{2+}-ions in the cytoplasm plays a primary role in the various stages of the platelet reaction [24,27–29]. However, Ca^{2+} from an internally releasable membrane pool, rather than external Ca^{2+} entering through the plasma membrane, would serve to initiate the activation by most agonists, at least for human platelets; indeed, the divalent cation ionophore A 23 187 induces platelet shape change and secretion in the presence, but also in the absence of extracellular Ca^{2+}; although requiring the presence of extracellular ionised Ca^{2+}, the primary aggregation induced by ADP is not associated with a simultaneous transmembrane uptake of the cation, but with a redistribution from intracellular pools, probably the dense tubular system. During the release reaction induced by thrombin, ADP and collagen, the permeability of the human platelet membrane for Ca^{2+} increases, but this change was proven to be the consequence rather than the cause of granule secretion. One exception to this system of intracellular Ca^{2+} translocation is the human platelet aggregation induced by epinephrine: human platelets isolated from the plasma take up Ca^{2+} during epinephrine-induced primary aggregation, but not during primary ADP reactions; antagonism of the platelet α-receptors with phentolamine results in inhibition of both epinephrine-induced Ca^{2+}-uptake and aggregation.

The reversibility, in suitable conditions, of the primary platelet activation implies the existence of a mechanism removing Ca^{2+} again from the cytoplasm; such a system would be provided by cAMP-dependent processes which, as a unidirectional mediator, activates a 'calcium pump' in the dense tubular system thus removing free Ca^{2+} again from the cytosol [see 24 for full review].

Inhibition of induction

Serotonergic antagonists

5-Hydroxytryptamine (5-HT) interacts with blood platelets of various species including man to produce *activation* and to be taken up by an energy-requiring transport system (*uptake*), both processes being regulated by two distinct surface membrane receptors [30–32]. The results of this receptor activation in

82

terms of subsequent platelet reactions depend upon the species involved and upon the experimental conditions: in contrast to pig, sheep and cat platelets, normal human platelets respond to 5-HT with a shape change and a weak reversible aggregation only, biphasic, release-associated irreversible aggregation occurring in a limited number of cases. However, 5-HT strongly amplifies the platelet response to low concentrations of other agonists in terms of enhanced reversible and irreversible aggregation, release of platelet products and biosynthesis of TXA_2 [30,33]. Moreover, in normal, but pre-sensitised, human platelets as well as in those from a substantial percentage of cardiovascular patients, 5-HT itself can induce a full irreversible aggregation/release reaction [30,33,34]. Additionally, intraplatelet 5-HT release together with adenine nucleotides and TXA_2, subsequent to a suitable platelet activation, may play a predominant role in the propagation of aggregation by additional platelet recruitment and release as evidenced by the inhibition obtained with serotonergic receptor antagonists of the biphasic, release-dependent aggregation wave induced by ADP in some normal human platelets and in all feline platelets, which are superreactive to 5-HT [33,35]. Therefore, in particular conditions of pre-sensitised platelets or amplification reactions between various agonists, 5-HT precipitates a full aggregation with release of vasoactive products; such a situation may also exist in migraineous platelets [36,37].

Platelet receptors for 5-HT involved in their activation resemble the $5-HT_2$ receptor subtype defined by Peroutka [38], as evidenced by the inhibition obtained with various drugs of the specific [^{3}H] ketanserin binding, a specific $5-HT_2$ receptor antagonist [39,40] in close correlation with the drug's potencies as inhibitors of the 5-HT induced platelet aggregation [30,33,35,40].

Radioligand binding experiments on brain membrane preparations [39,41, 42] show that methysergide, pizotifen and ergotamine are mixed inhibitors at both $5-HT_2$ and $5-HT_1$ receptor sites, be it with a higher potency on the former subpopulation (ratios $5-HT_2/5-HT_1$ of 8.2 and 230.7 for methysergide and pizotifen respectively). As found with the pure $5-HT_2$ receptor antagonist ketanserin [30,33], these compounds, through their effect at this receptor site, strongly inhibit the activation of normal human platelets induced by 5-HT in vitro (Table I). This inhibitory effect on platelet behaviour is specifically restricted to the reactions induced by $5-HT_2$ receptor activation, since neither the primary aggregation induced by ADP or epinephrine nor the release-dependent aggregation by collagen are significantly affected (Table I). At concentrations largely exceeding those inhibiting the functional platelet changes induced by 5-HT, these serotonergic antagonists do not markedly affect the uptake of the monoamine by the platelets [30,35]. Moreover, analysis of their effect on the metabolism of ^{14}C-arachidonic acid by washed human platelets [43] and on the generation of malondialdehyde (MDA) by thrombin-stimulated human platelets in plasma [30] indicates absence of marked effects on the generation of vasoactive prostanoids by platelets at concentrations up to 1×10^{-5} M (Table II);

83

TABLE I. Effect of antimigraine drugs on the aggregation of normal human platelets in vitro

Compounds (1 x 10^{-5} M, 5min)	Inhibition of aggregation induced by[1]			
	5-HT 5 x 10^{-6} M	ADP 5 x 10^{-6} M	Collagen 2μg/ml	Epinephrine 2 x 10^{-5} M
aspirin	29	21.3	19.5	0
ergotamine	100	9.8	11.2	91.9
pizotifen	100	9.7	5.1	13.8
methysergide	100	5.3	6.8	0.5
clonidine	0	20.1	0	72.8
propranolol	18.8	4.6	7.5	17.6
flunarizine	0	1.1	0	0
nimodipine	0	4.5	0	0
domperidone	93.2	1.6	1.7	0
ketanserin 1 x 10^{-7} M[2]	100	–		
VK 774 1 x 10^{-5} M		93.1		
aspirin 8 x 10^{-5} M			90.6	
suprofen 1 x 10^{-5} M			90.2	
yohimbine 1 x 10^{-6} M				82.9

1 Mean percentage inhibition (n=3) of the initial slope of the aggregation induced by 5-HT, ADP, collagen and epinephrine on normal human platelets (3.5 x $10^5/\mu$l) in citrated plasma at 37°C.

2 Inhibitor of 5-HT$_2$ receptors, phosphodiesterase activity, cyclo-oxygenase activity, α_2 receptors as reference compounds.

contrary to the stimulation of prostaglandin E production by ergotamine in isolated saphenous veins contributing to vasoconstriction [44], this compound is reported to inhibit specifically thromboxane A_2 synthetase in platelets, but only at subtoxic concentrations not practicable in vivo [45].

Adrenergic antagonists

Mitchell and Sharp [46] discovered that epinephrine and, less potently, norepinephrine causes human platelets, in contrast to those of other mammalian, non-primate species [47], to aggregate strongly in citrated plasma; in particular experimental conditions this response proceeds through biphasic, irreversible aggregation to completion with associated release of platelet intragranular

TABLE II. Effect of antimigraine drugs on the prostaglandin production by normal platelets in vitro

Compound (1 x 10^{-5} M, 5 min)	Arachidonic acid metabolism[1]							MDA[2]
	Ph. lipids	$PGF_{2\alpha}$	TXB_2	PGE_2	PGD_2	HHT	12-HTE	
solvent	1.1 ± 0.2	–	20.4 ± 0.9	–	–	27.0 ± 1.2	51.0 ± 1.8	–
aspirin	0.7 ± 0.3	–	3.4 ± 0.5	–	–	6.3 ± 0.19	89.4 ± 0.9	89.5
R 19 09_1[3]	2.8 ± 0.07	7.1 ± 0.01	1.5 ± 0.1	32.7 ± 0.2	9.3 ± 0.05	14.2 ± 0.03	32.1 ± 0.1	87
ergotamine	0.7 ± 0.2	–	19.6 ± 1.4	–	–	30.7 ± 2.7	48.9 ± 3.9	0
pizotifen	2.5 ± 0.2	–	24.6 ± 2.1	–	–	27.0 ± 1.7	45.0 ± 4.09	0
methysergide	0.9 ± 0.2	–	19.9 ± 1.1	–	–	30.6 ± 2.3	48.6 ± 3.1	0
clonidine	2.5 ± 0.2	–	23.9 ± 2.8	–	–	26.6 ± 3.0	47.0 ± 5.9	0
propranolol	2.3 ± 0.2	–	23.2 ± 2.4	–	–	24.0 ± 2.5	50.4 ± 4.2	0
flunarizine	2.6 ± 0.08	–	22.9 ± 2.0	–	–	27.1 ± 1.3	47.4 ± 3.3	2.1
nimodipine	2.05 ± 0.2	–	24.3 ± 2.0	–	–	29.0 ± 1.8	44.5 ± 3.4	0
domperidone	1.2 ± 0.7	–	21.6 ± 1.8	–	–	27.2 ± 2.6	49.9 ± 2.2	0

1 Washed human platelets (2 x 10^5 /µl) incubated for 5 min at 37°C with ^{14}C-arachidonic acid (A.A., 0.25µCi, 1.4µg/ml); TLC separation; quantification of metabolites in percentage (mean ± SEM; n=4) of the total A.A. radioactivity

2 Malondialdehyde (nM/2.5 x 10^8 platelets/30 min) generated by human platelets in citrated plasma, stimulated with thrombin 2-U/ml, 37°C; mean percentage inhibition, n=4

3 Specific inhibitor of thromboxane A_2 synthetase as reference compound

products including adenine nucleotides and 5-HT and biosynthesis of prostaglandins [48–50]. However the proportion of the total response which is *directly* (i.e. the primary, reversible wave of aggregation) dependent upon the interaction of the platelets with catecholamines is smaller than in the case of agonists such as ADP, secondary platelet recruitment after epinephrine-challenge being due to non-catecholamine platelet-released mediators [49–53]. The in vivo significance of a full aggregation/release response to catecholamines as sole stimulus remains unclear since it is not observed, or strongly reduced, in plasma with physiological Ca^{2+}-concentrations [54,55] or in samples anticoagulated with hirudin to exclude formation of traces of thrombin [55,56]. Nevertheless, epinephrine in human platelets, as well as in those of other species, retains a pro-aggregatory potential in terms of a positive amplification on the platelet response to other agonists as described for 5-HT [51,56–58].

Studies with antagonists in both physiological response [59–61] and radioligand binding experiments [62–64] show that the activation of human platelets results from the occupancy of α-adrenergic receptors. Human platelets contain both α_1- and α_2-adrenergic receptors at which phenylephrine and clonidine respectively, behaving as antagonists at higher concentrations [65,66], can act as partial agonists by inducing either aggregation (clonidine) or a pro-aggregatory state (phenylephrine), thus amplifying the response to other agonists [67]. However, the α_2-adrenergic receptor rather than the α_1 seems to be primarily responsible for mediating the response to the naturally occurring agonist, since α_2-selective antagonists such as yohimbine are much more effective as inhibitors of the aggregation response to epinephrine and of the reduction of adenylate cyclase activity in platelet lysates than the α_1-antagonists indoramin or prazosin [65,67].

In agreement with these concepts, we find (Table I) strong inhibition of the primary wave, and consequently, of the secondary irreversible aggregation and release reaction to epinephrine, with ergotamine [68], and clonidine [66] but not with prazosin at 1×10^{-5} M [66]. At the concentrations we tested, the former α_2-adrenergic receptor antagonists are selective for epinephrine-induced reactions, since they do not affect 5-HT-, ADP-, or collagen-induced aggregation (Table I), nor the production of ^{14}C-arachidonic acid metabolites by the platelets (Table II).

α-Adrenergic receptor activation with epinephrine inhibits the increase of platelet cAMP-levels produced by PGE_1 and directly inhibits adenylate cyclase activity in platelet membrane preparations [69–71]. On the other hand, it induces – contrary to ADP stimulation – a rapid transmembrane uptake of ^{45}Ca into the platelets [72]. Therefore, epinephrine has the capacity to enhance activatory Ca^{2+}-influx into the platelets and to inhibit the cAMP-related system for removal of activator-Ca^{2+} from the cytoplasm, mechanisms possibly involved in the induction of aggregation by this catecholamine [24].

By contrast, β-adrenergic receptor activation with, for example, isoprenaline

86

and the β_2-selective drugs salbutamol and terbutaline, stimulates in a dose-dependent way adenylate cyclase activity and – possibly by this virtue – reduces aggregation induced by non-catecholamine agonists [71,73,74,78]; these inhibitory effects of β_2-stimulation are blocked by non-selective β-adrenergic antagonists such as propranolol, timolol and the β_2-selective antagonist butoxamine, whereas the β_1-selective antagonist metoprolol does not interfere with the system; these findings suggest that β-adrenergic stimulation of the cAMP-related system in human platelets is mainly associated with β_2-adrenergic receptors [60,76–78].

While the three major effects of epinephrine on human platelets, namely the primary aggregation, the secondary irreversible aggregation associated with release and the amplification of other agonists can be prevented specifically by α_2-adrenergic receptor antagonists [59–61, 65–68], the effects of β-adrenergic receptor blocking drugs on platelet behaviour are more complex.

In platelets from normal human volunteers, propranolol in concentrations of 1×10^{-6} M or higher in vitro, mainly raises the ADP threshold for the occurrence of a second phase of release-associated irreversible aggregation. It reduces the second wave of aggregation and the extent of release induced by low concentrations of ADP, epinephrine, collagen or thrombin, the concentration of the antagonist required for this effect increasing with the strength of the stimulus [60,79–82].Primary aggregation as a reflection of direct receptor-agonist interaction is not affected (Table I) unless high concentrations are used which affect cell integrity, interfere with the uptake mechanisms of catecholamines by platelets and induce release of platelet intragranular material [80,82,83]. In these experiments d(+)-propranolol, which is about 40 times less effective as a β-blocker on vascular smooth muscle [84], is equally potent as a platelet inhibitor as the clinically used racemic mixture (d)(1)(+–)-propranolol; on the contrary the potent β-adrenergic receptor antagonist practolol, which lacks 'membrane-stabilising' activity, has virtually no effect on platelet behaviour; these findings suggest that propranolol alters the described platelet reactions by mechanisms other than β-adrenergic blockade [24,60,82,85].

Nevertheless, such an effect potentially may have clinical implications, be it limited to patients whose platelets display an increased sensitivity to aggregating stimuli; indeed it was shown that propranolol therapy (80–160mg daily) in patients with severe angina pectoris rendered their platelets, with low thresholds for aggregation by ADP and epinephrine, less sensitive to these agonists [86] and in post-myocardial infarction patients (40–320mg daily) progressively reduced the marginally increased number of circulating platelet aggregates [87]. Additionally – although not obvious in vitro at the 1×10^{-5} M concentration we tested (Table I) – (d)(1)(+–)-propranolol, as well as (d)(+)-propranolol treatment (640mg daily for four weeks) in hypertensive patients reduces the production of TXA_2 by thrombin-stimulated platelets as well as the secondary aggregation, by specifically inhibiting thromboxáne synthetase without affecting prostacyclin production by endothelial cells [88]; such an effect might increase its potential usefulness in controlling platelet reactions. However, by blocking the inhibitory effect of β_2-adrenergic stimulation, bearing upon the stimulation of platelet cAMP-related systems, propranolol unmasks the full α_2-agonistic properties of epinephrine, as reflected by the exaggerated response of platelets in its presence to low-dose challenge with this catecholamine [74,77,78]; such a finding precipitated a warning about the possible thrombotic hazards of therapy with non-selective β-blocking agents [77].

Dopaminergic antagonists

Dopamine alone, when added to human citrated platelet-rich plasma from normal volunteers, in concentrations between 2 to 5×10^{-5} M produces a weak, reversible aggregation response in some plasma preparations [89], but not in others [90] when tested between 1×10^{-6} M to 1×10^{-4} M. However it amplifies the aggregation and release reaction induced by low-dose ADP stimulation [90]. At concentrations between 1×10^{-4} M to 5×10^{-3} M dopamine progressively inhibits firstly the second wave of aggregation induced by epinephrine and, later on, the first wave without affecting the platelet response to ADP or to arachidonic acid [91].

Radioligand binding experiments with [^{3}H] dopamine showed that there is no evidence that it binds to specific receptors upon platelets which can be identified as a separate receptor population nor for a transport system analogous to the dopaminergic neurones [92]. The synergistic effect of dopamine on platelet reactions to other agonists such as ADP appears to be mediated through α_2-adrenoreceptors, because rauwolfia antagonises this effect and because dopamine specifically inhibits epinephrine-induced platelet activation [90,91]; this hypothesis is compatible with the known cross-reactivity of dopaminergic and α-adrenergic receptor blocking agents in some systems [93].

Domperidone, a peripheral dopamine-receptor antagonist [94] recently introduced for the prevention of migraine attacks [95] appears to be inactive at 1×10^{-5} M in vitro against platelet activation induced by ADP, collagen and epinephrine (Table I) as well as on the metabolisation of arachidonic acid by human platelets (Table II). At this comparatively high concentration it does block 5-HT-induced platelet aggregation (Table I), although a separate study on human platelets showed its potency in this respect (IC_{50} = 2.32×10^{-6} M) to be largely inferior to that of other serotonergic receptor antagonists such as spiperone (IC_{50} = 2.4×10^{-9} M) or methysergide (IC_{50} = 2.15×10^{-8} M). It is not known yet whether after oral intake in humans domperidone reaches high enough plasma levels to achieve the similar platelet effect ex vivo.

Inhibition of transmission

Inhibition of liberation of second messenger

Since Ca^{2+}, liberated from intracellular stores or traversing the plasma membrane in the case of stimulation with epinephrine, may be a primary agent acting as a second messenger in the various stages of platelet activation, Ca^{2+}-antagonists, interfering with one or both cation translocations, potentially can influence platelet function (see [24] for full review).

Inhibition by several Ca^{2+}-entry blockers of platelet functional changes induced by epinephrine, and by other agonists as well, are reported to occur both in vitro and in vivo; a number of these effects are difficult to explain on the basis of Ca^{2+}-channel blockade only.

At comparatively high concentrations (20–500μg/ml) verapamil as well as nifedipine inhibit the epinephrine-induced human platelet aggregation, formation of thromboxane A_2 and release of [^{14}C] 5-HT, but are ineffective against ADP- or thrombin-induced platelet activation [96,97]. This finding seems to be compatible with a drug-provoked inhibition of transmembrane Ca^{2+}-flux involved in epinephrine- but not ADP- or thrombin-induced platelet behavioural changes; the inhibition by verapamil of epinephrine-induced and -amplified reactions to ADP can be overcome by the addition of ionised Ca^{2+} to the sample [98,99] suggesting that the drug acts in this condition mainly by blockade of intracellular Ca^{2+}-translocations.

On the contrary in cat platelet-rich plasma, verapamil and nisoldipine (50μg/ml) but not nifedipine or nimodipine inhibit ADP-induced aggregation, verapamil only reducing additionally arachidonic acid-induced aggregation as well. Again, this inhibition by verapamil could be overridden by the addition of extracellular Ca^{2+} [100]. In human platelet-rich plasma verapamil, diltiazem and nifedipine (8 to 50μg/ml) in vitro inhibit both the primary and secondary aggregation induced by ADP, arachidonic acid, collagen and epinephrine, diltiazem being the most potent [101,102] while oral administration of nifedipine reduces ADP-, arachidonic acid- and collagen-induced aggregation but, paradoxically, does not affect epinephrine-induced reactions [101].

For the Ca^{2+}-entry blockers proposed for the treatment of migraine, namely flunarizine and nimodipine, we find no obvious inhibitory effect on the platelet activation induced by 5-HT, ADP, collagen or epinephrine (Table I) nor on the arachidonic acid metabolism by human platelets Table II), even at comparatively high concentrations of 1 x 10^{-5} M. With the former drug, the daily oral administration (10mg/daily x 14) to man also fails to affect ex vivo platelet aggregation induced by ADP, Thrombofax®, collagen, epinephrine or epinephrine reactions amplified by the other agents in platelet-rich plasma, suggesting absence of an obvious direct effect at therapeutic doses on the classic parameters of platelet function. However, platelets when suitably activated, release/produce vasoconstrictive mediators including 5-HT, TXA_2 and to a lesser extent $PGF_{2\alpha}$ [103,104]. Without interfering directly with the platelet activation itself flunarizine effectively inhibits the platelet-mediated vascular contractions, 5-HT as well as TXA_2 being affected at the level of the vascular smooth muscle cell reaction [104].

Inhibitors of cyclic phosphodiesterase

Platelets represent a bidirectional system since they respond positively to stimulatory agonists and negatively with reversal or inhibition of aggregation release to inhibitory antagonists. In this context, cAMP is currently considered to be a unidirectional regulator, the primary role of which would be to inhibit a number of Ca^{2+}-dependent intracellular activatory processes, including myosin phosphorylation required for action-myosin contraction, depolymerisation of microtubuli involved in early shape change and phospholipase A_2-induced liberation of arachidonic acid from membrane phospholipids required for the production of eicosanoids. This is done by modulating the removal of free Ca^{2+} from the cytosol through a 'calcium pump' contained in the dense tubular system of the platelets [24,105−108]. Although some aggregating agents (e.g. epinephrine and ADP) inhibit platelet adenylate cyclase activity in platelet lysates and reduce the increase of platelet cAMP caused by PGE_1, studies with intact platelets show that aggregating agents such as vasopressin, 5-HT, thrombin and collagen have little effect on the elevation of cAMP caused by PGE_1. Moreover, considerable ADP-induced aggregation still occurs in the presence of moderately elevated platelet cAMP levels induced by low PGE_1 concentrations, leading to the concept that aggregating agents do not have to reduce basal cAMP levels to induce aggregation [106,107].

However, elevation of cAMP levels by compounds stimulating platelet adenylate cyclase activity such as prostacyclin, PGD_2, PGE_1, adenosine and β-adrenergic agonists such as isoprenaline [105] and to some extent − by inhibitors of cyclic nucleotide phosphodiesterase or a combination of these two types of drugs [24,73,106], produces inhibition of platelet reactions to various agonists. Although some discrepancies exist between the inhibitory potential of some of these drugs and their effect on cAMP [105,109], it is generally accepted that, in this case, the changes in cAMP as a unidirectional mediator are largely responsible for the inhibitory potential of these compounds [105,106].

Dipyridamole, its active dosage depending upon the experimental conditions and the species involved, can affect various parameters of platelet activation including platelet retention to glass beads, aggregation induced by ADP, collagen, thrombin, noradrenaline, and release of 5-HT induced by collagen (for review see [100]).

When tested in vitro on platelet-rich plasma, dipyridamole is a comparatively weak inhibitor of human platelet aggregation requiring up to 50μg/ml or more for an effect [111,112]; its effect is largely potentiated by combining it with PGE_1 or adenosine stimulating cAMP-accumulation [73,113). At comparatively large concentrations, dipyridamole inhibits platelet cAMP phosphodiesterase activity [73,114], a mechanism which may be implicated in its increased effectiveness when tested in whole blood through potentiation of the effects of either prostacyclin [115] or RBC-derived adenosine [116] on the cAMP system of blood platelets.

Although potentially dipyridamole could thus correct abnormal platelet activation, the drug was reported to exacerbate the migraine attack, possibly because its vasodilator properties outweigh a possible beneficial action on platelet behaviour [21].

Inhibitors of extrusion

Acetylsalicylic acid (aspirin), both in vitro and after ingestion, affects mainly the release reaction of platelets, including ADP-, 5-HT- and PF_4-release, and the resulting aggregation induced by collagen, the irreversible aggregation induced by ADP or epinephrine, which are also associated with release of intraplatelet products [for review see 110,117]. The mechanism by which aspirin as well as other non-steroidal anti-inflammatory drugs act on platelets is still not completely understood. Aspirin does not affect the platelet surface charge, platelet nucleotides and cAMP levels or ADP degradation by plasma enzymes; however it inhibits fatty acid cyclo-oxygenase, the first enzyme involved in the cascade leading to the production of TXA_2, PGE_2 and $PGF_{2\alpha}$ by platelets and of prostacyclin by the vascular wall, but poorly affects thromboxane A_2 synthetase itself [24,110,118]. Such an effect has been proposed as a mechanism of action of these drugs [119], but, as demonstrated for flurbiproben and indomethacin, their effect on the release reaction does not always correlate closely with inhibition of cyclo-oxygenase, suggesting additional mechanisms of action [120]. Moreover, anti-inflammatory agents block the production of prostaglandins induced in platelets by thrombin or by collagen (compare aspirin 1×10^{-5} M on collagen-induced aggregation in Table I and on MDA production in Table II) without impairing the release reaction. Additionally, the drug inhibits the adherence of platelets to subendothelial tissue in vitro at low haematocrit values but fails to do so in the presence of a normal number of red blood cells [121].

Alternative mechanisms therefore exist which can bypass the inhibitory effect of aspirin on the platelet release reaction [122] leaving its inhibition of TXA_2 production by platelets as its only certain pharmacological effect in vivo.

Conclusion

The anti-migraine drugs discussed in this update can be classified according to their mechanism of action on platelets.

As inhibitors of the induction phase, $5-HT_2$ receptor antagonists such as methysergide, pizotifen, domperidone, ergotamine and α_2-adrenergic receptor antagonists such as ergotamine and clonidine specifically affect the platelet reactions subsequent to interaction of 5-HT and/or epinephrine with specific platelet membrane receptors; while β_2-adrenergic blockade with propranolol does not explicitly inhibit, but even enhances platelet reactions to catecholamines, this drug – by other non-receptor mediated mechanisms – can affect the platelet aggregation/release reaction and the production of TXA_2.

As inhibitors of the transmission phase, dipyridamole as a cyclic nucleotide phosphodiesterase inhibitor acting in synergism with prostacyclin and/or adenosine can inhibit platelet reactions to various agonists, but its vasodilator properties make it less suitable for the treatment of migraine; on the contrary, the Ca^{2+}-entry blockers flunarizine and nimodipine appear not to affect platelet function directly, but block the vasospastic effect of the platelet-derived mediators 5-HT and TXA_2 on the vascular tree.

As inhibitor of the extrusion phase, aspirin can reduce the release of intragranular platelet products induced by various agonists, but its effect can be bypassed by other mechanisms of platelet activation leaving inhibition of prostaglandin biosynthesis as its only established pharmacological effect in vivo. Since the relative importance of the various pathways or stages of platelet activation in the pathogenesis of migraine is still unclear, it is difficult to conclude whether the therapeutic effect of these drugs bears any relationship to their activity on the platelets. As platelets become exposed in vivo to a variety of stimuli, specific receptor blockade with a given drug is not liable to inhibit all platelet activatory pathways, unless of course a particular agonist would be of primary importance. If any relationship should exist between anti-migraine activity and anti-platelet effect, we speculate that drugs acting either on the release/production of prostaglandins and 5-HT and, even more, blocking the vascular effects of platelet-derived mediators, irrespective of the inducing stimulus, would stand the best chance to affect migraine through such an effect.

Summary

Antimigraine drugs can be classified according to their mechanism of action on platelets.

As inhibitors of the induction phase, the $5-HT_2$ receptor antagonists methysergide, pizotifen, ergotamine, domperidone and the α_2-adrenergic receptor antagonists ergotamine and clonidine specifically inhibit platelet reactions induced by 5-HT or 1-epinephrine only. The β-adrenergic receptor antagonist propranolol by inhibiting β_2-mediated stimulation of adenylate cyclase can enhance epinephrine-induced reactions but by non-receptor mediated mechanisms can reduce platelet aggregation/release and production of TXA_2 induced by non-catecholamine agonists.

As an inhibitor of the transmission phase dipyridamole, inhibiting platelet cyclic nucleotide phosphodiesterase and acting in synergism with prostacyclin and/or adenosine can inhibit platelet reactions to various agonists; on the contrary, the Ca^{2+}-entry blockers flunarizine and nimodipine do not directly affect platelet function but block the vasospastic effects of platelet-derived mediators on the vascular tree. As an inhibitor of the extrusion phase aspirin can reduce the release of intraplatelet products but its inhibitory effect can be bypassed by other mechanisms leaving inhibition of prostaglandin biosynthesis as its only established pharmacological effect in vivo.

It is concluded that drugs acting to inhibit the release/production of 5-HT and prostaglandins or to block the vascular effects of platelet-derived mediators, irrespective of the nature of the inducing stimulus, would stand the best chance to influence migraine through an 'anti-platelet' action.

References

1   Hanington E. Migraine: a blood disorder? *Lancet 1978; ii:* 501–502
2   Hanington E. Migraine: a platelet hypothesis. *Biomedicine 1979; 30:* 65–66
3   Hanington E. Migraine as a blood disorder: preliminary studies. *Adv Neurol 1982; 33:* 253–256
4   David JL, De Clerck F. Platelets and migraine. This volume
5   Hilton BP, Cummings JN. 5-Hydroxytryptamine levels and platelet aggregation responses in subjects with acute migraine headaches. *J Neurol Neurosurg Psychiatr 1972; 35:* 505–509
6   Kalendowsky L, Austin JH. Complicated migraine, its association with increased platelet aggregability and abnormal plasma coagulation factors. *Headache 1975; 15:* 8–35
7   Couch JR, Hassanein FR. Platelet aggregability in migraine. *Neurology 1977; 27:* 834–848
8   Deshmukh SV, Meyer JS. Cyclic changes in platelet dynamics and the pathogenesis and prophylaxis of migraine. *Headache 1977; 17:* 101–108
9   Oxman T, Hitzeman RJ, Smith R. Platelet membrane lipid composition and the frequency of migraine. *Headache 1982; 22:* 261–267
10 Deshmukh S, Meyer JS, Mouche RJ. Platelet dysfunction in migraine: effect of self-medication with aspirin. *Thromb Haemostas (Stuttg) 1976; 36:* 319–324
11 Gawel M, Burkitt M, Clifford Rose F. The platelet release reaction during migraine attacks. *Headache 1979; 19:* 323–327
12 D'Andrea G, Toldo M, Cortelazzo S, Milone FF. Platelet activity in migraine. *Headache 1982; 22:* 207–212
13 Glover V, Sandler M, Grant E et al. Transitory decrease in platelet monoamine-oxidase activity during migraine attacks. *Lancet 1977; i:* 391–393
14 Coppen A, Swade C, Wood K. Platelet 5-hydroxytryptamine accumulation and migraine. *Lancet 1979; ii:* 914
15 Mück-Seler D, Deanovic Z, Dupelj M. Platelet serotonin (5-HT) and 5-HT releasing factor in plasma of migrainous patients. *Headache 1979; 19:* 14–17
16 Carrol JD, Coppen A, Swade CC, Wood KM. Blood platelet 5-hydroxytryptamine accumulation and migraine. *Adv Neurol 1982; 33:* 233–235
17 Gawel MJ, Clifford Rose F. Platelet function in migraineurs. *Adv Neurol 1982; 33:* 237–242
18 Wachowicz B. Platelet activation: its possible role in the migraine mechanism. *Adv Neurol 1982; 33:* 243–246
19 Ryan RE, Ryan RE. The use of platelet inhibitors in migraine. *Adv Neurol 1982; 33:* 247–252
20 Dalessio DJ. Migraine, platelets, and headache prophylaxis. *JAMA 1978; 239:* 52–53
21 Hawkes CH. Dipyridamole in migraine. *Lancet 1978; i:* 153
22 Holmsen H. Classification and possible mechanisms of action of some drugs that inhibit platelet aggregation. *Ser Haematol 1976; 8:* 51–80
23 Vermylen J, de Gaetano G, Verstraete M. Platelets and thrombosis. In Poller L, ed. *Recent Advances in Thrombosis.* Edinburgh: Churchill Livingstone. 1973: 113–150

24 De Clerck F, David JL. Pharmacological control of platelet and red blood cell function in the microcirculation. *J Cardiovasc Pharmacol 1981; 3:* 1388–1412

25 White JG. Platelet morphology. In Johnson JA, ed. *The Circulating Platelet.* New York: Academic Press. 1971: 46–121

26 De Clerck F, Borgers M, Vermylen J, de Gaetano G. Human platelet aggregation of Thrombofax®. An electron-microscopic study of the sequences of events. *Scand J Haematol 1974; 12:* 93–103

27 Detwiler TC, Charo IF, Feinman RD. Evidence that calcium regulates platelet function. *Thromb Haemostas (Stuttg) 1978; 40:* 207–211

28 Lüscher EF, Massini P, Käser-Glanzmann R. The role of calcium ions in the regulation of platelet function and their pharmacological control. In *Advances in Pharmacology and Therapeutics. Prostaglandins–Immunopharmacology. Volume 4.* Oxford: Pergamon Press. 1978: 87–95

29 Massini P, Käser-Glanzmann R, Lüscher EF. Movements of calcium ions and their role in the activation of platelets. *Thromb Haemostas (Stuttg) 1978; 40:* 212–218

30 De Clerck F, David JL, Janssen PAJ. Inhibition of 5-hydroxytryptamine-induced and amplified human platelet aggregation by ketanserin (R 41 468), a selective 5-HT$_2$-receptor antagonist. *Agents Actions 1982; 12:* 388–397

31 Peters JR, Grahame-Smith DG. Human platelet 5-HT receptors: characterization and functional association. *Eur J Pharmacol 1980; 68:* 243–256

32 Lampugnani MG, de Gaetano G, Rossi EC. Functional distinction between serotonin uptake and serotonin-induced shape change receptors in rat platelets. *Biochem Biophys Acta 1982; 693:* 22–26

33 De Clerck F, Herman AG. 5-Hydroxytryptamine and platelet aggregation. *Fed Proc 1983; 42:* 228–232

34 Leempoels J, De Cock W, De Cree J, Verhaegen H. The effect of ketanserin on 5-HT-induced irreversible platelet aggregation in patients with cardiovascular diseases. *First Eur Meeting on Hypertension, Milan 1983, May 29–June 1 (Abstract)*

35 De Clerck F, Xhonneux B, Leysen J, Janssen PAJ. The involvement of 5-HT$_2$ receptor sites in the activation of platelets. *Thromb Res 1983:* in press

36 Hilton BP, Cumings JN. An assessment of platelet aggregation induced by 5-hydroxytryptamine. *J Clin Pathol 1971; 24:* 250–258

37 Dalsgaard-Nielsen T, Genefke IK. Serotonin (5-HT) and release and uptake in platelets from healthy persons and migrainous patients and attack-free intervals. *Headache 1974; 14:* 26–32

38 Peroutka SO, Snyder SH. Multiple serotonin receptors: differential binding of [³H] 5-hydroxytryptamine, [³H] lysergic acid diethylamide and [³H] spiroperidol. *Mol Pharmacol 1974; 16:* 687–694

39 Leysen J, Awouters F, Kennis L et al. Receptor binding profile of R 41 468, a novel antagonist at 5-HT$_2$ receptors. *Life Sci 1981; 28:* 1015–1022

40 Leysen JE, Gommeren W, De Clerck F. Demonstration of S$_2$-receptor binding sites in cat blood platelets using [³H] ketanserin. *Eur J Pharmacol 1983; 88:* 125–130

41 Leysen JE, Tollenaere JP. Biochemical models for serotonin receptors. *Ann Rep Med Chem 1982; 17:* 1–10

42 Leysen JE, Niemegeers CJE, Van Nueten JM, Laduron PM. [³H] Ketanserin (R 41 468) a selective ³H-ligand for serotonin$_2$ receptor binding sites. Binding sites, brain distribution, and functional role. *Mol Pharmacol 1982; 21:* 301–314

43 De Clerck F, Van Nueten JM. Platelet-mediated vascular contractions: inhibition of the serotonergic component by ketanserin. *Thromb Res 1982; 27:* 713–727

44 Müller-Schweinitzer E, Brundell J. Enhanced prostaglandin synthesis contributes to the venoconstrictor activity of ergotamine. *Blood Vessels 1975; 12:* 193–205

45 Zijlstra FJ, Spierings ELH, Vincent JE. Effect of ergotamine on platelet prostaglandin synthesis – *in vitro* and *in vivo* experiments. *Cephalalgia 1981; 1:* 25–27

46 Mitchell JRA, Sharp AA. Platelet clumping *in vitro. Br J Haematol 1964; 10:* 78–93

47 Mills DCB. Platelet aggregation and platelet nucleotide concentration in different species. *Symp Zool Soc Lond 1970; 27:* 99–107

48   O'Brien JR. Some effects of adrenaline and anti-adrenaline compounds on platelets *in vitro* and *in vivo*. *Nature (London) 1963; 200:* 763–764
49   Mills DCB, Robb IA, Roberts GCK. The release of nucleotides, 5-hydroxytryptamine and enzymes from human blood platelets during aggregation. *J Physiol 1968; 195:* 715–729
50   Best LC, Holland TK, Jones PBB, Russell RGG. The interrelationship between thromboxane biosynthesis, aggregation and 5-hydroxytryptamine secretion in human platelets *in vitro*. *Thromb Haemostas (Stuttg) 1980; 43:* 38–40
51   Cameron HA, Ardlie NG. The facilitating effects of adrenaline on platelet aggregation. *Prostaglandins Leukotrienes Med 1982; 9:* 117–128
52   Belleau B, Benfey BG, Melchiorre C, Mowtambault M. Inhibition of adrenaline-induced platelet aggregation by the α-adrenoceptor blocking drug benextramine. *Br J Pharmacol 1982; 76:* 253–257
53   MacMillan DC. Secondary clumping effect in human citrated platelet-rich plasma produced by adenosine diphosphate and adrenaline. *Nature 1966; 211:* 140–144
54   Lages B, Weiss HJ. Dependence of human platelet functional responses on divalent cations: aggregation and secretion in heparin- and hirudin-anticoagulated platelet-rich plasma and the effects of chelating agents. *Thromb Haemostas (Stuttg) 1981; 45:* 173–179
55   Glusa E, Markwardt F. Adrenaline-induced reactions in hirudin plasma. *Haemostasis 1980; 9:* 188–192
56   Cazenave JP, Sutter A, Hemmendinger S et al. Adrenaline activates human platelets but does not cause primary aggregation if thrombin generation is inhibited by hirudin. *Thromb Haemostas (Stuttg) 1981; 46:* 95 (Abstract)
57   Mei Huang E, Detwiler TC. Characteristics of the synergistic actions of platelet agonists. *Blood 1981; 57:* 685–691
58   Patscheke H. Role of activation in epinephrine-induced aggregation of platelets. *Thromb Res 1980; 17:* 133–142
59   Barthel W, Markwardt F. Aggregation of blood platelets by biogenic amines and its inhibition by antiadrenergic and antiserotonergic agents. *Biochem Pharmacol 1974; 23:* 37–45
60   Mills DCB, Roberts GCK. Effects of adrenaline on human blood platelets. *J Physiol 1967; 193:* 443–453
61   O'Brien JR. Some effects of adrenaline and anti-adrenaline compounds on platelets *in vitro* and *in vivo*. *Nature 1963; 200:* 763–764
62   Shattil S, McDonough M, Turnbull J, Insel PA. Characterization of alpha-adrenergic receptors in human platelets using [^{3}H] clonidine. *Mol Pharmacol 1981; 19:* 179–183
63   Elliot JM, Grahame-Smith DG. The binding characteristics of [^{3}H]-dihydroergocryptine on intact human platelets. *Br J Pharmacol 1982; 76:* 121–130
64   Alexander RW, Cooper B, Hunden RI. Characterization of the human platelet α-adrenergic receptor. Correlation of [^{3}H] dihydroergocryptine binding with aggregation and adenylate cyclase inhibition. *J Clin Invest 1978; 61:* 1136–1144
65   Lasch P, Jakobs KH. Agonistic and antagonistic effects of various α-adrenergic agonists in human platelets. *Naunyn-Schmiedebergs Arch Pharmacol 1979; 306:* 119–125
66   Jakobs KH. Synthetic α-adrenergic agonists are potent α-adrenergic blockers in human platelets. *Nature 1978; 274:* 819–820
67   Grant JA, Scrutton MC. Novel α_2-adrenoreceptors primarily responsible for inducing human platelet aggregation. *Nature 1973; 277:* 659–661
68   Glusa E, Markwardt F, Barthel W. Studies on the inhibition of adrenaline-induced aggregation of blood platelets. *Pharmacology 1979; 19:* 196–201
69   Robinson GA, Arnold A, Hartmann RC. Divergent effects of epinephrine and prostaglandin E_1 on the level of cAMP in human blood platelets. *Pharmacol Res Commun 1969; 1:* 325–332
70   Jakobs KH, Saur W, Schultz G. Reduction of adenylate cyclase activity in lysates of human platelets by the alpha-adrenergic component of epinephrine. *J Cycl Nucleotide Res 1976; 29:* 381–392

71   Haslam RJ, Taylor A. Effects of catecholamines on the formation of adenosine 3':5'-cyclic monophosphate in human blood platelets. *Biochem J 1971; 125:* 377–379

72   Owen NE, LeBreton GC. The involvement of calcium in epinephrine or ADP potentiation of human platelet aggregation. *Thromb Res 1980; 17:* 855–863

73   Mills DCB, Smith JB. The influence on platelet aggregation of drugs that affect the accumulation of adenosine 3':5'-cyclic monophosphate in platelets. *Biochem J 1971; 121:* 185–196

74   Yu SK, Latour JG. Potentiation of α and inhibition by β-adrenergic stimulation of rat platelet aggregation. A comparative study with human and rabbit platelets. *Thromb Haemostas (Stuttg) 1977; 37:* 413–422

75   Mills DCB, Roberts GCK. Effect of adrenaline on human blood platelets. *J Physiol 1967; 193:* 443–453

76   Scrutton MC, Wallis RB. Catecholamine receptors. In Gorden JL, ed. *Platelets in Biology and Pathology–2.* Amsterdam: Elsevier North-Holland Biomedical Press. 1981: 179–210

77   Winther-Hansen K, Klysner R, Geisler A et al. Platelet aggregation and beta-blockers. *Lancet 1982; i:* 224–225

78   Abdulla YJ. β-Adrenergic receptors in human platelets. *J Atheroscler Res 1969; 9:* 171–177

79   Gibelli A, Montanati C, Bellani D et al. Beta-blocking drugs and human platelet aggregation *in vitro. Experientia 1973; 29:* 186–187

80   Dvilansky A, Korczyn D, Sage J, Nathan I. Effect of propranolol and pindolol on platelet aggregation and release of serotonin. *Isr J Med Sci 1976; 12:* 1529

81   Bucher HW, Stucki P. The effect of various beta-receptor blocking agents on platelet aggregation. *Experientia 1969; 25:* 280–282

82   Weksler B, Gillick M, Pink J. Effect of propranolol on platelet function. *Blood 1977; 49:* 185–196

83   Bygdeman S, Johnson Ø. Studies on the effect of adrenergic blocking drugs on catecholamines and 5-hydroxytryptamine. *Acta Physiol Scand 1969; 75:* 129–138

84   Howe R, Shanks RG. Optimal isomers of propranolol. *Nature 1966; 210:* 1336–1338

85   Lemmer B, Wiethold G, Hellenbrecht D et al. Human blood platelets as cellular models for investigation of membrane active drugs: Beta-adrenergic blocking agents. *Naunyn-Schmiedebergs Arch Pharmacol 1972; 275:* 299–313

86   Frishman WK, Weksler B, Christodoulou JP et al. Reversal of abnormal platelet aggregability and change in exercise tolerance in patients with angina pectoris. *Circulation 1974; 50:* 887–898

87   Green D, Rossi EC, Haring O. The β-blocker heart attack trial: studies of platelets and Factor VIII. *Thromb Res 1982; 28:* 261–267

88   Campbell WB, Johnson AR, Callahan KS, Graham RM. Anti-platelet activity of beta-adrenergic antagonists: inhibition of thromboxane synthesis and platelet aggregation in patients receiving long-term propranolol treatment. *Lancet 1981; ii:* 1382–1384

89   Boullin DJ, Green AR, Grimes RPJ. Human blood platelet aggregation induced by dopamine, 5-hydroxytryptamine and analogous. *J Physiol 1975; 252:* 46P–47P

90   Glusa E. Interaction of lisuride with monoamine receptors on human blood platelets. *Biochem Pharmacol 1983:* in press

91   Sharma HM, Panganamala RV, Geer JC, Cornwell DG. Inhibition of platelet aggregation induced by either epinephrine or arachidonic acid. *Thromb Res 1975; 7:* 879–884

92   Boullin DJ, Molyneux D, Roach B. The binding of haloperidol to human blood platelets and interactions with 5-hydroxytryptamine and dopamine. *Br J Pharmacol 1978; 63:* 561–566

93   Willems JL. Dopamine-induced inhibition of synaptic transmission in lumbar paravertebral ganglia of the dog. *Naunyn-Schmiedebergs Arch Pharmacol 1973; 279:* 115

94   Van Nueten JM, Schuurkes JAJ. Animal pharmacology of domperidone, anti-emetic and gastrokinetic properties. In Towe G, ed. *Progress with Domperidone, a Gastrokinetic and Anti-emetic Agent.* London: Royal Society of Medicine. 1981: 21–27

95 Waelkens J. Domperidone in the prevention of complete classical migraine. *Br Med J 1982; 284:* 944

96 Addonizio VP, Fischer CA, Edmonds LH. Effects of verapamil and nifedipine on platelet activation. *Circulation 1980; 62 (Suppl III):* III-326

97 Addonizio VP, Fischer CA, Strauss JF, Edmonds LH. Inhibition of human platelet function by verapamil. *Thromb Res 1982; 28:* 545–556

98 Owen NE, LeBreton GC. The involvement of calcium in epinephrine or ADP production of human platelet aggregation. *Thromb Res 1980; 17:* 855–863

99 Owen NE, Feinberg H, LeBreton GC. Epinephrine induces Ca^{2+} uptake in human platelets. *Am J Physiol 1980; 239:* H483–H488

100 Schmunk GA, Lefer AM. Anti-aggregatory actions of calcium channel blockers in cat platelets. *Res Commun Chem Pathol Pharmacol 1982; 35:* 179–187

101 Johnsson H. Effects of nifedipine (ADALAT®) on platelet function *in vitro* and *in vivo*. *Thromb Res 1981; 21:* 523–528

102 Kiyomoto A, Sasaki Y, Odawaza A, Morita T. Inhibition of platelet aggregation by diltiazem. Comparison with verapamil and nifedipine and inhibitory potencies of diltiazem metabolites. *Circ Res 1983; 52 (Suppl I):* 115–119

103 De Clerck F, Van Nueten J. Platelet-mediated vascular contractions: inhibition of the serotonergic component by ketanserin. *Thromb Res 1982; 27:* 713–727

104 De Clerck F, Van Nueten J. Platelet-mediated vascular contractions. Inhibition by flunarizine, a calcium-entry blocker. *Biochem Pharmacol 1983; 32:* 765–771

105 Haslam RJ, Davidson ML, Davies T et al. Regulation of blood platelet function by cyclic nucleotides. *Adv Cycl Nucleotide Res 1978; 9:* 633–553

106 Haslam RF, Davidson MML, Fox JEB, Lynham JA. Cyclic nucleotides in platelet function. *Thromb Haemostas (Stuttg) 1978; 40:* 232–240

107 Feinstein MB, Rodan GA, Cutler LS. Cyclic AMP and calcium in platelet function. In Gorden JL, ed. *Platelets in Biology and Pathology–2.* Amsterdam: Elsevier-North Holland Biomedical Press. 1981: 437–472

108 Vermylen J, Badenhorst PM, Deckmyn H, Arnout J. Normal mechanisms of platelet function. *Clin Haematol 1983; 12:* 107–151

109 Tsien WH, Sass SP, Sheppard H. The lack of correlation between inhibition of aggregation and cAMP levels with canine platelets. *Thromb Res 1982; 28:* 509–519

110 Vermylen J, de Gaetano G, Verstraete M. Platelets and thrombosis. In Poller L, ed. *Recent Advances in Thrombosis.* Edinburgh: Churchill Livingstone. 1973: 113–150

111 Eliason R, Bygdeman S. Effect of dipyridamole and two pyrimido-pyrimidine derivatives on the kinetics of human platelet aggregation and on platelet adhesiveness. *Scand J Clin Lab Invest 1969; 24:* 145–151

112 Emmons PR, Harrison MJG, Honour AJ, Mitchell JRA. Effect of dipyridamole on human platelet behaviour. *Lancet 1965; ii:* 603–606

113 Born GVR, Mills DCB. Potentiation of the inhibitory effect of adenosine on platelet aggregation by drugs that prevent its uptake. *J Physiol 1969; 202:* 41P–42P

114 Lam SCT, Guccione MA, Packham MA, Mustard JF. Effect of cAMP phosphodiesterase inhibitors on ADP-induced shape change, cAMP and nucleotide diphosphokinase activity of rabbit platelets. *Thromb Haemostas 182; 47:* 90–95

115 Moncada S, Korbut R. Dipyridamole and other phosphodiesterase inhibitors act as antithrombotic agents by potentiating endogenous prostacyclin. *Lancet 1978; i:* 286–289

116 Gresele P, Zoja C, Deckmyn H et al. Dipyridamole inhibits platelet aggregation in whole blood *in vitro* and *in vivo*. *Thromb Haemostas (Stuttg) 1983; 50:* 132 (Abstract)

117 Holmsen H. Platelet secretion (Release reaction) – mechanism and pharmacology. *Adv Pharmacol Ther 1979; 4:* 97–109

118 Moncada S, Vane JR. Arachidonic acid metabolites and the interactions between platelets and blood-vessel wall. *N Engl J Med 1979; 300:* 142–147

119 Vane JR. Inhibition of prostaglandin biosynthesis as a mechanism of action for aspirin-like drugs. *Nature 1971; 231:* 232–235

120 Cockbill SA, Meptinstall S, Taylor PM. A comparison of the abilities of acetylsalicylic acid, flurbiprofen and indomethacin to inhibit the release reaction and prostaglandin biosynthesis in human blood platelets. *Br J Pharmacol 1979; 67:* 73–78

121 Cazenave JP, Kinlough-Rathbone RL, Packham MA, Mustard JF. The effect of acetylsalicylic acid and indomethacin on rabbit platelet adherence to collagen and the subendothelium in the presence of low or high hematocrit. *Thromb Res 1978; 13:* 971–981

122 Vargaftig BB, Chignard M, Benveniste J. Present concepts on the mechanisms of platelet aggregation. *Biochem Pharmacol 1981; 30:* 263–271

7

THE AUTONOMIC NERVOUS SYSTEM AND MIGRAINE PATHOGENESIS

M J Biggs, E S Johnson

No single theory has yet been proposed that adequately explains the cause, or causes, of migraine. The pulsating quality of the headache and its deep-seated 'visceral' character indicate that intracranial blood vessels are involved. But difficulties arise when attempts are made to link the changes in blood vessel tone to the symptoms of the migraine attack. The vessels are richly innervated so, in theory, changes in vascular tone might be neurological in nature. Alternatively the changes might reflect increases in the plasma concentrations of a number of vasoactive substances known to occur early on in an attack.

Some of the earliest theories on migraine pathogenesis involved the autonomic nervous system as is evident from the following description by Rothlin [1] of his early experiments with ergotamine: "In 1925, faced with a severe and intractable case of migraine, a condition which was thought, at that time, to be related to a state of sympathicotonia, I had the idea of administering ergotamine tertrate by subcutaneous injection, as it was known to exert a sympatholytic effect." This idea was carried further by Sicuteri [2] who suggested that the initial vasoconstrictor element of migraine was due to the transiently increased release of the transmitter noradrenaline to the vessels involved. All other manifestations of the disease followed this initial vasoconstriction. Most of the evidence in favour of this 'autonomic theory' was reappraised by Johnson [3] in 1978.

Any plausible theory on the causes of migraine should satisfy a number of criteria [3]. In particular it should permit or explain the symptomatology and the underlying vascular and/or neurological pathology; the function of the vasomotor innervation to the vasculature involved; the mechanism of action of migraine-inducers such as tyramine, phenylethylamine, contraceptive steroids and other trigger factors; the prediction of drugs likely to be useful in the management of the disease enabling the theory to be challenged in clinical practice; the basis for the modes of action of apparently dissimilar therapeutic

99

agents and explain why migraine is more likely to respond to treatment instituted in the prodromal phase of the syndrome. The latter will not be considered further in the present paper. But probably the most important criterion of all for a theory to be tenable is that it must explain the unilateral nature of the symptoms experienced by some 70 per cent of individuals.

This article explores how far the autonomic noradrenergic hypothesis fulfills these criteria. It will not include discussion on autonomic nerves known to release acetylcholine or neuropeptides.

Symptoms and pathology

The neurological symptoms that augur the migraine attack have been attributed for many years to the constriction of cerebral blood vessels [4] and the headache phase has similarly been associated with a vasodilatation [5] especially of extra-cranial arteries. According to the autonomic theory, the neurological symptoms of the prodromal phase result from vasoconstriction due to the neurally released noradrenaline acting on vascular α_1-adrenoceptors. Neurological sequelae would be expected to occur if perfusion were to fall to a level critical for adequate oxygenation. If this noradrenaline-induced constriction is not modified by pharmacological intervention then the vessels will ultimately dilate, possibly assisted by the presence of vasodilator metabolites accumulated during the constrictor phase [2] and also perhaps by a reflex inhibition of the constrictor drive — a form of reactive hyperaemia [3].

In contrast to some of the older isotope wash-out experiments [6, 7] recent [133] Xenon blood flow studies made during the aura of classical migraine (see Oleson, Chapter 1) have shown a decrease in cortical flow which outlasts the prodromal symptoms. The hypoperfusion may occur in both occipital cortices and this makes it difficult to attribute the cause of the aura to a localised vascular spasm; yet many of the symptoms are consistent with a transient episode of focal cerebral hypoxia. Certainly the rebreathing of expired CO_2 or administration of 10 per cent CO_2 in air, manoeuvres known to cause cerebral cortical vaso-dilatation, will reverse the progression of the visual disturbances in some patients.

During the headache phase Oleson could not find evidence for a measurable increase in cerebral blood flow in patients with either common or classical migraine. Indeed in classical migraine the hypoperfusion that persisted after the prodromal state was always present on the headache side and bilateral headache sometimes occurred with a unilateral decrease in flow. Thus changes in cerebro-vascular tone do not readily account for the siting of the headache although the two could be linked indirectly, for example, if the vasoconstriction were to lead to the release of pain-inducing or pain-potentiating substances such as kinins, prostaglandins, serotonin and histamine.

Dilatation of scalp vessels has been said to contribute to the headache [5] but this cannot be solely responsible for the pain associated with migraine as it

100

has been shown in migraine patients that scalp vessel dilatation by immersion of the body in hot water [5] or by the injection of methacholine [8] is not usually painful, and does not produce the other focal features of an attack [9].

Innervation of blood vessels

In order to establish the presence of a significant noradrenergic neurogenic control of cerebral blood vessels, several factors should be demonstrable:

i) There must be an adrenergic innervation of these vessels;

ii) The vessels must be capable of responding to the transmitter noradrenaline;

iii) The reversal of noradrenergic cerebral vasoconstriction should be brought about by α_1-adrenoceptor blockade if the constriction of cerebral vessels results from the activation of α_1-adrenoceptors as it does in the periphery and provided that the α_1-receptor antagonist can cross the blood-brain barrier.

i) There is some evidence that adrenergic nerves make contact with the cerebral vessels, probably capillaries, and that these nerves have their origin in cell bodies within the locus coeruleus in the brain stem [10], some fibres from which also relay in the hypothalamus. Thus it is conceivable that the vasoconstrictor phase of migraine might be centrally mediated and this would avoid objections to the adrenergic hypothesis based on the apparent inability of catecholamines to cross the blood-brain barrier. Sympathetic nerve fibres originating in the superior cervical ganglia innervate cerebral arteriolar smooth muscle.

ii) Decreases in cerebral blood flow have been observed in man following intravenous infusion of noradrenaline [11] and scotomata have been induced [12] although it is said that amines have very little effect on cerebral blood flow when assessed by the ^{133}Xe technique.

iii) There is evidence that cerebral adrenergic vascular receptors are largely of the alpha variety [13]. Interestingly Corbett et al [13] have also demonstrated that intracranial vessels do not seem to be under continuous neurogenic vaso-constrictor tone as is the case in other blood vessels. This implies that the cerebral vasoconstriction of classical migraine is possibly due to an abnormal adrenergic drive which ought to prove responsive to post-synaptic α_1-adrenoceptor antagonism. This abnormal drive need not be very marked as atonic vessels are likely to be sensitive to small amounts of noradrenaline. From this it can be predicted that centrally acting α_1-blockers given early in the constrictor phase, and in low doses unlikely to influence vessels normally under sympathetic constrictor tone, will prevent the vascular changes.

Peripheral sympathetic activity

When nerve impulses pass along the peripheral sympathetic nerves they release noradrenaline and DβH from storage vesicles by exocytosis [14]. There is limited evidence that plasma noradrenaline concentration is more significantly increased during the three hours preceeding patients' awakening with migraine than in the similar three hours in those awakening without migraine [15]. Furthermore plasma catecholamine levels were significantly higher in the three hours preceding a migraine than in the corresponding three hours when the same subject did not awaken with migraine. These results are consistent with the 'autonomic' hypothesis in which a noradrenaline-induced vasoconstriction precedes the headache phase. Further evidence favouring an increased activity of the sympathetic nervous system in migraine sufferers was provided by Gotoh et al [16] who showed the DβH activity was significantly higher in serum from untreated patients (taken during a headache-free interval) than in that from normal controls. There were no significant differences in serum DβH activity between patients with classicial and common migraine.

More recently Anthony [17] demonstrated a rise in plasma levels of noradrenaline, cAMP, free fatty acids and DβH during the headache period above those measured before and after the headache phase. This was taken to indicate sympathetic overactivity concomitant with a migraine attack.

In headache-free periods migraine patients demonstrate enhanced peripheral vasoconstrictor tone [18] consistent with an overactive sympathetic system. Ellertson [19] found that migraine patients had more pronounced cardiovascular responses to auditory stimuli and became tolerant to such stimuli more slowly than did control subjects. Migraine sufferers may be trained with biofeedback techniques to reduce their sympathetic tone and thus abort an attack [20]. Mathew et al [21] related the anti-migraine action of biofeedback to the demonstrable fall in plasma catecholamines. It is conceivable that the unilateral nature of migraine can be explained on the basis of enhanced hypersensitivity to NA at the level of the cerebral arteries, as there is some evidence that hypersensitivity is asymmetrical and similar to the phenomenon of denervation hypersensitivity [21].

Migraine trigger factors

Tyramine

In 1967, Hanington [23] noted that foods especially those containing tyramine and known to interact with monoamine oxidase inhibitors (MAOIs) corresponded to those foods that could precipitate migraine. She postulated that some individuals demonstrate an especially sensitive localised vascular response to amines such as tyramine and she provided evidence for this by inducing migraine attacks by means of the oral administration of 100mg tyramine in patients showing a clear history of migraine provocation by diet. More recently Boisen et al [24], in a double-blind crossover trial carried out over two consecutive eight week periods, found that daily doses of 125mg tyramine administered to migraine sufferers produced no more headaches than did placebo. The results from those patients with a history of food-provoked migraine were analysed separately but no significant differences were found between the number of headaches experienced on tyramine or placebo administration.

Shaw [25] gave even higher doses of tyramine orally (200mg) to those sufferers whose headaches were triggered by cheese but was unable to produce an attack unless a MAOI was taken simultaneously in which case doses of only 20mg of tyramine were effective in producing a migraine. When tyramine alone was administered, none was found in the plasma and there were no changes in plasma levels of glucose, lactate, pyruvate, free fatty acids or ketone bodies.

This and other contradictory evidence has been appraised by Kohlenberg [26] who concluded that on balance tyramine probably will precipitate a migraine attack and that differing results reflect variations in subject selection and procedure. A possible source of confusion might be that the placebo itself provokes a stress reaction and thus will induce attacks.

In those patients who are sensitive to tyramine there is evidence of a deficiency in the enzyme responsible for sulphate conjugation of the amine [27] thus potentiating its action. Since it is capable of releasing noradrenaline from sympathetic nerve endings, a possible mechanism emerges for tyramine's alleged ability to induce migraine, viz a noradrenergic vasoconstriction of intra- and extracranial vessels in susceptible individuals.

Another factor to be taken into consideration is that platelet MAO has been reported to be less in migraine patients at the time of attacks than between attacks [28]. It is just possible that in diet-susceptible patients sufficient tyramine escapes first-pass degradation and is capable of reaching the brain. Monoamines in general are known for their relative inability to cross the blood-brain barrier. However it has been reported that in many regions of the brain the barrier is not so impenetrable [29].

Thus Willoughby in 1981 [29] drew attention to the potential significance of the circumventricular organs such as the median eminence, area postrema, subfornical organ, vascular organ of the lamina terminalis and subcommissural organ. These areas seem devoid of a blood-brain barrier and receive a fenestrated capillary supply which provides a route for the ready diffusion of substances into the brain. Furthermore many of these structures receive both serotoninergic and/or adrenergic innervations from the brain stem. Consequently the circumventricular organs are receptive to serotonin and catecholamines and should the concentration of these substances increase in the systemic circulation there will be a parallel increase in these areas and the autonomic functions which they subserve may be disturbed producing for example nausea, vomiting, changes in fluid intake or vasomotor instability, all of which commonly occur with migraine. This attractive hypothesis of Willoughby provides a basis for the mechanism of action of the aforementioned monoamines in foods said to precipitate migraine attacks.

Reserpine

Reserpine is well known to deplete the monoamines dopamine, noradrenaline and serotonin from neuronal and extraneuronal sites. Kimball et al [30] induced a migraine-like syndrome in nine out of ten known migraine sufferers by the intramuscular injection of 2.5mg reserpine.

Reserpine-induced headaches closely resemble those of spontaneous migraine whereas prodromal visual symptoms are rare [31]. Vasodilatation, the intensity of which is not simply related to that of the headache, is extremely prominent after reserpine in contrast to the spontaneous migraine attacks in which the patient is usually pale. One possible explanation of these aspects of reserpine's action might be that the noradrenaline released by reserpine from the nerve-endings causes a relatively short-lived vasoconstriction of cerebral and extra-cranial vessels insufficient in intensity to cause visual disturbances but enough to cause the accumulation of acid metabolites. The noradrenaline, after its surge, is itself metabolised, and the neuronal depletion leads to passive vasodilatation which the ischaemic metabolites potentiate by active vascular smooth muscle relaxation.

Steroid hormones

Migraine is more common in women and frequently begins with the onset of ovulation. This has led to speculation that female hormones may be involved in the generation of migraine attacks [32]. Consistent with this are the observations that the attacks are often less frequent during pregnancy, may be provoked by use of the combined oral contraceptive pill paradoxically more commonly in the seven pill-free days, and that migraine tends to lessen in intensity and fre-quency after the menopause.

There is evidence that the relationship is mediated by the actions of the ovarian hormones on the sympathetically mediated responses. Endometrial monoamine oxidase activity increases after ovulation or under the influence of certain oral contraceptives [33, 34]. Furthermore the contractile effects of noradrenaline, adrenaline and tyramine on the rabbit isolated aorta were poten-tiated by both 17β-oestradiol and progesterone [35]. It has been suggested that these steroids exert their action by the inhibition of the enzyme catechol-O-methyltransferase, although an uptake inhibitory mechanism has also been postulated [30]. In either case the noradrenergic response is potentiated.

In women, there appears to be menstrual cycle-related changes in sympathetic nervous activity. Ghose et al [34] demonstrated an increase in peripheral adrenergic function, as assessed by the tyramine pressor test, at the end of the follicular phase and beginning of the luteal phase. Meanwhile, Wineman [38] who assessed autonomic nervous activity during the menstrual cycle by using oral temperature, heart rate, diastolic blood pressure, galvanic skin resistance and salivary output as indices, found high levels of sympathetic activity during menstruation and the follicular and ovulatory phases, but low levels during the luteal phase.

That ovarian steroids potentiate the vascular responses of the sympathetic nervous system is consistent with the hypothesis that noradrenergic mechanisms are involved with the genesis of menstrually-linked migraine.

Others

Many dietary triggers of migraine are known [39] apart from those such as cheese which contains tyramine. They include chocolate, citrus fruit, alcohol, yeast extracts and seafoods. Smoking is also a powerful trigger in some individuals and nicotine is known to stimulate the release of catecholamines [40]. Chocolate contains large amounts of phenylethylamine [41] which stimulates vascular α_1-adrenoceptors directly [42].

Glyceryl trinitrate [43, 44] and amphetamine [45] will also precipitate migraine in susceptible patients and both are believed to be acting in a way similar to tyramine.

Prediction of drugs likely to be useful for the treatment of migraine

If a vasoconstrictor action of noradrenaline on vascular α_1-adrenoceptors is the fundamental factor initiating migraine attacks, and this is still an open question, then selective blockade of these receptors provides both the basis for the prophylactic therapy of the condition and a clinical challenge for the present hypothesis.

The choice of a suitable α_1-adrenoceptor antagonist should satisfy the following criteria:

a) It must be active when taken by mouth;

b) It should preferably have a duration of action following oral administration of at least four to six hours;

c) It should preferably be a reversible competitive antagonist;

d) It must cross the blood-brain barrier;

e) The drug should not cause agonist constrictor side-effects as do many of the currently used agents such as the ergot alkaloids.

It has been argued that only very low doses of an α_1-antagonist drug will be required to overcome the slight increase in the noradrenergic activity presently postulated to occur in migraine. Therefore the successful use of a competitive α_1-blocker in migraine will predictably be with sub-hypotensive doses thus minimising troublesome side-effects such as postural hypotension and failure of ejaculation.

Summary

A number of observations have been linked together to suggest that adrenergic activity is involved in migraine pathogenesis. A story can be made out but the vast majority of the evidence needs confirming. There can be no question that the migraine syndrome includes symptoms of both vascular and neurological origin but the contributions of catecholamines to the two systems remain unresolved, as do their possible link with other neurotransmitters and local hormones.

References

1   Rothlin E. Historical development of the ergot therapy of migraine. *Int Arch Allergy Appl Immunol 1955; 7:* 205–209

2   Sicuteri F. Vasoneuroactive substances and their implication in vascular pain. *Res Clin Stud Headache 1967; 1:* 6

3   Johnson ES. A basis for migraine therapy – the autonomic theory reappraised. *Postgrad Med J 1978; 54:* 231–242

4   Dalessio DJ. On migraine headache: serotonin and serotonin antagonism. *JAMA 1962: 181:* 318

5   Lance JW. *Mechanism and Management of Headache 2nd edition.* London: Butterworths. 1973

6   O'Brien MD. Cerebral blood flow changes in migraine. *Headache 1971; 10:* 139

7   Skinhoj E. Hemodynamic studies within the brain during migraine. *Arch Neurol 1973; 29:* 95

8   Ostfeld AM. Migraine headache. Its physiology and biochemistry. *JAMA 1960; 174:* 1188

9   Chapman LR, Ramos AO, Goodell H et al. A humoral agent implicated in vascular headache of the migraine type. *Arch Neurol 1960; 3:* 223

10   Raichle ME, Hartman BK, Eichling JO, Sharpe LG. Central noradrenergic regulation of cerebral blood flow and vascular permeability. *Proc Natl Acad Sci 1975; 72:* 3726–3730

11   Sensenbach W, Madison L, Ochs L. Comparison of the effects of L-norepinephrine, synthetic L-epinephrine and U.S.P-epinephrine upon cerebral blood flow and metabolism in man. *J Clin Invest 1953; 32:* 226

12   Tunis MM, Wolff HG. Studies on headache: long-term observations of the reactivity of the cranial arteries in subjects with vascular headache of the migraine type. *Arch Neurol Psychiatry 1953; 70:* 551

13   Corbett JL, Eidelman BH, Debarge O. Modification of cerebral vasoconstriction with hyperventilation in normal man by thymoxamine. *Lancet 1972; ii:* 461

14   Schanberg SM, Stone RA, Kirshner N et al. Plasma dopamine B-hydroxylase: a possible aid in the study and evaluation of hypertension. *Science 1974; 183:* 523

15   Hsu LKG, Crisp AH, Kalucy RS et al. Early morning migraine. Nocturnal plasma levels of catecholamines, tryptophan, glucose and free fatty acids and sleep encephalographs. *Lancet 1977; i:* 447

16   Gotoh F, Kanda T, Sakai F et al. Serum dopamine-B-hydroxylase activity in migraine. *Arch Neurol 1976; 33:* 656

17   Anthony M. Biochemical indices of sympathetic activity in migraine. *Cephalalgia 1981; 1:* 83–89

18   Appenzeller O. Reflex vasomotor function. Clinical and experimental studies of migraine. *Res Clin Stud Headache 1978; 6:* 160–166

19   Ellertsen B, Hammerborg D. Psychophysiological response patterns in migraine patients. *Cephalalgia 1982; 2:* 19–24

20   Dalessio DJ, Kunzel M, Sternbach R, Sorak M. Conditioned adaptation-relaxation reflex in migraine therapy. *JAMA 1979; 242:* 2102–2104

21   Mathew RJ, Ho BT, Kralik P et al. Catecholamines and migraine: evidence based on biofeedback induced changes. *Headache 1980; 20:* 247–252
22   Yamamoto M, Meyer JS. Hemicranial disorder of vasomotor adrenoceptors in migraine and cluster headache. *Headache 1980; 20:* 321–335
23   Hanington E. Preliminary report on tyramine headache. *Br Med J 1967; 1:* 550
24   Boisen E, Deth S, Hubbe P et al. Clonidine in the prophylaxis of migraine. *Acta Neurol Scand 1978; 58:* 288–295
25   Shaw SWJ, Johnson RH, Keogh HJ. Oral tyramine in dietary migraine sufferers. In Greene R, ed. *Current Concepts in Migraine Research.* New York: Raven Press. 1978: 31–39
26   Kohlenberg RJ. Tyramine sensitivity in dietary migraine, a critical review. *Headache 1982; 22:* 30–34
27   Smith I, Kellow AH, Mullen PE, Hanington E. Dietary migraine and tyramine metabolism. *Nature 1971; 230:* 246
28   Sandler M. Transitory platelet monoamine oxidase deficit in migraine: some reflections. *Headache 1977; 17:* 153–158
29   Willoughby JO. The pathophysiology of vegetative symptoms in migraine. *Lancet 1981; Aug 29:* 445–446
30   Kimball RW, Friedman AP, Vallejo E. Effect of serotonin in migraine patients. *Neurology 1960; 10:* 107
31   Curzon G, Barrie M, Wilkinson MIP. Relationships between headache and amine changes after administration of reserpine to migraineous patients. *J Neurol Neurosurg Psychiatry 1969; 32:* 555
32   Greene R. The endocrinology of headache. In Pearce J, ed. *Modern Topics in Migraine.* London: William Heinemann Medical Books Ltd. 1975: Chapter 7
33   Southgate J, Grant ECG, Pollard W et al. Cyclic variations in endometrial monoamine oxidase: Correlation of histochemical and quantitative biochemical assays. *Biochem Pharmacol 1968; 17:* 721
34   Grant ECG, Carroll JD, Goodwin P, Pryce-Davies J. Effect of oral contraceptives on depressive mood changes and on endometrial monoamine oxidase and phosphatases. *Br Med J 1968; 3:* 777
35   Kalsner S. Steroid potentiation of responses to sympathomimetic amines in aortic strips. *Br J Pharmacol 1969; 36:* 582
36   Iversen LL, Salt PJ. Inhibition of catecholamine uptake by steroids in the isolated rat heart. *Br J Pharmacol 1970; 40:* 528
37   Ghose K, Coppen A, Carroll D. Intravenous tyramine response in migraine before and during treatment with indoramin. *Br Med J 1977; 1:* 1191
38   Wineman EW. Autonomic balance changes during the human menstrual cycle. *Psychophysiology 1971; 8/1:* 1–6
39   Hanington E, Horn M, Wilkinson M. Further observations on the effects of tyramine. In Cochrane AL, ed. *Background to Migraine, the Third Migraine Symposium.* London: Heinemann. 1970: 113–119
40   Grant ECG , Alburquerque M, Steiner TJ, Rose FC. Oral contraceptives, smoking and ergotamine in migraine. *Abstracts of the Migraine Trust International Symposium.* London, September 1976: 8–9
41   Sandler M, Youdim MBH, Hanington E. A phenylethylamine oxidising defect in migraine. *Nature 1974; 250:* 335
42   Gonsalves A, Johnson ES. Possible mechanism of action of B-phenylethylamine in migraine. *J Pharm Pharmacol 1977; 29:* 646
43   Campus S, Fabris, Rapelli A et al. Escrezione urinaria di acido 5-idrossiindolacetico durante crisi cefalalgia indotta da trinitroglicerina. *Bollettino della Societa di Biologia Sperimentale 1967; 43:* 1844
44   Henderson WR, Raskin NH. "Hot-dog" headache: individual susceptibility to nitrite. *Lancet 1972; ii:* 1162
45   Smith I, Kellow AH, Hanington E. A clinical and biochemical correlation between tyramine and migraine headache. *Headache 1970; 10:* 43

8

ADRENOCEPTOR MECHANISMS AND MIGRAINE THERAPY

L Edvinsson

Introduction

The acute migraine attack is often associated with clinical symptoms such as paleness of the skin, alterations in blood pressure and heart rate. It can be triggered by stress and by dietary substances, e.g. tyramine, which suggests an increase in the activity of the sympathetic nervous system. Plasma noradrenaline, dopamine β-hydroxylase, cyclic AMP and free fatty acids, are all increased during migraine attacks, reflecting the enhanced sympathetic activity [1]. A change in the activity of the sympathetic system during migraine attacks is likely to affect not only the extracranial but also the intracranial blood vessels since both vascular beds are supplied with dense plexuses of perivascular noradrenergic nerves originating in the superior cervical ganglion (Figure 1) as well as α-adrenoceptors and β-adrenoceptors (Figure 2).

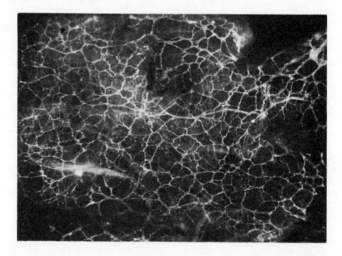

Figure 1. Fluorescence photomicrograph of a human pial artery. The vessel has been cut open longitudinally, mounted flat on a microscope slide and exposed to formaldehyde gas under dry conditions for visualisation of the green-fluorescent noradrenaline transmitter. Magnification x 100 (reduced for publication)

108

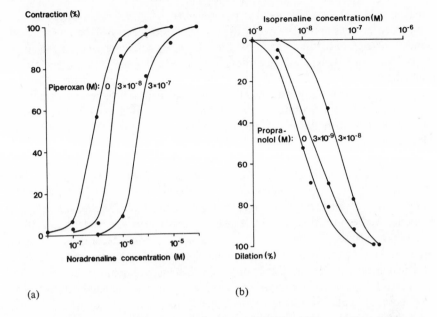

Figure 2. Noradrenaline-induced contractions (a) and isoproterenol-induced dilations (b) of human pial arteries during in vitro conditions. The responses are in (a) blocked by the α-adrenoceptor antagonist piperoxan and (b) by the β-adrenoceptor blocker propranolol. For further technical details see reference [36]

In the past, several drugs that are known to interact with the autonomic nervous system (via adrenoceptors) have been used to alleviate migraine symptoms, e.g. ergotamines and propranolol. The present paper will review, firstly, the present knowledge of adrenoceptor classification and, secondly, the current use of these agents in the pharmacotherapy of migraine.

Classification of α-adrenoceptors

Recent advances in the knowledge and understanding of the various steps and processes involved in adrenergic transmission have been responsible for a renaissance of interest in α-adrenoceptors and their role in the regulation of the cardiovascular bed. It has been shown that noradrenaline released from sympathetic nerve terminals may regulate its own release through a negative feedback mechanism, mediated by pre-junctional α-adrenoceptors that are independent of the nature of the post-junctional adrenoceptors on the effector cells [2–4]. This is an essential component of a comprehensive and integrated system for local control of transmitter release, operating at the terminal ramifications of the autonomic nervous system. This concept of a local control of transmitter release has enabled a pharmacological distinction to be made from those α-adrenoceptors

109

that are located post-junctionally. Furthermore, when it became apparent that major differences existed between the pre- and post-junctional α-adrenoceptors, and consequently that some agonists and antagonists acted preferentially in either pre- or post-junctional α-adrenoceptors, it raised exciting therapeutic possibilities. Investigation of differences between pre- and post-synaptic α-adrenoceptors was clouded when receptors resembling the presynaptic ones were encountered post-synaptically. Therefore, at present the prefixes α_1 and α_2 are solely used for receptors with different sensitivity to adrenoceptor agents regardless of location or function.

Definition

It is now generally regarded, based on results from both functional and ligand binding studies in various tissues, that α_1-adrenoceptors can be defined as those that have affinity for antagonists with a potency that declines in the order prazosin, corynanthine $\gg$ yohimbine, rauwolscine, and α_2-adrenoceptors as those for which the affinity declines in order rauwolscine, yohimbine $\gg$ corynanthine, prazosin (Table I). A definition of the adrenoceptors on agonist data seems to be more difficult. α_1-adrenoceptors appears to prefer (−) noradrenaline over (−) erytho-α-methylnoradrenaline, whereas it is the other way around for α_2-adrenoceptors. Clonidine has a higher affinity and potency than phenylephrine for α_2-adrenoceptors whereas it is the opposite case for α_1-adrenoceptors [4].

The mechanism or mechanisms by which α-adrenoceptors elicits activation in various tissues is not yet known in full detail. It has been suggested that cyclic

TABLE I. Comparison of effects of antagonists at pre- and post-synaptic α-adrenoceptors in the pulmonary artery of the rabbit. The quotient EC_{30} pre/K_B post has been taken as index of preferences for α_1-adrenoceptors and α_2-adrenoceptors [4]

Antagonists	EC_{30} pre/K_B post
Prazosin	>50
Corynanthine	40
Clozapine	27
Azapetine	12
Phentolamine	2.7
Mianserin	2.2
Piperoxan	0.69
Dihydroergocristine	0.47
Tolazoline	0.18
Dihydroergotamine	0.14
Yohimbol	0.12
Yohimbine	0.020
Rauwolscine	0.0039

guanosine $3'-5'$monophosphate (cyclic GMP) might play a role in effects mediated via α-adrenoceptors, similar to that of cyclic AMP in β-adrenoceptor mediated responses [5]. However, available data do not support this assumption [6]. There is evidence which suggests that α-adrenoceptor activation involves a net increase in transmembrane calcium movements [7, 8] and an increase in intracellular calcium concentration. This may explain the increase in cyclic GMP concentration in response to administration of α-adrenoceptor agonists as observed in some tissues [5]. Since activation of α-adrenoceptors is associated with an influx of calcium through the cell membrane, the combination of α-adrenoceptor antagonists and drugs that specifically block calcium influx offers an interesting and potentially potent way to influence vascular smooth muscle tone in various vascular disorders [9].

Alpha-adrenoceptor drugs used in the pharmacotherapy of migraine

Since α-adrenergic mechanisms have been implied in the pathophysiology of migraine, the noradrenaline reactivity of human temporal arteries from common migraine sufferers has been compared with those of control patients [10]. Noradrenaline constricts both types of vessels in a concentration-dependent manner and the response is blocked by phentolamine in a competitive manner. There is no statistically significant difference between migraine patients and controls either with respect to maximum contraction or sensitivity. The affinity of phentolamine for the α-adrenoceptors (pA_2 value) was 8.3 in vessels from controls and 7.6 in arteries from migraine sufferers ($p>0.05$). There is thus clear evidence for the presence of α-adrenoceptors in human temporal arteries (Figure 3) but no indication that there is a change in the sensitivity of the vascular α-adrenoceptors in common migraine [10].

Agonists

Classically, stimulation of α-adrenoceptors give rise to excitation and contraction of most smooth muscles, e.g. vasoconstriction of arteries and veins. It has, therefore, been logical to suggest α-adrenoceptor antagonists as useful agents to control hypertension. The interesting exception from this general role is clonidine, an α-adrenoceptor agonist, which causes hypotension. Studies during the last decade have shown that the cardiovascular inhibitory effect of clonidine is due to stimulation of central α-adrenoceptors [11]. Clonidine is a partial α_2-adrenoceptor agonist with both stimulating and blocking properties of central and peripheral α-adrenoceptors. This hypotensive effect appears to be a general pharmacological pattern of α-adrenoceptor agonists, with selectivity towards α_2-adrenoceptors, provided they can pass the blood-brain barrier in sufficiently high concentrations [12].

Clonidine is the only α-adrenoceptor agonist that at present is used in the pharmacotherapy of migraine [13, 14] (for literature review, see [15]). It

111

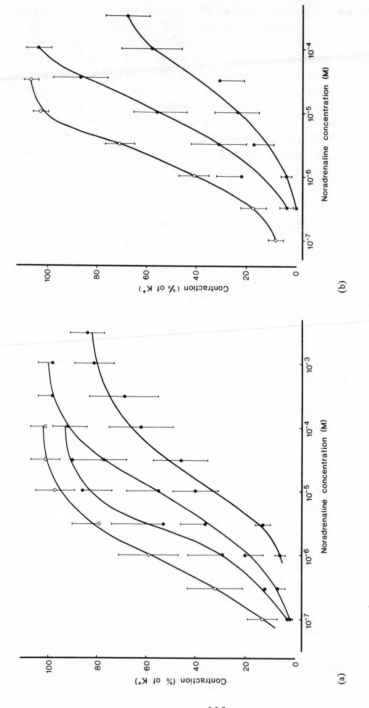

Figure 3. Contractile response to noradrenaline (○) and effect of varying concentrations of phentolamine (●) on human temporal arteries in (a) control patients ($10^{-8}-10^{-6}$ M) and in (b) migraine sufferers ($10^{-7}-10^{-6}$ M). There was no significant difference between the two patient groups in sensitivity to noradrenaline or in the dissociation constant of phentolamine (control, $pA_2 = 8.3$; migraine group, $pA_2 = 7.6$). For details see [10]

112

may produce weak contractions of human intracranial and extracranial arteries. Since there is no other α-adrenoceptor agonist that has been noted to have a beneficial effect in migraine, we are tempted to believe that clonidine interacts with central vasomotor functions to alleviate the migraine symptoms. The doses used in the treatment of migraine appear to be approximately half those used for treatment of hypertension. Clonidine is not the strongest prophylactic agent in severe migraine but has a satisfactory effect in milder migraine cases [15]. In the future we might expect to see clinical trials with other centrally acting sympathomimetics, e.g. guanfacin and clonidine-like imidazolidines, not only in the treatment of hypertension but also as anti-migraine drugs.

Antagonists

The first group of agents which has been reported to block α-adrenoceptors is ergot alkaloids [16]. Several α-adrenoceptor antagonists have since been tested both in animal experiments and clinically. Of the first generation of α-adrenoceptor antagonists, only phentolamine and phenoxybenzamine are still available for limited therapeutic use. Prazosin is the first α-adrenoceptor blocking drug which is effective for the treatment of high blood pressure. It differs from the classical α-adrenoceptor antagonists in possessing a high degree of selectivity, estimates ranging from 10,000–100,000 to 1 for post-junctional (α_1), as opposed to pre-junctional (α_2) adrenoceptors [17]. The effectiveness of prazosin as an antihypertensive agent, not only serves to illustrate the importance of the local control of noradrenaline release in man, but also suggests that the primary pharmacological reason for the failure of the original non-selective α-adrenoceptor antagonists in the treatment of hypertension is, as has been predicted, the loss of the pre-junctionally mediated inhibitory feedback look.

Ergotamine and dihydroergotamine are the only α-adrenoceptor antagonists that are in common use in the pharmacotherapy of migraine. Both drugs are non-selective with regard to α-adrenoceptor subtypes (Table I). The effects of these ergot alkaloids on intracranial and extracranial vessels are complex and have been studied in great detail by Müller-Schweinitzer and colleagues [18, 19]. It has been found that both ergotamine and dihydroergotamine, though the latter to a somewhat lesser extent, can induce vasoconstriction. This effect is mainly due to stimulation of vascular 5-hydroxytryptamine (5-HT) receptors in cranial arteries, and activation of 5-HT receptors and α-adrenoceptors in peripheral arteries. In cranial arteries ergotamine has been shown to potentiate the vasoconstrictor effect of noradrenaline, while in limb arteries it acts as a competitive antagonist. Dihydroergotamine appears only to inhibit noradrenaline induced contractions in the two types of arteries and does not cause any potentiation [19]. Furthermore, ergotamine and dihydroergotamine block vasoconstrictor responses induced by 5-HT in both types of vessels in a non-competitive way. i.e. reduction of maximum and slope of the concentration response curves. It

113

has been suggested therefore that the efficiency of ergotamine and dihydro-ergotamine to abort a migraine attack is due, firstly, to the ability to reinforce noradrenaline-induced contractions and secondly, to their direct vasoconstrictor effects. Methysergide, another ergot derivative, is only effective as a prophylactic agent in migraine. This might be due to its negligible vasoconstrictor ability.

Characterisation of β-adrenoceptors

The pharmacological classification of adrenoceptors by Ahlquist [20], the synthesis of β-adrenoceptor blockers [21, 22] and the subdivision of the receptors into the β_1 and β_2 subtypes [23] have led to an intense development in the field of adrenoceptor research with multiple clinical applications. Most effects that are mediated via β-receptors (both β_1 and β_2) are believed to result from the stimulation of membrane bound adenylate cyclase, giving rise to an increase in the production of intracellular cyclic AMP. Stimulation of vascular β-adrenoceptors usually causes relaxation, probably due to several mechanisms. One of these is through a hyperpolarisation of the cell membrane, which reduces the net influx of extracellular calcium, the other is by stimulation of adenylate cyclase. The resultant increase in cyclic AMP provides energy for the removal of calcium from the contractile proteins into intracellular storage sites, or for an active extrusion of calcium through the cell membrane. Since no β-adrenoceptor agonist has been found to be of value in migraine therapy, we will only discuss the β-adrenoceptor antagonists.

Definition

Beta-adrenoceptor blockers are usually classified on the basis of well known pharmacodynamic properties like selectivity, intrinsic sympathomimetic activity (ISA) and membrane stabilising effect. Another property which influences the

TABLE II. Pharmacological properties and effects of α-adrenoceptor antagonists when tested for migraine prophylaxis. For further literature see [27, 35]

Drug	Cardioselectivity (β_1-antagonism)	Intrinsic sympathomimetic activity (ISA)	Membrane stabilising activity	Anti-migraine activity
Alprenolol	−	+	+	−
Oxprenolol	−	+	+	−
Pindolol	−	+	(+)	−
Propranolol	−	−	+	+
Sotalol	−	−	−	n.d.
Timolol	−	−	(+)	n.d.
Practolol	+	+	−	(+)
Atenolol	+	−	−	+
Metoprolol	+	−	(−)	+

+ = positive effect shown; − = no effect; n.d. = not determined

114

pharmacokinetics is lipid solubility, a phenomenon that has clinical relevance (Table II). It has been suggested that cardioselective drugs are preferable to non-selective for treatment of, for example, hypertension, but not for the treatment of patients with migraine. Whether cardioselective agents (β_1-adrenoceptors) are more effective than non-selective substances in reducing blood pressure is not yet established. In some situations, e.g. in hypertension associated with increased secretion of adrenaline such as in insulin-induced hypoglycaemia, mental stress and smoking, non-selective agents might be more appropriate. Similarly, ISA and lipid solubility are still discussed whether or not they are of benefit in various clinical situations [24].

Beta-adrenoceptor antagonists in the treatment of migraine

The only β-adrenoceptor blocker that has a well established migraine prophylactic effect is propranolol, a non-selective antagonist. The interest in this agent started when patients receiving propranolol for cardiovascular disorders were at the same time relieved of a co-existing migraine [25]. Subsequent clinical studies have amply confirmed this [26, 27]. Trials with other β-blockers have generally been less convincing [27, 28] (Table II). From the literature only selective β_1-adrenoceptor antagonists have, in addition to propranolol, shown some effect. Practolol seems to have a weak antimigraine effect [29], whereas atenolol and metoprolol have been reported to be as effective as propranolol [27, 30]. It is interesting to note that cerebral blood vessels are supplied with the β_1 type of adrenoceptors as opposed to the β_2 type, which predominates in peripheral blood vessels [31]. There is thus no clear relation between the pharmacological properties of β-blockers and their migraine prophylactic effect, and further clinical trials are needed, since factors other than β-adrenoceptor antagonism may be of importance. Propranolol has, in its racemic form, been compared with D-propranolol and placebo [32]. Both forms of propranolol have similar effects in migraine prophylaxis. It has, therefore, been thought that factors not necessarily due to β-adrenoceptor blockade also contribute to the beneficial effects. The reason behind the prophylactic effect of propranolol is thus still not clear. However, since it readily passes the blood-brain barrier and may reduce the cerebral blood flow and metabolism [33], it has been speculated that this explains part of its action. Future studies with propranolol-like agents will further our understanding of its prophylactic effect and may give new insight into the pathophysiology of migraine.

Summary and conclusion

To summarise, only few drugs with activity on adrenoceptors are at present in use for the treatment of migraine. Clonidine and propranolol appear to have their main actions on receptors in the central nervous system, whereas ergot derivatives interact with both α-adrenoceptors and 5-hydrotryptamine receptors in the cranial circulation. The recent demonstration of the co-existence and co-operation of neuropeptide Y (NPY) in sympathetic nerves (with noradrenaline) around cerebral and peripheral blood vessels [34] opens exciting possibilities for future developments in the understanding and treatment of migraine.

Acknowledgments

I gratefully acknowledge the excellent secretarial assistance of Miss Gunvor Nilsson.

The work was supported by the Swedish Medical Research Council (No. 5958) and the Swedish Association Against Heart and Lung Diseases.

References

1   Anthony M. Biochemical indices of sympathetic activity in migraine. *Cephalalgia 1981; 1:* 83–89
2   Langer SZ. Presynaptic regulation of the release of catecholamines. *Pharmacol Rev 1981; 32:* 337–362
3   Starke K. Presynaptic receptors. *Ann Rev Pharmacol Toxicol 1981; 21:* 7–30
4   Starke K, Docherty JR. Recent development in alpha-adrenoceptors research. *J Cardiovasc Pharmacol 1980; Suppl 3,* S269–S286
5   Schultz G, Schultz K, Hardman JG. Effects of norepinephrine on cyclic nucleotide levels in the ductus deferens of the rat. *Metabolism 1975; 24:* 429–437
6   Wikberg JES. The pharmacological classification of adrenergic alpha$_1$ and alpha$_2$ receptors and their mechanisms of action. *Acta Phsyiol Scand 1979; Suppl 468:* 1–99
7   Drew GM. The effect of different calcium concentrations on the inhibitory effect of presynaptic alpha-adrenoceptors in the rat vas deferens. *Br J Pharmacol 1978; 63:* 417–419
8   Karlsner S, Nickerson M, Boyd GN. Selective blockade of potassium-induced contractions of aortic strips by beta-diethylaminoethyl-diphenylprophylacetate (SKF 525 A). *J Pharmacol Exp Ther 1970; 174:* 500–508
9   Fleckenstein A. *Calcium Antagonism in Heart and Smooth Muscle.* New York: John Wiley. 1983
10 Edvinsson L, Tfelt-Hansen P, Skärby T et al. Presence of alpha-adrenoceptors in human temporal arteries. Comparison between migraine patients and controls. *Cephalalgia 1983.* In press
11 Schmitt H, Schmitt H, Fénard S. New evidence for an alpha-sympathomimetic component in the effects of catapresan on vascular centers: antagonism by piperoxane. *Eur J Pharmacol 1971; 14:* 98–100
12 Van Zwieten PA. Pharmacology of centrally acting hypotension drugs. *Br J Clin Pharmacol 1980; 10:* 13S–20S
13 Heathfield KWG, Raiman JD. The long-term management of migraine with clonidine. *The Practitioner 1972; 208:* 644–648
14 Shafar J, Tallet ER. Evaluation of clonidine in prophylaxis of migraine. *The Lancet 1972; i:* 403–406
15 Hakkarainen H, Hokkanen E, Kallanranta T. The role of clonidine in the treatment of migraine. A review of the literature and personal experience. *Ups J Med Sci 1980; Suppl 31:* 16–19
16 Dale HH. On some physiological actions of ergot. *J Phsyiol 1906; 34:* 163–206

17 Cambridge D, Davey MJ, Massingham R. Prazosin, a selective antagonist of post-synaptic alpha-adrenoceptors. *Br J Pharmacol 1977; 59:* 514P–515P

18 Müller-Schweinitzer E, Weidmann H. Basic pharmacological properties. In Berde B, Schild HO, eds. *Ergot Alkaloids and Related Compounds Handb Exp Pharm 49.* Berlin–Heidelberg: Springer Verlag. 1978: 87–232

19 Müller-Schweinitzer E, Fanchamps A. Effects on arterial receptors of ergot derivatives used in migraine. In Critchley M, Friedman AP, Gorini S, Sicuteri F, eds. *Advances in Neurology, Vol 33, Headache Physiopathological and Clinical Concepts.* New York: Raven Press. 1982: 343–356

20 Ahlquist RP. A study of the adrenotropic receptors. *Am J Physiol 1948; 153:* 586–600

21 Moran NC, Perkins ME. Adrenergic blockade of mammalian heart by a dichloro analogue of isoproterenol. *J Pharmacol Exp Ther 1958; 124:* 223–237

22 Powell CE, Slater IH. Blocking of inhibitory adrenergic receptors by a dichloro analogue of isoproterenol. *J Pharmacol Exp Ther 1958; 122:* 480–488

23 Lands AM, Luduena FP, Buzzo JH. Differentiation of receptors responsive to isoproterenol. *Life Sci 1967; 6:* 2241–2249

24 Cruickshank JM. The clinical importance of cardioselectivity and lipophilicity in beta-blockers. *Am Heart J 1980; 100:* 160–178

25 Rabkin R, Leven NW, Stables DP, Suzman MM. The prophylactic value of propranolol in angina pectoris. *Am J Cardiol 1966; 18:* 370–383

26 Weber RB, Reinmuth OM. The treatment of migraine with propranolol. *Neurol 1972; 22:* 366–369

27 Stensrud P, Sjaastad O. Comparative trial of tenormin (atenolol) and inderal (propranolol) in migraine. *Ups J Med Sci 1980; Suppl 31:* 37–40

28 Bruyn GW. Cerebral cortex and migraine. In Critchley M, Friedman AP, Gorini S, Sicuteri F, eds. *Advances in Neurology, Vol 33, Headache Physiopathological and Clinical Concepts.* New York: Raven Press. 1982: 151–169

29 Kallanranta T, Hakkarainen H, Hokkanen E, Tuovinen T. Clonidine in migraine prophylaxis. *Headache 1977; 17:* 169–172

30 Ljung O. Treatment of migraine with metoprolol. *N Engl J Med 1980; 303:* 156–157

31 Edvinsson L, Owman C. Pharmacological characterisations of adrenergic alpha and beta receptors mediating the vasomotor responses of cerebral arteries in vitro. *Circ Res 1974; 35:* 835–849

32 Stensrud P, Sjaastad O. Short-time clinical trial of propranolol in racemic form (Inderal), D-propranolol and placebo in migraine. *Acta Neurol Scand 1976; 53:* 229–232

33 MacKenzie ET, McCulloch J, Harper AM. Influence of endogenous norepinephrine on cerebral blood flow and metabolism. *Am J Physiol 1976; 231:* 489–494

34 Moghimzadeh E, Edvinsson L, Wahlstedt C et al. Neuropeptide co-exists and co-operates with noradrenaline in perivascular nerve fibres. *Nature 1983.* Submitted

35 Waal-Manning JH. Hypertension: which beta-blocker? *Drugs 1976; 12:* 412–441

36 Edvinsson L, Owman C, Sjöberg N-O. Autonomic nerves, mast cells and amine receptors in human brain vessels. A histochemical and pharmacological study. *Brain Res 1976; 115:* 377–393

9

CEREBRAL HYPOXIA AND MIGRAINE

W K Amery

Some time ago, I hypothesised [1] that a brief episode of focal cerebral hypoxia occurs in every attack of migraine. The present paper is an attempt at re-evaluating this hypothesis. In order to keep the reference list of this paper within reasonable limits, most references used for the original paper are not included again here. The interested reader, therefore, is referred to the original publication for more information in this respect.

In evaluating the potential pivotal role of cerebral hypoxia in the pathophysiology of the migraine attack, three basic questions come to mind:

a) Can the clinical syndrome, represented by a migraine attack, be explained if it is due to cerebral hypoxia?

b) If cerebral hypoxia indeed leads to the attack, what causes the hypoxia?

c) Is there any evidence that hypoxia actually occurs during a migraine attack and is there any evidence that migraineurs may be more susceptible to hypoxic brain damage than other subjects are?

These three questions will be dealt with in the following three sections.

Can hypoxia explain the migraine attack?

A distinction must be made here between the aura of the classic migraine attack and the subsequent headache phase.

The aura

Every physician knows that hypoxic insults to the brain can cause neurological symptoms. It is, therefore, no surprise that the neurologic aura is often considered to be the consequence of a cerebral vasospasm. Yet, the slow spreading of the

118

neurological phenomena, which are so typical of an attack of classical migraine, may argue against such a mechanism, since it would require a similar (rather slow) rate of expansion of the hypoxic insult itself.

Recently, growing attention has, therefore, been paid to spreading cortical depression since this neurophysiologic mechanism could provide a much better explanation of the neurological phenomena of the aura (see elsewhere in this volume). The possible presence of a spreading cortical depression during the aura phase, does not rule out the presence of cerebral hypoxia, however:

1. To start with, as summarised in Table I, there are very striking biochemical similarities between spreading depression and cerebral hypoxia. In fact, one could argue that spreading depression may be considered a peculiar (i.e. a spreading) type of neuronal hypoxia.

2. Furthermore, in the experimental lab, spreading depression is usually provoked by a drastic, topical increase of the extracellular K^+ concentration in the cerebral cortex. It is likely that a focus of neuronal hypoxia may lead to sufficiently high extracellular K^+ levels to initiate a similar spreading depression wave.

Cerebral hypoxia may thus conceivably trigger a spreading depression phenomenon, whilst, biochemically at least, the spreading depression may be considered a wave-like expansion from the hypoxic focus.

TABLE I. Similarities between spreading depression and cerebral hypoxia

Variable	Spreading depression	Cerebral hypoxia
Intracellular pO_2 ↓	LK Lukyanova & J Bures (1967) [8] M Tsacopoulos & A Lehmenkühler (1977) [9]	By definition
Intracellular lactic acid ↗	J Krivanek (1961) [7]	ES Gurdjian et al (1949) [2] + other authors
Neuronal glycogen content ↓	J Krivanek (1958) [6]	Various authors
Neuronal creatine phosphate ↓	J Krivanek (1961) [7]	ES Gurdjian et al (1949) [2]
$[K^+]e$ ↗ early during the process*	AJ Hansen et al (1980) [4] RP Kraig & C Nicholson (1978) [5]	AJ Hansen et al (1982) [3] RP Kraig & C Nicholson (1978) [5] ME Morris (1974) [10]

* $[K^+]$ only rises to more than 10–12mM in spreading depression and in anoxia, according to Kraig & Nicholson (1978) [5]

119

The potential mechanisms linking the cerebral hypoxia to the full-blown migraine attack have been discussed at length in the original paper [1]. But is there any clinical evidence that cerebral hypoxia may *cause* headache anyhow? The answer is yes, although it must be admitted that only few investigators appear to have studied the occurrence of headache in patients presenting with an episode of cerebral hypoxia.

There is, first, the case of transient ischaemic attacks (TIA). In a retrospective study of 240 TIA patients, Grindal and Tool [11] found headache to be a prominent symptom in about one-quarter of them. Sometimes, the headache was even the presenting complaint. As is the case during an attack of classical migraine, the headache usually accompanied or followed the TIA; in only a few cases did it precede the onset of the neurological symptoms. The authors further comment that their report probably underestimates the true frequency of the described association. One could argue that these investigators may have wrongly included a certain number of attacks of classical migraine amongst their TIA cases. This is not very likely, however, since both the mean age (56.4 years) and the sex distribution (26 men, 14 women) of the patients presenting with the association, are reminiscent of a TIA population rather than of a group of migraine patients. Actually, both the age and the sex ratio were very similar to those of the TIA patients who reportedly had no headache in this study (57 years and 107 men/53 women).

Headaches may also occur in association with a stroke. According to Miller-Fisher quoted by Heyck [12], depending upon the affected cerebral artery, both an embolism and a thrombosis may be associated with a headache in 20–70 per cent of the cases. More specifically, it was noted that headaches are not infrequently complained of in occlusions of even a small artery. Of further interest is the author's comment that a variety of other accompanying symptoms – such as nausea, vomiting, visual disturbances and hemianopia – can be responsible for confusing such a stroke with a migraine attack.

It would thus appear that cerebral hypoxia – even if due to an obstruction in a small cerebral artery – may indeed give rise to headache complaints.

What is the cause of the cerebral hypoxia in migraine?

There are a variety of factors that may cause an episode of cerebral hypoxia in apparently normal subjects such as migraine sufferers. Several of these factors are discussed elsewhere in this volume and will, therefore, be dealt with only briefly here. In addition, it should be clear from the outset that it is not mandatory that only one and the same cause would be operative in all migraineurs: different causes may be the culprit in different patients, and more than one cause may be operative at the same time as well. Also, the following discussion must not be considered an exhaustive listing of all potential causes since other mechanisms may well have been overlooked.

Vasospasm and/or vasoconstriction

This mechanism is mentioned first, because it is commonly believed to play a role in the triggering of the migraine attack. If true, a further aspect to be considered under this heading is the potential role of the sympathetic nervous system, but this is also discussed at greater length elsewhere in this volume.

At this moment, the evidence confirming a role of vasospasm in the pathogenesis is scarce [1]. Yet, in view of recent observations that angiospastic diseases such as Raynaud's phenomenon and coronary vasospasm seem to occur more frequently in migraineurs [13, 14], it may be hoped that this potential mechanism will be studied more carefully in the years to come.

Arteriovenous (A V) blood shunting

There is no evidence that AV shunting would give rise to the aura symptoms [15], although it may play a role during the headache phase of the migraine attack [1].

Mismatching of cerebral oxygen need and blood supply

In normal circumstances, cerebral blood flow follows the metabolic needs of the brain tissue. The question may arise, however, as to whether cerebral autoregulation is normal in migraine sufferers or not. Little information is available on this point. Perhaps of interest in this respect are Olesen's observations [16] in certain patients with classical migraine; he observed that cortical blood flow was not activated by finger movements during a migraine attack and that hyperaemia, occurring early in an attack, was short-lived and paradoxically followed by (spreading) hypoperfusion. This might indicate that such patients may fail to initiate or, respectively, to maintain a normal hyperaemic reaction to increased cerebral oxygen demands. A further case report, reported by Bousser and Baron [17], is of even greater interest in this context. These authors, using positron emission tomography (PET) found evidence of uncoupling of flow and metabolism in the brain of a migraine sufferer, who had been hospitalised because of a stroke that had occurred during a migrainous episode. Such an uncoupling, occurring at distance from the infarct zone, had never been observed before by these authors in their rather extensive experience in strokes due to cerebral atherosclerosis.

Autoregulation may also be weakened and, therefore, may become deficient under critical circumstances. As discussed elsewhere in this volume, there is reasonably good evidence that migraineurs may show sympathetic nervous system

121

over-activity. Sympathetic tone and catecholamines may modulate cerebro-vascular autoregulation under certain conditions, according to experimental findings. The issue is complex, however. On the one hand, experimental findings have shown that catecholamines or sympathetic nerve stimulation can reduce the normal vasodilatory response to local tissue acidosis and to hypercapnia or hypoxia [18–22]. On the other hand, however, Kuschinsky and co-workers [23] have reported evidence to suggest that norepinephrine may *in*crease the normal activation of local cerebral blood flow in the presence of increased (by the same amine) local cerebral glucose utilisation. These findings, in turn, contrast with those of King and his group [24] who reported that an i.v. infusion of the same amine caused a marked increase in cerebrovascular resistance, associated with a decreased cerebral blood flow, while the cerebral oxygen consumption remained unaltered. Although these seemingly contradictory results could be a consequence of the use of different experimental techniques, they can also be explained by a dual effect of norepinephrine on cerebrovascular resistance:

- norepinephrine may directly activate adrenergic receptors, present on the endothelium of the cerebral arteries and responsible for vasoconstriction. In order to induce vasoconstriction, norepinephrine does not have to diffuse across the endothelium and this is thus the first, normal response to circulating norepinephrine [25];

- it is only when sufficient amounts of norepinephrine reach the brain tissue that this amine will activate cerebral metabolism. In this case, the auto-regulation mechanisms prevail, but there is a resetting of the coupling mech-anism, the reason of which, however, is poorly understood [23].

Further evaluation of the possibility that excess sympathetic drive and/or hypersensitivity of the cerebrovascular adrenergic receptors may, via a reduction of cerebral blood flow, lead to hypoxic episodes in at least part of the migraine sufferers, could thus prove to be a fruitful avenue for further research.

Platelet aggregation

Localised platelet aggregation in cerebral blood vessels could, at least theoretically, be a cause of cerebral hypoxia. Whether or not regular migraine patients show platelet abnormalities which may facilitate platelet aggregation is a matter of debate and this topic is more extensively discussed in another chapter of this volume. It must be kept in mind, however, that possibly all platelet changes, observed in the course of a migraine attack and which are absent in the headache-free periods, do not necessarily represent a causal mechanism but may as well be explained as a consequence of the proposed brain hypoxia [1].

Still, in those cases where a primary platelet disorder is present, platelet aggregation may be a mechanism of brain hypoxia in patients with migraine attacks. This may apply to patients with thrombocytopenia who suffer migraine-like headaches during periods of low platelet count [26] and to patients with thrombocytaemia, whose TIAs are very similar to migraine attacks [27].

Increased cerebral metabolism

The presence of a high metabolic rate in the brain will increase the likelihood of an hypoxic episode. Increased brain metabolism may be the consequence of a variety of factors.

Crisp has advanced the concept of stressful overloading of the brain, in particular of one hemisphere, as a cause of migraine [28]. Stress is commonly considered a triggering factor in migraine and Graham has suggested that the migraineur may handle stressful events in an exaggerated or inappropriate manner, although there is much to suggest that he or she, while under stress, acts very well, perhaps too well [29]. With his psychiatric background, Crisp considers [28] that stressful overloading of the brain may arise if (a) there is an excess of information, (b) if information is conflictive, (c) if the individual's nature is such that he or she cannot side-step such conflictive information with secondary neurotic devices, (d) if the individual's nature is such that the assimilation process is stifled. The latter two mechanisms may provide a more psychophysiologic translation of the popular belief that part of the migraine problem is to be found in the migraineur's peculiar psychological structure.

From a more somatic point of view one may point to a general arousal, which is often associated with excessive sympathetic activity, on the one hand, and to an increased sensorial input to the brain, on the other hand, as possible causes of stressful overloading of the cerebrum. General arousal brings to mind stress, a known trigger of migraine attacks, and may also cover different types of effort headache, a migraine-like syndrome that occurs during various types of physical exercise [30–32] or during a sexual orgasm [30, 33, 34]. Regarding the sensorial input to the brain, certain observations may indeed suggest that migraineurs, as a group, seem to be hypersensitive to sensorial stimulation. As Graham has pointed out [29], many observers have been struck by the unusual sensitivity of the migraine sufferer to light, noise, smells, and, to a certain extent, tastes. These individuals are unusually sensitive at all times to such stimuli, and at the time of onset and during an attack of migraine this sensitivity reaches even greater heights [29]. In addition, Klee has found that perceptual disturbances are common features of the migraine attack; usually, visual perception is affected, but alterations in auditory perception and distortion of the body image have also been described [35]. Klee feels that there is little doubt that these perceptual disturbances are organic in nature. More objective evidence of abnormal handling of sensorial information by the migraine sufferer has also been reported. According to Ellertsen and Hammerborg [36], migraine patients show increased heart rate changes and heightened pulse amplitude responses in the superficial temporal artery, when exposed to auditory stimuli. In addition, Gawel and colleagues found that migraineurs showed several abnormalities in visually evoked potentials, the amplitude of these potentials often being larger and their peak latency tending to be delayed [37]. Such an increased amplitude has also been observed by Nyrke and Lang [38]. It may be speculated that the increased amplitude of the latter potentials, being a sign of a synchronous depolarisation of a larger number of neurones, may facilitate the likelihood of a regional hypoxia in the brain areas where these depolarisations occur.

Another type of increased neuronal activity occurs in epilepsy. Such an increased activity could play a role in certain cases of migraine, particularly of childhood migraine perhaps, since Kinast and co-workers [39] found that focal epileptiform discharges were more common in children with migraine than in the normal population (9% against 1.9% respectively).

Deficient supply of 'fuel'

Hunger, missing a meal during a busy day, exertion 'on an empty stomach', prolonged sleeping (and skipping breakfast), all have been considered by migraineurs as well as by headache specialists to be factors that may provoke a migraine attack. Although these observations may suggest that the common factor is hypoglycaemia, systematic investigations have failed to confirm that hypoglycaemia is involved indeed [40]. Yet, it must be borne in mind that, when sugar levels drop in the blood, compensatory mechanisms come into play to correct the glycaemia. One of the important mechanisms involved is a release of epinephrine and an associated activation of the autonomic nervous system. The role of the latter in the pathogenesis of migraine is discussed at more length elsewhere in this volume and, also, in the present paper (see *Mismatching of cerebral oxygen need and blood supply*).

Apart from glucose, also the supply of oxygen may be insufficient in the presence of an adequately functioning cerebral circulation. Lack of oxygen is the probable explanation of a migraine-like headache occurring at high altitude [30], during decompression [30] and during chronic carbon monoxide poisoning [41].

Evidence of cerebral hypoxia in migraineurs

As stated in the introduction to this paper, this section is meant to evaluate whether there is any evidence suggesting that (a) cerebral hypoxia occurs indeed during a migraine attack, and that (b) migraine sufferers are more prone to hypoxic brain damage than other subjects are.

Findings indicative of cerebral hypoxia during a migraine attack

The relevant information has been summarised in the original paper [1]. There is suggestive evidence from a variety of sources, including clinical observations,

TABLE II. Cerebrovascular complications in migraineurs (literature survey)

Type of complication	Source of information	Total number of patients	Sex and age* distribution	Type of migraine†
Stroke‡	18 publications (1933–1982)§	77	Male (n = 26) 34 (7–58) years Female (n = 51) 35 (10–68) years	Classical migraine: 23 Hemiplegic migraine: 8 Ophthalmic migraine: 8 *Migraine accompagnée*: 6 Basilar migraine: 2 Common migraine: 15 Orgasmic migraine: 1 Not specified: 14
	Gardner et al (1968) [42]	15	Female (all 15) 32 (22–51) years	Not specified
	Orgogozo et al (1982) [43]	15	Male (n = 6) 9 Female (n = 9) 42 (24–60) years	Not specified
TGA	Caplan et al (1981) [44]	12	Male (n = 6) 46 (27–66) years Female (n = 6) 61 (53–67) years	Classical migraine: 6 Common migraine: 6
	Staehelin Jensen and de Fine Olivarius (1980) [45]	8	Female (all 8) 51 (28–67) years	Classical migraine: 7 Common migraine: 1
TIA	Moretti et al (1980) [46]	2	Female (both) 39 (33 and 45) years	Not specified

* Figures for age give average (and extremes)

† The authors' diagnosis is used; in case of mixed forms (common + other type), the more severe type is listed

‡ Including seven cases of stupor reported by Lee and Lance (1977) [47]

§ References: Bousser et al (1980) [27]; Lee and Lance (1977) [47]; Boisen (1975) [48]; Bradshaw and Parsons (1965) [49]; Castaldo et al (1982) [50]; Centonze et al (1980) [51]; Critchley and Ferguson (1933) [52]; Crowell et al (1982) [53]; Ferguson and Robinson (1982) [54]; Gilbert (1982) [55]; Guest and Woolf (1964) [56]; Kalendovsky and Austin (1975) [57]; Levy (1981) [58]; Prendes (1980) [59]; Rascol et al (1982) [60]; Shafey and Scheinberg (1966) [61]; Solomon and Spaccavento (1982) [62]; Stone and Burns (1982) [63]

125

CSF changes, EEG findings and CT scans. The more recent literature has provided a few scattered reports that expand the, largely circumstantial, evidence that did already exist, but truely new facts or observations do not seem to have been reported in this respect since the original publication appeared.

Are migraineurs more prone to developing hypoxic cerebral damage?

There is a wealth of reports in the literature showing that cerebrovascular complications, though not frequent, do occur from time to time in migraineurs. Table II gives a survey of the reports, available to us. The survey covers 107 cases of stroke, 20 cases of transient global amnesia (TGA) and two cases of transient ischaemic attack (TIA). In at least one of the studies, it has been shown

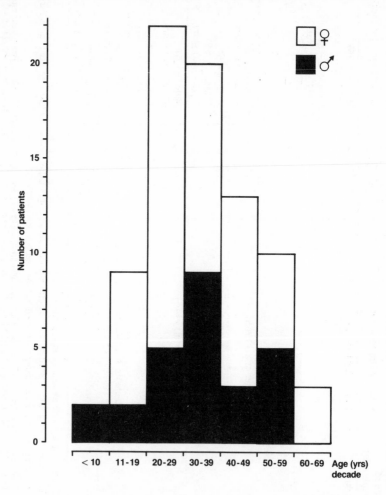

Figure 1. Age distribution of 77 migraineurs presenting with a stroke

that the strokes are mainly (9/10 cases) due to an arterial occlusion (Rascol et al [60]). It is apparent from Table II that the age range of the patients concerned is very similar to that of a regular group of migraine sufferers and is significantly lower than the age range at which strokes normally tend to occur. This is further illustrated by Figure 1 which shows the age distribution of the 77 stroke cases reported in the 18 publications that give detailed information in this regard. The data summarised in Table II also show that the sex distribution is similarly reminiscent of that of a migraine population, showing a preponderance of females (91 women against 38 men). Finally, this survey suggests that cerebrovascular complications may occur more frequently in those types of migraine, that are associated with neurological symptoms, than in common migraine, although such complications clearly do not fail to occur in the latter type of migraine as well.

All of this provides circumstantial evidence that migraineurs may be more at risk of developing cerebrovascular problems, but it does not prove the point. Further circumstantial evidence of (hypoxic) brain damage comes from the finding that serial psychometric data have revealed deterioration of specific cognitive and motor skills and marked behaviour change in a child with severe migraine accompagnée [64] and from EEG changes found in about three-quarters of children with the diagnosis of migraine [65]. The latter findings probably also apply to adults, since Jonkman and Lelieveld [66] found that the interictal EEG was abnormal in 55—75 per cent of 20 migraineurs, in contrast to five per cent of 20 matched controls. Much may depend upon the criteria used to evaluate the EEG though, since Slevin and co-workers [67], using different criteria, found an abnormal interictal EEG in only 20 per cent of 55 adults with classical or common migraine.

That migraine is not as benign a disease as it is often supposed to be, particularly with regard to its effects on the brain, is further suggested by the findings reported by Ruiz and co-workers [68] who found that signs of cerebral atrophy, as studied by CT scans, are more frequent among (common and classical) migraine sufferers than in controls, and especially so in the younger age groups. This is illustrated in Figure 2.

Finally, there is some epidemiologic evidence, coming from three independent studies, showing that migraine may be an independent risk factor for developing a stroke, especially in the younger age ranges. In 1975, the 'Collaborative Group for the Study of Stroke in Young Women' [69] reported that, in young (15—44 years) women, a history or symptoms indicative of migraine increase the likelihood of a subsequent stroke and independently so from other known risk factors. That the same may also hold true for young men, was suggested by Spaccavento and co-workers [70] who reported that 4 of 15 (= 27%) male stroke patients, aged 20—40 years, were migraineurs who had no other known risk factor for stroke. Finally, Maxion and Dorn-Schomburg [71] recently published their findings related to 174 consecutive ischaemic stroke patients.

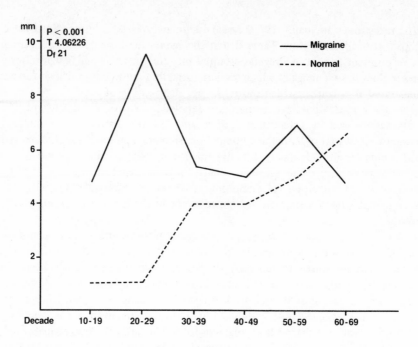

Figure 2. Third ventricular width in migraineurs as compared with normal controls. The 'paired t-test' shows significant difference between the two groups, principally in the younger decades. Reproduced with permission from Ruiz et al [68]

TABLE III. Risk factors in 174 consecutive patients with a first stroke. Results from Maxion and Dorn-Schomburg [71]

	Women (n = 85)		Men (n = 89)		Total group (n=174)	
	Age <60	Age >60	Age <60	Age >60	Age <60	Age >60
No risk factor	7 (−2)*	43	18 (−4)	28	25 (−6)	71
Migraine	12 ⎫	10 ⎫	3 ⎫	0 ⎫	15 ⎫	10 ⎫
	⎬ 14	⎬ 10	⎬ 3	⎬ 0	⎬ 17	⎬ 10
Migraine + cigarette smoking	2 ⎭	0 ⎭	0 ⎭	0 ⎭	2 ⎭	0 ⎭
	⎫ 11	⎫ 2	⎫ 30	⎫ 10	⎫ 41	⎫ 12
Risk factors, other than migraine	9 ⎭	2 ⎭	30 ⎭	10 ⎭	39 ⎭	12 ⎭
Total	30	55	51	38	81	93

* Between brackets: the number of patients with hypertension

128

The results are summarised in Table III. Of the 27 migraineurs, represented in this study, 63 per cent suffered their stroke before the age of 60. This contrasts with only 26 per cent of the patients, having no risk factor (apart from hypertension), who had their first stroke before that age.

Discussion and conclusions

As it is the case for every hypothesis related to the pathogenesis of migraine, the present cerebral hypoxia-hypothesis remains unproven. There are certainly a series of arguments and observations that favour the hypothesis but it also remains clear that, in order to have a conclusive evaluation, much elaborative clinical research work is still needed. Hopefully, the availability of clinically useful NMR scanners will provide us with a technically feasible approach. Still, even then the problems will remain formidable, since this equipment will have to be used at the right moment (i.e. in the very beginning of, and preferably even immediately before, the migraine attack), in a sufficiently large number of patients suffering from the most representative types of migraine (i.e. classical and common migraine – and we must not forget about the fact that the diagnosis of common migraine may be subject to serious controversy) and by properly trained investigators. In addition, we must not forget about the tremendous cost that will be involved in carrying out this enterprise. It seems likely, therefore, that the hypoxia hypothesis will remain unproven for several more years.

Meanwhile, this hypothesis provides a basis which may be helpful in unifying most other hypotheses regarding the pathogenesis of migraine into a single entity, since it obviously shows many interfaces with these other theories. In addition, the hypothesis will hopefully help researchers, clinical as well as pharmacological, in designing their migraine-related activities, so that eventually better strategies can be developed for helping the migraine sufferers in dealing with their disease.

If correct, the hypoxia hypothesis may also have consequences for the use of medicines in treating migraine patients. Is the repetitive use, for example, of drugs, that potentially may interfere with the blood supply to the brain, really a good choice? Or should we pay more attention to prophylactic treatments that not only prevent migraine attacks (or make them less severe), but that, preferably, also offer some protection against ischaemic and/or hypoxic brain injury? Clearly, long-term well-controlled clinical trials could be very instructive in this context.

Summary

Based on a triple argumentation, a recension is made of the previously developed hypothesis that a brief episode of focal cerebral hypoxia occurs in every migraine attack. First, it is shown that the migraine attack can be well explained if it is due to cerebral hypoxia. In fact, hypoxia may trigger a spreading cortical depression which is a serious candidate for causing the neurological symptoms of the aura. The headache itself may also be caused by cerebral hypoxia, as inferred from observations in patients with transient ischaemic attacks or a stroke. Second, several factors are pinpointed which may underly cerebral hypoxia in migraine: vasospasm and/or vasoconstriction, with increased sympathetic activity, imbalance between oxygen need and blood supply, a localised platelet aggregation, an increased cerebral metabolic rate consequent to stress or due to a hypersensitivity to sensorial stimuli, and a deficient supply of glucose or oxygen. Third, clinical, instrumental and/or epidemiologic evidence is summarised which suggests that hypoxia does occur during a migraine attack and that migraineurs may be particuarly prone to developing hypoxic brain damage. By definition, the hypoxia hypothesis leaves many questions unanswered, but one should not lose sight of its possible relevance to the patient.

References

1   Amery WK. Brain hypoxia: the turning-point in the genesis of the migraine attack? *Cephalalgia 1982; 2:* 83–109
2   Gurdjian ES, Webster JE, Stone WE. Cerebral constituents in relation to blood gases. *Am J Physiol 1949; 156:* 149–157
3   Hansen AJ, Hounsgaard J, Jahnsen H. Anoxia increases potassium conductance in hippocampal nerve cells. *Acta Physiol Scand 1982; 115:* 301–310
4   Hansen AJ, Quistorff B, Gjedde A. Relationship between local changes in cortical blood flow and extracellular K^+ during spreading depression. *Acta Physiol Scand 1980; 109:* 1–6
5   Kraig RP, Nicholson C. Extracellular ionic variations during spreading depression. *Neuroscience 1978; 3:* 1045–1059
6   Křivánek J. Changes of brain glycogen in the spreading EEG-depression of Leão. *J Neurochem 1958; 2:* 337–343
7   Křivánek J. Some metabolic changes accompanying Leão's spreading cortical depression in the rat. *J Neurochem 1961; 6:* 183–189
8   Lukyanova LK, Bureš J. Changes in pO_2 due to spreading depression in the cortex and nucleus caudatus of the rat. *Physiol Bohemoslov 1967; 16:* 449–455
9   Tsacopoulos M, Lehmenkühler A. A double-barrelled Pt-microelectrode for simultaneous measurement of PO_2 and bioelectrical activity in excitable tissues. *Experientia 1977; 33:* 1337–1338
10 Morris ME. Hypoxia and extracellular potassium activity in the guinea-pig cortex. *Can J Physiol Pharmacol 1974; 52:* 872–882
11 Grindal AB, Toole JF. Headache and transient ischemic attacks. *Stroke 1974; 5:* 603–606
12 Heyck H. *Headache and Facial Pain. Differential Diagnosis/Pathogenesis/Treatment.* Stuttgart and New York: Georg Thieme Verlag. 1981: 207
13 Kuritzky A. Prevalence of Raynaud's phenomenon and chest pain in migraineurs. *Personal communication.* 1981
14 Miller D, Waters DD, Warnica W et al. Is variant angina the coronary manifestation of a generalised vasospastic disorder? *N Engl J Med 1981; 304:* 763–766
15 Spierings ELH. Arterial vasoconstriction versus arteriovenous shunting in the migraine aura. In Rose FC, Amery WK, eds. *Cerebral Hypoxia in the Pathogenesis of Migraine.* London: Pitman Books Limited. 1982: 12–22

16   Olesen J, Larsen B. Cerebral blood flow in migraine. Is ischaemia involved? In Rose FC, Amery WK eds. *Cerebral Hypoxia in the Pathogenesis of Migraine*. London: Pitman Books Limited. 1982: 53–73

17   Bousser MG, Baron JC. Intérèt de la tomographie par émission de positions pour l'étude de l'ischémie cérébrale. *Ann Méd Int 1981; 132:* 449–455

18   Busija D, Heistad D. Sympathetic nerves reduce cerebral blood flow during hypercapnia (abstract). *Circulation 1981; 64:* IV–232

19   Deshmukh VD, Harper AM, Rowan JO, Jennett WB. Studies on neurogenic control of the cerebral circulation. *Eur Neurol 1971–72; 6:* 166–174

20   James IM, Millar RA, Purves MJ. Observations on the extrinsic neural control of cerebral blood flow in the baboon. *Circ Res 1969; 25:* 77–93

21   Lavyne M, Wurtman RJ, Moskowitz M, Zervas N. Brain catecholamines and cerebral blood flow. *Life Sci 1975; 16:* 475–486

22   Zervas NT, Lavyne MH, Negoro M. Neurotransmitters and the normal and ischemic cerebral circulation. *N Engl J Med 1975; 293:* 812–816

23   Kuschinsky W, Suda S, Bünger R, Sokoloff L. The influence of IV norepinephrine on the local coupling between brain metabolism and blood flow. In Heistad DD, Marcus ML, eds. *Cerebral Blood Flow: Effects of Nerves and Neurotransmitters*. Amsterdam: Elsevier North-Holland. 1982: 169–175

24   King BD, Sokoloff L, Wechsler RL. The effects of l-epinephrine and l-nor-epinephrine upon cerebral circulation and metabolism in man. *J Clin Invest 1952; 31:* 273–279

25   Aubineau P, Sercombe R, Lusamvuku NAT, Seylaz J. Can the response to circulating vasoactive substances be initiated by endothelial receptors of cerebral arteries? In Heistad DD, Marcus ML, eds. *Cerebral Blood Flow: Effects of Nerves and Neurotransmitters*. Amsterdam: Elsevier North-Holland. 1982: 47–56

26   Damasio H, Beck D. Migraine, thrombocytopenia, and serotonin metabolism. *Lancet 1978; i:* 240–242

27   Bousser MG, Conard J, Lecrubier C, Bousser J. Migraine ou accidents ischémiques transitoires au cours d'une thrombocytémie essentielle. Action de la ticlopidine. *Ann Méd Int 1980; 131:* 87–90

28   Crisp AH, Hall A. Information overload: increased brain metabolism and migraine. In Rose FC, Amery WK, eds. *Cerebral Hypoxia in the Pathogenesis of Migraine*. London: Pitman Books Limited. 1982: 23–27

29   Graham JR. The migraine connection. *Headache 1981; 21:* 243–250

30   Dalessio DJ. Effort, high altitude, and decompression headaches. In Rose FC, Amery WK, eds. *Cerebral Hypoxia in the Pathogenesis of Migraine*. London: Pitman Books Limited. 1982: 28–35

31   Massey EW. Effort headache in runners. *Headache 1982; 22:* 99–100

32   Powell B. Weight lifter's cephalalgia. *Ann Emerg Med 1982; 11:* 449–451

33   Porter M, Jankovic J. Benign coital cephalalgia. Differential diagnosis and treatment. *Arch Neurol 1981; 38:* 710–712

34   Schmidt D. Koitale Kopfschmerzen. *Schweiz Med Wochenschr 1982; 112:* 1068–1069

35   Klee A. Perceptual disorders in migraine. In Pearce J, ed. *Modern Topics in Migraine*. London: W Heinemann. 1975: 45–51

36   Ellertsen B, Hammerborg D. Psychophysiological response patterns in migraine patients. *Cephalalgia 1982; 2:* 19–24

37   Gawel M, Connolly JF, Rose FC. Migraine patient exhibit abnormalities in the visual evoked potential. *Headache 1983; 23:* 49–52

38   Nyrke T, Lang AH. Spectral analysis of visual potentials evoked by sine wave modulated light in migraine. *Electroencephalogr Clin Neurophysiol 1982; 53:* 436–442

39   Kinast M, Lueders H, Rothner AD, Erenberg G. Benign focal epileptiform discharges in childhood migraine. *Neurology 1982; 32:* 1309–1311

40   Hockaday JM, Williamson DH, Whitty CMW. Blood-glucose levels and fatty-acid metabolism in migraine related to fasting. *Lancet 1971; i:* 1153–1156

41   Dalessio DJ. Carbon monoxide (CO) and headache. *Headache 1982; 22:* 89

42   Gardner JH, Hornstein S, van den Noort S. The clinical characteristics of headache during impending cerebral infarction in women taking oral contraceptives. *Headache 1968; 8:* 108–111

43   Orgogozo JM, Henry PY, Pellerin R. Ischaemic strokes during migraine attacks. Consequence or coincidence. *4th International Symposium of The Migraine Trust. Abstract Book.* London. 1982: 44–45

44   Caplan L, Chedru F, Lhermitte F, Mayman C. Transient global amnesia and migraine. *Neurology 1981; 31:* 1167–1170

45   Staehelin Jensen T, de Fine Olivarius B. The syndrome of transient global amnesia in migraine: a follow-up study. *Upsala J Med Sci 1980; Suppl 31:* 34–36

46   Moretti G, Manzoni GC, Carpeggiani P, Parma M. Attacchi ischemici transitori, emicrania e progestinici. Correlazioni etiopatogenetiche. *Minerva Med 1980; 71:* 2125–2129

47   Lee CH, Lance JW. Migraine stupor. *Headache 1977; 17:* 32–38

48   Boisen E. Strokes in migraine: report on seven strokes associated with severe migraine attacks. *Can Med Bull 1975; 22:* 100–106

49   Bradshaw P, Parsonson M. Hemiplegic migraine, a clinical study. *Q J Med 1965; 34:* 65–85

50   Castaldo JE, Anderson M, Reeves AG. Middle cerebral artery occlusion with migraine. *Stroke 1982; 13:* 308–311

51   Centonze V, Amat G, Loisy C et al. Considérations sur les accidents vascularies cérébraux chez les migraineux. *Sem Hôp Paris 1980; 56:* 1908–1910

52   Critchely M, Ferguson FR. Migraine. *Lancet 1933; i:* 123–126 and 182–187

53   Crowell GF, Carlin L, Biller J. Neurologic complications of migraine. *Am Fam Physician 1982; 26:* 139–148

54   Ferguson KS, Robinson SS. Life-threatening migraine. *Arch Neurol 1982; 39:* 374–376

55   Gilbert GJ. An occurrence of complicated migraine during propranolol therapy. *Headache 1982; 22:* 81–83

56   Guest IA, Woolf AL. Fatal infarction of brain in migraine. *Br Med J 1964; 1:* 225–226

57   Kalendovsky Z, Austin JH. 'Complicated migraine' its association with increased platelet aggregability and abnormal plasma coagulation factors. *Headache 1975; 15:* 18–35

58   Levy RL. Stroke and orgasmic cephalgia. *Headache 1981; 21:* 12–13

59   Prendes JL. Considerations on the use of propranolol in complicated migraine. *Headache 1980; 20:* 93–95

60   Rascol A, Clanet M, Rascol O. Cerebrovascular accidents complicating migraine attacks. In Rose FC, Amery WK, eds. *Cerebral Hypoxia in the Pathogenesis of Migraine.* London: Pitman Books Limited. 1982: 110–116

61   Shafey S, Scheinberg P. Neurological syndromes occurring in patients receiving synthetic steroids (oral contraceptives). *Neurology 1966; 16:* 205–211

62   Solomon GD, Spaccavento LJ. Lateral medullary syndrome after basilar migraine. *Headache 1982; 22:* 171–172

63   Stone GM, Burns RJ. Cerebral infarction caused by vasospasm. *Med J Austr 1982; 1:* 556–559

64   Ferguson KS, Robinson SS. Acquired learning problems secondary to migraine. *Dev Behav Pediatr 1982; 3:* 247–248

65   Prensky AL, Sommer D. Diagnosis and treatment of migraine in children. *Neurology 1979; 29:* 506–510

66   Jonkman EJ, Lelieveld MJH. EEG computer analysis in patients with migraine. *Electroencephalogr Clin Neurophysiol 1981; 52:* 652–655

67   Slevin JT, Faught E, Hanna GR, Lee SI. Temporal relationship of EEG abnormalities in migraine to headache and medication. *Headache 1981; 21:* 251–254

68   Ruiz JS, du Boulay GH, Zilkha KJ, Rose FC. The abnormal CT scan in migraine patients. In Rose FC, Amery WK, eds. *Cerebral Hypoxia in the Pathogenesis of Migraine.* London: Pitman Books Limited. 1982: 105–109

69   Collaborative Group for the Study of Stroke in Young Women. Oral contraceptives and stroke in young women. *JAMA 1975; 231:* 718–722

70   Spaccavento LJ, Solomon GD, Mani S. An association between strokes and migraine in young adults. *Headache 1981; 21:* 121

71   Maxion H, Dorn-Schomburg J. Migräne, ein Risikofaktor für den ischämischen zerebralen Insult. *Med Welt 1983; 34:* 233–234

10

PROTECTION AGAINST CEREBRAL HYPOXIA BY ANTIMIGRAINE DRUGS

A Wauquier, D Ashton, H L Edmonds

Introduction

Migraine is the result of a constellation of events including prodromal symptoms (scotoma, peripheral dysfunction, etc), local cerebral vasospasm, ischaemia, hypoxia, spreading depression, headache. Since no single pharmacological model involves all of these events, it was decided to examine the effects of a series of antimigraine drugs on single aspects of the migraine attack. The actions of drugs on vasospasm itself, and spreading depression, have been covered by Van Nueten et al and Hansen et al respectively in this volume.

Two important events remain to be examined. The first is cerebral ischaemia. We have therefore studied the actions of several antimigraine drugs in a model of ischaemia. The second, hypoxia, may precipitate the spreading depression which causes the prodromal signs; both may ultimately produce the headache [1]. Therefore, we tested antimigraine agents in an in vivo and in an in vitro model of hypoxia.

ANTI-ISCHAEMIC EFFECTS

Different animal models have been developed to study global brain ischaemia [for example see 2]. These are often complicated and involve not only the brain, but also the cardiovascular system, which in its turn can worsen brain hypoxia and attenuate possible outcome. Cardiac arrest followed by resuscitation is an example of such a test [3].

In different models, brain ischaemia is induced by applying common carotid artery occlusion. In such experiments gerbils are often used because of their incomplete circle of Willis. Using such a model the efficacy of the hypnotic etomidate has been demonstrated [4]. The mortality rate following common carotid ligation is highly species dependent. In preliminary experiments, it was found that adult or aged (more than 10 months) Wistar rats and spontaneous hypertensive rats of the Okamoto strain were not very suitable, since a large variability in mortality rate was observed. In mice, a more predictable outcome exists, suggesting that bilateral common carotid ligation in mice is a useful method to study the efficacy of drugs. In recent experiments Izumi and Yasuda [5] showed a marked increase in survival rate following carotid ligation in mice pretreated with pentobarbital. In the present experiments, the following anti-migraine drugs were tested: clonidine, domperidone, ergotamine, flunarizine, methysergide, pizotifen and propranolol, in order to find out whether an anti-ischaemic effect could be demonstrated.

Materials and methods

Adult mice weighing 25 ± 5g were anaesthetised with ether. Through a ventral approach a midline incision was made and the bilateral common carotid arteries were exposed and ligated. Thereafter, the wounds were sutured and the animals were placed in an observation cage. Mice were pretreated i.p. 60min before surgery with either saline (control group) or with clonidine, domperidone, ergotamine, flunarizine, methysergide, pizotifen or propranolol, at doses of 0.63, 2.5 or 10mg/kg. The time of survival was noted up to 24hr after the induction of ischaemia. The Mann Whitney U-test (two tailed probability) was used as a test for significance between saline- and drug-treated mice.

Results

Of the 21 saline-treated mice, 19 died within the first and two within the second hour after the induction of ischaemia. At the 0.63mg/kg dose a significant protection was seen with clonidine ($p < 0.01$). At 2.5mg/kg, a significant protection was obtained with flunarizine ($p < 0.01$) and methysergide ($p < 0.001$). At 10mg/kg a significant protection was found with ergotamine ($p < 0.05$), flunarizine ($p < 0.05$), propranolol ($p < 0.05$) and with methysergide ($p < 0.05$).

For illustrative purposes Figure 1 represents the percentage survival in mice treated with 2.5mg/kg of the different compounds. As seen, flunarizine and methysergide appeared to afford the best protective effect. With both compounds, survival for more than 24 hours was obtained in two out of the seven mice treated. After pizotifen one mouse survived for more than 24 hours, but this was the only mouse protected throughout the whole experiment. With both flunarizine and methysergide a biphasic effect was obtained, in that the intermediate dose was more effective than the higher dose.

Discussion

If bilateral carotid ligation in the mouse leads to death as a result of ischaemia in vital centres, then active compounds must interfere with the series of events

135

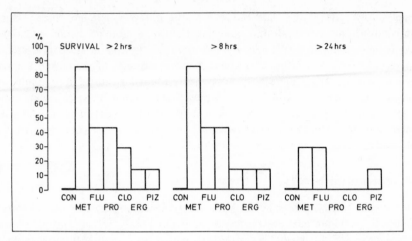

Figure 1. Percentage mice surviving for more than two, four and 24 hours following bilateral carotid ligation. Mice were treated i.p. 30min before the ligation with either saline (control, CON), methysergide (MET), flunarizine (FLU), propranolol (PROP), clonidine (CLO), ergotamine (ERG) or pizotifen (PIZ)

immediately following ligation. These events must include altering the mismatch between delivery of glucose and oxygen and its consumption. All seven compounds produced some increase in survival time. The most effective compounds were flunarizine and methysergide, which still showed some activity at 24 hours.

One possible explanation for the beneficial effects of these compounds is antagonism to vasoconstriction. This explanation is most likely for methysergide because of its well known antiserotonergic activity; cerebral vessels are particularly sensitive to the vasoconstrictive properties of a number of substances, including serotonin [6]. However, pizotifen which is also an antiserotonergic agent displayed weak activity. Thus other factors may be involved in the anti-ischaemic effect obtained with methysergide. Alternatively agents could prolong survival by preserving neuronal function in the vital centres. Both mechanisms have been suggested for flunarizine [7].

ANTIHYPOXIC EFFECTS OF ANTIMIGRAINE DRUGS

Most of the experimental models of brain hypoxia do not aim to replicate a clinical situation, but they can be used to select compounds possessing potential antihypoxic properties. It appears advantageous to apply several of these tests, mainly because the origin and consequences of the induction of the insults are highly diverse. For quantitative purposes, multiple doses have to be used, instigating the use of very simple tests. Many substances have been tested in hypoxic situations [7,8]. These tests are: hypobaric hypoxia in mice; hypoxic hypoxia caused by bringing rats into a 100 per cent nitrogen environment; histotoxic hypoxia by injecting potassium cyanide in rats. The heterogeneity of activity appears quite large, yet a number of specific agents was found active: hypnotics, like etomidate [8], the calcium entry blocker flunarizine [7,9]; anticonvulsants like carbamazepine [7]. Of these tests the nitrogen hypoxia seems most suitable for evaluation of the antihypoxic properties of antimigraine compounds. Hypoxia involves reduction of oxygen content below the requirements for the maintenance of tissue structure, function or metabolism. Hypoxic hypoxia involves low oxygen tension in the presence of normocapnia. The nitrogen test fulfils this definition; in addition the heart remains beating, suggesting that ischaemia is relatively unimportant.

Materials and methods

The detailed methodology has been described by Wauquier et al [8]. For the nitrogen hypoxia test, the subjects were male Wistar rats, deprived of food overnight, weighing 200 ± 10g. They were placed in a container through which pure nitrogen flowed during a period of one minute. Thereafter they were removed and placed in an observation cage. Survival was scored two hours after removal from the closed container.

In each test the following compounds were given orally one hour before the hypoxic challenge: clonidine, domperidone, ergotamine, flunarizine, methysergide, pizotifen and propranolol. At least three doses of the substances were given, which allowed ED_{50}-values to be calculated. When substances were inactive, the highest dose tested is also indicated. In addition, the dose producing neurological disturbances (e.g. ataxia, tremor, . . .) is indicated for those compounds found active against hypoxia.

Results

In the nitrogen hypoxia test, none of the 1604 saline treated rats survived. Table I shows the results obtained with the different drugs tested. One hour after treatment, only flunarizine was found active. Four hours after treatment, flunarizine, clonidine and ergotamine were found active. It is also evident that the dose protecting against hypoxia is only two to three times lower than the dose producing neurological disturbances for ergotamine and clonidine respectively. With flunarizine neurological disturbances are caused at a dose more than 10 times the antihypoxic dose.

Discussion

In the hypoxic hypoxia test the combination between low oxygen tension and normocapnia appears to be insufficient to stimulate respiratory reflexes in control animals. Protection by drugs in this model could result from physical or cellular effects. Amongst the physical effects would be shallow ventilation,

137

TABLE I. ED$_{50}$-values (limits) in mg/kg, of antihypoxic properties of antimigraine drugs obtained in the nitrogen hypoxia test in rats. Drugs were given orally either one hour or four hours before the hypoxic challenge

Compound	Hypoxic hypoxia rats		Neurological disturbances
	−60 min	−240 min	
clonidine	>2.5	0.858 (0.497−1.48)	⩾2.5
domperidone	>40	>40	−
ergotamine	>40	20.0 (11.6−34.5)	⩾40
flunarizine	35.7 (20.7−61.5)	14.0 (8.83−22.3)	⩾160
methysergide	>40	>40	−
pizotifen	>40	>40	−
propranolol	>40	>40	−

reduced respiratory rate and increasing oxygen carrying capacity. Amongst the cellular effects would be decreasing high energy phosphate utilisation and blocking of depolarisation via 'membrane stabilisation'.

In this situation survival can be achieved by increasing carbon dioxide tension (e.g. 10% CO_2 in nitrogen environment of intravenous injection of bicarbonate). In order to discover which factors might be involved in the mechanisms by which active drugs increase survival, an additional experiment was performed.

Rats were treated with either saline or a protective dose of clonidine (2.5mg/kg), ergotamine (40mg/kg) or flunarizine (40mg/kg) four hours prior to, or after exposure to the nitrogen environment, in different groups of rats (n=7 in each group). Both before and after nitrogen exposure rectal temperature was taken. The trachea was clamped and arterial blood was removed by intracardiac puncture. Blood gases were measured using an ABL 3 Acid-base Laboratory System.

Figure 2 shows the changes in rectal temperature and in pCO_2 occurring in rats before and after a one minute exposure to nitrogen. Marked hypoxia was seen in all groups. Untreated control rats apparently responded to the hypoxic stimulus with the classic 'fight or flight' reaction. Massive sympathetic outflow no doubt led to an increase in peripheral vascular resistance (PVR), cardiac output, pulmonary blood flow (PBF) and minute ventilation. Hypoxia-induced decrease in rectal temperature seems to be a consequence of elevated PVR. Diminished pCO_2 followed the increases in PBF and ventilation. Ultimately this loss of pCO_2 removed the necessary stimulus to breathe.

138

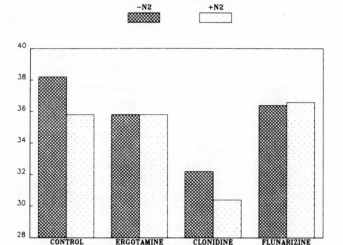

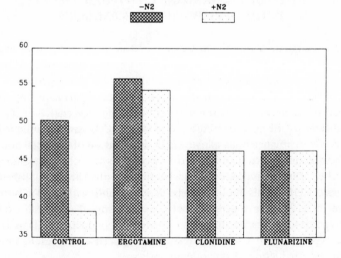

Figure 2. Rectal temperature (upper part) and pCO_2 (lower part) measured before or after exposure to 100 per cent nitrogen for one minute, in rats (n=7 in each group), orally treated four hours before with either saline, ergotamine (40mg/kg), clonidine (2.5mg/kg) or flunarizine (40mg/kg)

The peripheral vasoconstriction during hypoxia does not involve serotonergic mechanisms since methysergide and pizotifen, both potent antiserotonergics, were inactive.

Protection against hypoxia was uniformly related to a maintenance of normocapnia. Interestingly, each of the drug groups appeared to provide this protective action in a different way. In all probability, ergotamine's well known vasoconstrictive properties blocked the increase in PBF which prevented the lowering of pCO_2. Blockade of augmented myocardial stimulation by clonidine likewise limited PBF and maintained adequate CO_2 tension. PVR still increased, however, as indicated by a further decrease in rectal temperature. In contrast, flunarizine minimised the development of peripheral vasoconstriction. Rectal temperature in this group remained unchanged during the hypoxic period. In the face of an elevated cardiac output and normal vascular resistance, flow to the periphery must have increased. Increases in the elimination of CO_2 coincident with an augmented PBF were offset by enhanced CO_2 production associated with stimulation of metabolic activity.

The anti-vasoconstrictive properties of flunarizine may thus explain a portion of the protective action in the nitrogen hypoxia test. In order to explore a possible direct cellular effect independent of its vascular activity, the in vitro brain slice technique was also employed.

ACTION OF FLUNARIZINE ON HYPOXIC INSULTS
IN THE IN VITRO HIPPOCAMPAL SLICE

In order to eliminate the problem encountered in in vivo models of ischaemia/hypoxia, we studied flunarizine in the in vitro hippocampal slice. This has the advantage of removing 'physical' behavioural variables and questions of cardiovascular effects. In this in vitro technique thin slices of guinea-pig hippocampus are placed on a metal grid at the interface between oxygenated artificial cerebrospinal fluid (ACSF) and humidified 95% O_2/5% CO_2 gas. The unique lamellar structure of the hippocampus allows direct visualisation of both cell body layers and their afferent inputs. The action of hypoxia has scarcely been studied in the in vitro slice. During hypoxia electrical activity in the slice is abolished within three minutes [10]. This abolition became irreversible within 10 minutes [11]. Hansen et al [12] have suggested that the reduction of nerve cell excitability during hypoxia is primarily due to increased K^+ conductance. Thus the nerve cells are hyperpolarised and input resistance reduced which results in a higher threshold and a reduction of synaptic potentials.

In the present study pyramidal cells in the CA_1 region were activated monosynaptically by stimulation of the Schaffer collaterals. Extracellular recordings were made before, during and after a five minute hypoxic insult in the presence or absence of flunarizine.

Materials and methods

Three hundred gram male guinea-pigs were decapitated and $500\mu M$ slices of the hippocampus were made in the usual way [13]. Slices were placed in the chamber at the interface between oxygenated ACSF (composition: NaCl 134M, KCl 4mM, KH_2PO_4 1.25mM, $MgSO_4$ 1.1mM, $CaCl_2$ 2.0mM, $NaHCO_3$ 16mM, glucose 0.01M) and humidified gas (95% O_2/5% CO_2) for one hour prior to penetration. The chamber used was a laminar flow one, which allowed rapid and complete changes of incubation media and humidified gas. Chamber temperature was 35°C. Tungsten or platinum bipolar stimulation electrodes were placed in Schaffer collaterals, stimulus parameters were 0.1Hz, $<200\mu S$, <12 V. Glass recording electrodes (2−10M) were filled with 2M NaCl and placed in the CA_1 soma. Signals were recorded using a WPI KS 700 electrometer, via two WPI gold microprobes and displayed on a Tectronix oscilloscope.

Experimental protocol

After setting recording and stimulating electrodes, the stability of the signal was assessed for 15 minutes. In all experiments two recording electrodes were placed in CA_1. Since the two recordings came from the same slice, they share many common variables. For those reasons channels 1 and 2 of the electrometer were grouped and assessed separately. The criterion for inclusion in the study was a population spike of $>3mV$. Slices were then perfused for one hour with normal ACSF, or ACSF and flunarizine $10^{-7}M$.

During the five minute hypoxic period the humidified gas above the slice was changed to 95% N_2/5% CO_2. In addition, the slices were perfused with ACSF, or ACSF with flunarizine $10^{-7}M$, saturated with 95% N_2/5% CO_2 during the hypoxic period. After the hypoxic period normal gas and ACSF were started. Drug-treated slices continued to receive $10^{-7}M$ flunarizine during the 30 minute post-hypoxic observation period. Every minute oscilloscope tracings were made. The latency to the population spike was assessed at the time between the beginning of the stimulation artefact and the most negative peak to a point midway between the preceding and following positive deflections. All values were converted to a percentage of the pre-hypoxic values. The Mann-Whitney U-test, two-tailed, was applied to assess differences.

Results

The extracellular evoked response consisted of a population excitatory post-synaptic potential (EPSP) going in the positive direction and a superimposed brief negative potential variation reflecting the population spike (see Figure 3) [13,14]. During control recordings the response was shown to remain constant for several hours. Flunarizine at a concentration of $10^{-7}M$ did not alter either

141

the latency or amplitude of the response during the one hour period prior to the induction of hypoxia. Hypoxia abolished the population spike in both flunarizine and control groups within 40 seconds. The population EPSP gradually decreased over a period of one to three minutes (Figure 3).

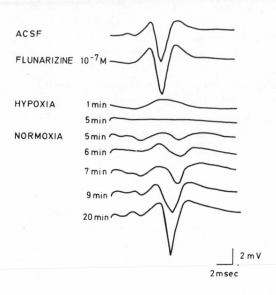

Figure 3. Extracellular evoked response recorded in the CA_1 region of the hippocampal brain slice following electrical stimulation of Schaffer collaterals during perfusion with artificial cerebrospinal fluid (ACSF), flunarizine $10^{-7}M$ and at different times following the induction of hypoxia

After resumption of normal oxygenation in medium and humidified gas the evoked response gradually returned. The population EPSP always returned before the population spike. The latency of the population spike and the population EPSP was increased in both groups (control site 1, (mean ± SD) 130 ± 10%, site 2, 130 ± 15%; flunarizine site 1, 128 ± 17%, site 2, 129 ± 16%). The latency of the signal gradually returned to normal over the following minute. No differences were seen in latency between control- and flunarizine-treated groups. The time required after hypoxia for the population spike amplitude to return to 10 per cent of the pre-hypoxic values was similar in the two groups (mean ± SD control site 1, 12 ± 9min, site 2, 9 ± 3min, flunarizine site 1, 6 ± 2 min, site 2, 6 ± 1min). The time required for the population spike amplitude to reach 50 per cent of the pre-hypoxic levels was also similar in the two groups (see Figure 4). However, the time required for the population spike to reach 90 per cent of the control value was significantly different between the flunarizine- and the control groups for both electrode sites. This result was caused by

142

CUMULATIVE PERCENTAGE OF HIPPOCAMPAL SLICES REACHING 50%
OF PRE-HYPOXIC POPULATION SPIKE AMPLITUDE

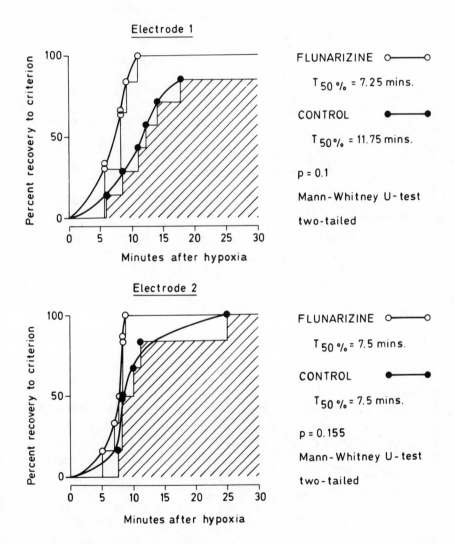

Figure 4. Time required for the population spike amplitude to return to 50 per cent of the pre-hypoxic values

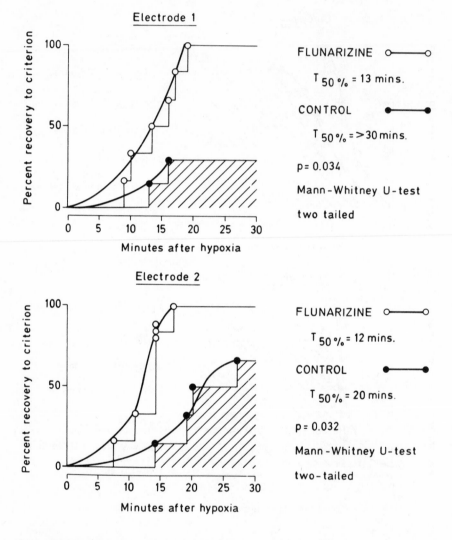

CUMULATIVE PERCENTAGE OF HIPPOCAMPAL SLICES REACHING 90% OF PRE-HYPOXIC POPULATION SPIKE AMPLITUDE

Electrode 1

FLUNARIZINE ○————○
$T_{50\%}$ = 13 mins.

CONTROL ●————●
$T_{50\%}$ = >30 mins.

p= 0.034
Mann-Whitney U-test
two tailed

Electrode 2

FLUNARIZINE ○————○
$T_{50\%}$ = 12 mins.

CONTROL ●————●
$T_{50\%}$ = 20 mins.

p= 0.032
Mann-Whitney U-test
two-tailed

Figure 5. Time required for the population spike amplitude to return to 90 per cent of the pre-hypoxic values

144

the failure of many control slices to return to the pre-hypoxic level. This is illustrated in Figures 5 and 6.

MEDIAN POPULATION SPIKE AMPLITUDE AS PERCENT OF CONTROL AFTER 5 mins. HYPOXIA

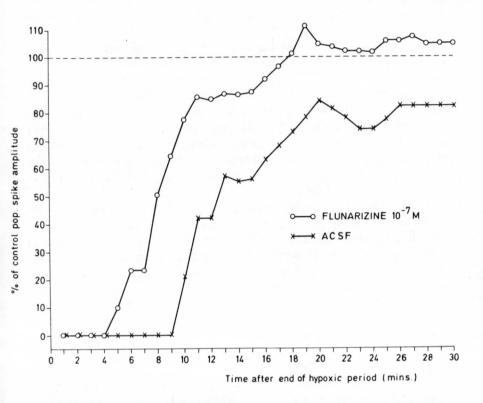

Figure 6. Median population spike amplitude as a percentage of the control values at different times following re-oxygenation after a five minute hypoxic period

In most control and drug experiments two recording electrodes were placed in CA_1. In the different slices tested there was only one control slice in which the signal did not return on one site, whilst it did at the other. Differences between sites are also apparent in Figure 6. These results indicate some degree of inhomogeneity in the response to hypoxia between different recording sites at the same slice.

Discussion

Intra- [15] and extracellular [14] studies have shown that the population spike corresponds to the spiking discharge of individual pyramidal cells. The amplitude of the population spike depends on the synchronism, tissue resistance, and the number of discharging cells. In the present study the amplitude of the population spike was measured from the height before and after positive deflections of the population EPSP which reflects the excitatory post-synaptic potentials of individual cells. In addition, the amplitude of the population spike obviously depends on the number of the synchronism and degree of activation of the Schaffer collaterals.

In the present experiments the population spike disappeared at the same times in the flunarizine and control groups. However, the amplitude of the population spike returned to control levels in all the flunarizine-treated slices, whilst it failed to do so in the majority of the control slices. Bearing in mind the preceding description of the origin of the population spike, a failure of the amplitude of the population spike to return to baseline levels in the control group could be caused by the following: decrease of tissue resistance, decrease in synchronism of pyramidal cell discharge, decrease in the number of pyramidal cells firing, decrease in the amplitude of the population EPSP or reduction in the number of Schaffer collaterals activated.

The width of the population spike at half the amplitude divided by the area of the population spike provides a measure of the synchrony of the pyramidal cells. In both groups there was no indication of a decrease in synchronism. In addition, the height of the population EPSP did not appear to be altered at the end of the recovery phase. Three possibilities thus remain: a decrease in tissue resistance, a decrease in the number of cells firing or a reduction of the number of Schaffer collaterals activated.

Assuming that the activation of the Schaffer collaterals remains constant the two remaining conclusions are not mutually exclusive, since a selective decrease of tissue resistance will also reduce the number of cells firing. Hansen et al [12] and Krnjević [16] have suggested that the increase of intracellular Ca^{2+} mediates the increased K^+ permeability seen during hypoxia. Flunarizine might thus be expected to alter either of these processes. Further studies will be necessary to determine which of these possibilities is true.

These experiments show for the first time that flunarizine given at a low dose improved the recovery of synaptic activity in nerve cells after a hypoxic insult in the absence of circulation.

Conclusion

The present experiments concentrated on two important aspects of a theory of migraine, namely ischaemia and particularly hypoxia. Firstly, all the drugs with the exception of domperidone, which lacks central effects and probably acts on peripheral vegetative dysfunction, were found to be active in the models presented. This confirms the suggestion that ischaemia and hypoxia are pivotal events in the mechanism of action of these antimigraine drugs.

The most active compounds against ischaemia in the mouse were flunarizine and methysergide. In the hypoxic hypoxia test the two most active compounds were clonidine and flunarizine. Flunarizine seems thus to possess both anti-ischaemic and antihypoxic properties. In the in vitro hippocampal slice flunarizine was shown to increase recovery from a hypoxic insult in the absence of circulation, thus demonstrating for the first time direct protective effects on neurones.

Taken as a whole the data from these experiments are consistent with the migraine hypothesis. However, these studies do not demonstrate whether or not the temporal progression of events suggested in the hypothesis actually occurs.

Summary

Ischaemia and hypoxia are pivotal points of the migraine theory suggested by Amery et al [1]. The present paper reports on the activity of seven antimigraine drugs (clonidine, domperidone, ergotamine, flunarizine, methysergide, pizotifen, propranolol) in three models of hypoxia or ischaemia. These models were cerebral ischaemic by bilateral carotid ligation in mice, hypoxic hypoxia by placing mice in a 100 per cent nitrogen environment, and hypoxia in in vitro hippocampal slices. All the drugs, with the exception of domperidone, were found to be active in the first two models, suggesting that antihypoxic/ischaemic effects are part of the mechanism of action of antimigraine drugs. Although domperidone has been successfully used against migraine, it lacks central effects, and probably acts on peripheral vegetative dysfunction. In the ischaemia test in mice the two most active compounds were methysergide, probably because of its antiserotonergic properties, and flunarizine which probably prevents vasoconstriction and/or preserves neuronal function. In the hypoxic hypoxia test in rats ergotamine, clonidine and flunarizine were the most active compounds. All three compounds acted in different ways so as to preserve normocapnia after the insult, and hence induce the gasping-reflex. In order to examine whether flunarizine had direct antihypoxic effects on nerve cells, in addition to its anti-vasoconstrictive action, the influence of hypoxia on the monosynaptic pathway between Schaffer collaterals and CA_1 pyramidal cell soma was studied in slices of hippocampus held in vitro. In the majority of control slices the population spike amplitude failed to return to its pre-hypoxic baseline. In all slices treated with flunarizine $10^{-7}M$ complete recovery was seen after hypoxia.

Flunarizine thus prevented a post-hypoxic decrease in tissue resistance or kept the number of pyramidal cells activated by stimulation constant. These experiments are thus consistent with a role for antihypoxic activity in the mechanism of action of antihypoxic drugs, and strengthen the migraine theory suggested by Amery et al [1].

Acknowledgments

We are much indebted to G Clincke and R Marrannes for valuable discussions. Thanks are also due to J Fransen and C Hermans for expert technical assistance.

References

1   Amery W, Wauquier A, Van Nueten J, De Clerck F et al. The anti-migrainous pharmacology of flunarizine (R 14 950), a calcium antagonist. *Drug Exp Clin Res 1981; 7:* 1–10

2   Safar P, Gisvold SE, Vaagenes P, Hendrickx HHL et al. Long-term animal models for the study of global brain ischemia. In Wauquier A, Borgers M, Amery WK, eds. *Protection of Tissues against Hypoxia.* Amsterdam: Elsevier Biomedical Press. 1982: 147–170

3   Mullie A, Vandevelde K, Van Belle H, Jageneau A et al. A dog model to evaluate post-cardiac arrest neurological outcome. In Wauquier A, Borgers M, Amery WK, eds. *Protection of Tissues against Hypoxia.* Amsterdam: Elsevier Biomedical Press. 1982: 311–314

4   Hermans CFM, Fransen JF, Wauquier A. Survival and neurological outcome after bilateral carotid ligation in the Mongolian gerbil treated with ether, thiopental or etomidate. In Wauquier A, Borgers M, Amery WK, eds. *Protection of Tissues against Hypoxia.* Amsterdam: Elsevier Biomedical Press. 1982: 299–303

5   Izumi N, Yasuda H. A convenient cerebral ischemia model using mice. *J Cer Blood Flow Metab 1983; 3 (Suppl 1):* S391–S392

6   Van Nueten JM, De Ridder W, Van Beek J. Hypoxia and spasms in the cerebral vasculature. *J Cer Blood Flow Metab 1982; 2 (Suppl 1):* S29–S39

7   Wauquier A, Ashton D, Clincke G, Van Reempts J. Pharmacological protection against brain hypoxia: the efficacy of flunarizine, a calcium entry blocker. In Clifford Rose F, Amery WK, eds. *Cerebral Hypoxia in the Pathogenesis of Migraine.* London: Pitman. 1982: 139–154

8   Wauquier A, Ashton D, Clincke G, Niemegeers CJE. Anti-hypoxic effect of etomidate, thiopental and methohexital. *Arch Int Pharmacodyn Ther 1981; 249:* 330–334

9   Wauquier A, Clincke G, Ashton D, Van Reempts J. Considerations on models and treatment of brain hypoxia. In Van Hof MW, Mohn S, eds. *Recovery from Brain Damage.* Amsterdam: Elsevier North-Holland Biomedical Press. *Devel Neurosci 1981; 13:* 95–114

10 Lipton P, Whittingham TS. The effect of hypoxia on evoked potentials in the in vitro hippocampus. *J Physiol 1979; 287:* 427–438

11 Kass IS, Lipton P. Metabolic changes and irreversible loss of synaptic transmission due to severe hypoxia in the rat hippocampal slice. *Proc Soc Neurosci 1982; 8:* 992

12 Hansen AJ, Hounsgaard J, Jahnsen H. Anoxia increases potassium conductance in hippocampal nerve cells. *Acta Physiol Scand 1982; 115:* 301–310

13 Langmoen TA, Anderson P. The hippocampal slice. In Kerkut JA, Wheal HV, eds. *In Vitro. A Description of the Technique and some Examples of the Opportunities it offers in Electrophysiology of Isolated Mammalian C.N.S. Preparations.* London: Academic Press. 1981: 51–107

14 Anderson P, Bliss TVP, Skrede KK. Unit analysis of hippocampal population spikes. *Exp Brain Res 1971; 13:* 208–221

15 Schwartzkroin PA. Characteristics of CA_1 neurons recorded intracellularly in the in vitro hippocampal slice preparation. *Brain Res 1975; 85:* 423–436

16 Krnjević K, Puil D, Worman R. Significance of 2–4 dinitrophenol action on spinal motoneurones. *J Physiol 1978; 275:* 225–239

11

SPREADING CORTICAL DEPRESSION IN MIGRAINE

M Lauritzen

The idea of a functional disturbance of cortical neuronal elements as the primary mechanism in classical migraine is neither new nor original. The first observations leading to such a proposition stem from the neurological clinic!

The typical migraine prodrome is a sensory disturbance preceding the headache by 20 to 30 minutes. When vision is involved, the prodrome manifests as a zig-zag pattern (scintillations) near the centre of vision, and propagates to the periphery of the visual field, followed by dimmed acuity within the zig-zag area (scotoma). When the prodromal symptoms refer to an extremity, usually a tingling commences in the hand slowly ascending to the arm, leaving behind a numb and sometimes clumsy extremity. The propagation of the scintillation-scotoma corresponds to the ascending paraesthesia, reflecting the same patho-physiological event in different regions of the brain [1].

Several investigators have themselves observed migraine prodromes. On more than one occasion Lashley [2] mapped his scotomas of ophthalmic migraine at brief intervals. The scotomas were symmetrically placed in the visual fields indicating cortical origin. The character of the prodrome suggested a wave of intense excitation that moved at the speed of 3mm/min across the visual cortex. This wave seemed to be followed by complete inhibition of neuronal activity recovering with the same speed. Lashley noted that the prodrome was confined to the primary visual cortex and raised the question of communication between different cyto-architectonic regions. Did the spread of the migraine disturbance depend on the number and interactions of different cell types in the cortical tissues? The answer to the question appeared to be affirmative, indicating propagation of the migraine prodrome along established neuronal connections.

Spreading depression (SD) of electroencephalographic activity was identified and intensively studied by Leão [3]. However, little attention was paid to its possible clinical significance, though Leão and Morrison noted the possible implications of SD in epilepsy and migraine [4]. The parallel between the wave

149

of intense excitation followed by complete inhibition as described by Lashley [2] and the phenomenon of SD was addressed by Milner [5] and later by a multitude of researchers in the migraine field.

In contrast, Wolff and co-workers [6] advanced the now commonly held view that migraine was a disease caused by dysfunction of brain blood vessels: an arterial vasospasm giving rise to transient cerebral ischaemia and the premonitory focal symptoms. The ensuing headache appeared to be related to an extra- and/or intracranial vasodilation, probably accompanied by a local sterile inflammatory reaction lowering the stimulation threshold of the pain sensitive blood vessels to subnormal levels.

We are by pragmatic means slaves of the available technique. The two viewpoints could therefore not be investigated until atraumatic techniques for measuring blood flow of the brain were developed.

In the present text, I would like to propose a synthesis of the two views. The function of blood vessels and brain cortex are certainly disturbed in migraine. The causal relationship seems, however, to be the opposite of what has hitherto been proposed.

Characteristics of spreading depression

Spreading depression is a common response of the cerebral cortex to different noxious stimuli. It sometimes develops during the course of an experiment in which the cerebral cortex is exposed.

Conditioning the brain to SD initiation can be accomplished by application to the brain cortex of:

1. Saline solutions containing high levels of potassium (20mM or more);

2. Depolarising amino acids (e.g. glutamate);

3. Agents which block the Na-K pump; or

4. Solutions containing decreased concentrations of Cl⁻.

SD may then be elicited by local electrical stimulation. SD can be initiated, without conditioning, by local application of concentrated potassium, focal injury (needle stab), mechanical stimulation and microinjections of homologous blood in the subarachnoid space [7]. The increase of extracellular potassium associated with a volley of incoming activity may, in the metrazol treated animal, be sufficient to initiate a SD [8].

The event itself is characterised by depression of spontaneous EEG activity, spreading at a rate of 3mm/min across the cortical surface [3]. Prior to cessation of activity, an intense burst of action potentials is seen lasting for one to three seconds [9]. At each cortical point, the EEG decreases to the level of maximal depression in 20 to 30 seconds. The maximal depression lasts up to 10 minutes, but EEG activity is never completely abolished and reaches predepression

150

amplitudes during the recovery period. Both neurones and glial cells are depolarised during SD [10]. Accompanying the SD wave front is a change in the local tissue potential consisting of a surface positive wave of 1–2mV of amplitude (1–2min), a surface negative wave of 15–30mV (1–2min) and a surface positive wave of 1–2mV (1–2min) [11]. Evoked potentials and direct cortical responses are impaired during SD and may be of reduced form and size up to one hour after SD.

The SD front is accompanied by transient local changes in the extracellular composition of ions. These last as long as the duration of the negative wave of the extracellular potential change and move with the same speed [12]. The extracellular potassium activity increases to 60mM, sodium and chloride activity decreases to approximately 60mM, and calcium activity decreases from 1.0 to 0.1mM. At the same time the volume fraction of the extracellular space decreases by 50 per cent [13], as is also evidenced by an increase of tissue resistance. The extracellular ionic changes suggest that cortical membrane function during SD is transiently abolished: the ions run along their electrochemical gradients with the result that concentration differences disappear between intra- and extracellular compartments [12]. The slow velocity of SD propagation precludes normal mechanisms of neuronal information transfer and indicates that diffusion of substances is involved in the process. The most probable mediator of SD appears to be potassium as proposed by Grafstein [9]. Enhanced neuronal activity in a localised region leads to build-up of potassium in the extracellular space with depolarisation of neighbouring inactive neurones, leading to further increase of potassium activity. Hence, propagation of the SD appears to be accomplished by a combination of electrical conduction of neuronal activity, and diffusion of potassium in the extracellular space.

SD is more easily elicited in lower animals, such as rodents, than in primates. This property is probably due to the higher density of neural elements in lower mammals. SD remains within the architectonic structure where it is elicited. An SD in the neocortex does not spread to the archi- or paleocortex or subcortical structures in the same hemisphere or to the opposite hemisphere. Within the neocortex, SD stops at the cytoarchitectonic borders of the surface when the surface of neural membranes per unit volume of tissue suddenly decreases, e.g. at the central sulcus in the primate, or at the parasagittal sulcus of the rabbit. These properties of SD propagation constitute important criteria for SD identification in brain imaging studies in man. Furthermore in experimental studies comparison of the SD hemisphere with the contralateral control hemisphere within the same animal can be made [14].

The recovery of extracellular ion concentrations to normal values is an energy-dependent process, since active transport across the cell membranes is needed to restore the electrothermical gradients. The glucose consumption increases by 200 per cent [15,16], and oxygen tension drops for one to two minutes leading to activation of the glycolytic pathway with a consequent rise in lactate production by more than 100 per cent. The accelerated energy metabolism is accompanied by a drop of NADH by approximately 20 per cent [17]. The concentrations of lactate, glucose and NADH normalise within the following 10 minutes of recovery, while glycogen remains reduced by 40 per cent for the following 45 minutes [18]. Cortical SD may induce a variety of behavioural effects ranging from long-lasting hemiparaesthesia, impairment of memory and tendency to yawning and abnormal intake of food [14,19]. Pain reactions have not been observed.

The electrophysiological, metabolic, ionic and behavioural aspects of SD have been reviewed in a book by Bures et al [12] and a paper by Nicholson and Kraig [20] to which the reader is referred.

Blood flow changes in spreading depression

The SD wave is accompanied by a brief period of hyperperfusion (1–2min) (Figure 1a). The mechanism underlying the hyperperfusion probably relates to the increased oxygen demand during the rapidly inserting, increased glucose metabolism [21,22].

What happened to the cortical perfusion following the SD wave front was unknown until recently when cerebral blood flow was studied up to one hour after the passage of the SD. The post-SD period proved to be characterised by a protracted decrease of cortical blood flow by 25 to 35 per cent lasting an hour or more (Figure 1b and 2). This delayed hypoperfusion was strictly confined to the cortex [23]. The hypoperfusion was independent of whether barbiturate or halothane anaesthesia was employed, and was also observed in unanesthetised rats. Blood pressure autoregulation was intact in the post-SD period while CO_2 reactivity was markedly decreased in the SD cortex, only half of control values [24]. In summary, SD is followed by a persistent, moderate hypoperfusion and abnormal vasoreactivity, strictly confined to the cortex. The functional disturbance underlying the flow changes is at present unknown.

Spreading depression and the EEG of classical migraine

Identification of SD in man by electrophysiological technique is hampered by a) its short duration, b) the non-steady state character of the condition, and c) the small area of EEG depression. The wavelength of the severely impaired EEG activity is only 1.5–2cm and therefore escapes detection by scalp electrodes, and measurements of changes of the DC potential is not routine in clinical neurophysiology. These limitations of the EEG technique may help to explain our own failure to record EEG abnormalities during uncomplicated attacks of classical and common migraine [25]. The development of techniques for blood flow measurements in small ($1.7cm^2$) regions of the human brain has, however, allowed descriptions of vascular phenomena related to SD as described in the following.

152

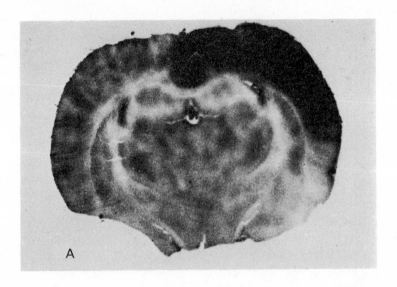

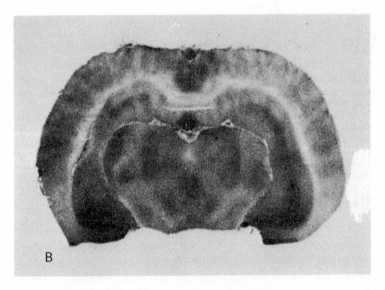

Figure 1. Cerebral blood flow autoradiograms of rat brain. Spreading depression (SD) was elicited by 30-second application of 1M KCl to the cerebral cortex. At selected times after the elicitation of SD, regional CBF was measured by the indicator fractionation method [33]. The rat received 150Ci/kg of 4-(N-methyl-^{14}C) iodoantipyrine in 200 1 of saline rapidly injected into one femoral vein. The autoradiograms shown are coronal 17.5m sections through parietal cortex: (A) one minute after SD showing the hyperperfusion of the SD front in the barbiturate anaesthetised rat; (B) 45 minutes after SD showing the post-SD hypoperfusion. Note that alterations of blood flow are restricted to neocortex where SD was elicited. Reproduced from *Ann Neurol 1982; 12:* 469–474

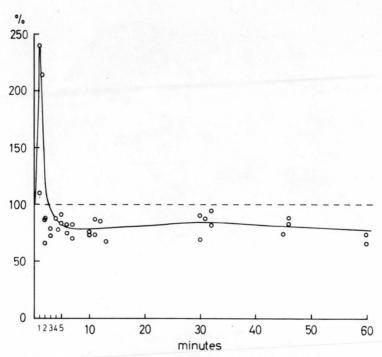

Figure 2. Compiled autoradiographic data of rat brains. Change in cortical blood flow at different times after spreading depression (SD), expressed as percentage of cortical blood flow in the control hemisphere. Rats were treated as described in legend to Figure 1. Frozen brain was cut in 17.5m slices every 35mm through the brain and autoradiographed. Cortical blood flow values for approximately 10 slices covering one minute (at SD speed of 3.5mm min^{-1}) were averaged and normalised against averaged cortical blood flow values of control hemisphere. The figure demonstrates the protracted hypoperfusion in the period following SD of approximately 25 per cent, succeeding the hyperperfusion of the SD wave front. Reproduced from *Ann Neurol 1982; 12:* 469–474

Cerebral blood flow in classical migraine

The prolonged decrease of cortical perfusion, and the specific disturbances of cerebral vasomotor reactivity in SD proved useful in our clinical studies of regional cerebral blood flow (rCBF) of migraine patients during attacks. Two- and three-dimensional approaches for the study of brain perfusion were employed. The techniques are described in detail elsewhere [26,27]. rCBF was measured in a total of 42 patients with common and classical migraine from the onset of attack and up to eight hours thereafter. In 20 patients, suffering from migraine with hemiplegic manifestations, carotid angiography was carried out as part of the clinical evaluation. Fourteen of the patients had migraine attacks induced by the arteriography and were examined during the subsequent, ongoing rCBF study. In these patients rCBF was measured during the development of pro- dromes and headache.

In our second study, 22 patients with spontaneous common and classical migraine attacks who applied to the Copenhagen acute headache clinic had rCBF measured with an atraumatic technique, employing Xenon-133 inhalation and single photon emission tomography. The three-dimensional approach circumvented tissue layer superposition and allowed distinction of rCBF in cortical and subcortical regions. Patients in the latter study were usually examined corresponding to the phase of the attack when measurements were terminated in the former study. By compiling the data of the two series a rather detailed pattern of the pathophysiological events during the acute migraine attack emerged.

The concept of 'spreading oligaemia' and its relationship to the development of premonitory focal neurological symptoms in classical migraine

In our first (retrospective) study of six patients with classical migraine it appeared that a specific change of rCBF accompanied the development of symptoms [28]. The decrease in blood flow (25–30%) always started in the posterior aspect of the brain and progressed anteriorly in a wave-like fashion, independent of the territorial supply of the large arteries. The phenomenon was termed 'spreading oligaemia'. In the following study of nine patients who developed classical migraine attacks after the arteriography, the reduction of rCBF also started in the posterior part of the brain, the occipito-parietal region, and progressed anteriorly. It was possible to estimate the velocity of propagation of the 'spreading oligaemia' to 2.2mm/min. The calculated rate was probably an underestimation, since we were unable to take the convolutions of the human brain into consideration. The 'spreading oligaemia' did not cross the central or lateral sulcus, but appeared in the frontal lobe apparently independent of the posterior oligaemia corresponding to the frontal or orbital operculum, indicating that its way of progression to the frontal regions probably occurred through the insula. That is, the oligaemia propagated according to the architecture of the cortex, and not to the supply territories of major branches of the carotid or vertebral artery [29].

The oligaemia usually occupied some part of the posterior aspect of the brain before the symptoms began. The focal neurological symptoms from the contralateral side of the body then appeared when most of the temporal and parietal lobes exhibited hypoperfusion. The oligaemia persisted on the other hand in the same regions when the symptoms had vanished, and sometimes continued to spread in the frontal lobe during the development of headache [28,29]. This dissociation in time between focal symptoms and hypoperfusion strongly indicated that the symptoms were not caused by the hypoperfusion per se, but by a disturbance of tissue function which was not causally related to the perfusion changes. The hypoperfusion persisted during the development of unilateral pain. Regions of absolute or relative hyperperfusion were not observed.

155

The abnormalities of blood flow regulation of the partly hypoperfused brain in migraine

The occurrence of the 'spreading oligaemia' was taken as an opportunity to examine cerebral blood flow regulation during the migraine attack, i.e. blood pressure autoregulation, CO_2 reactivity and metabolic autoregulation. Blood pressure autoregulation was intact in all parts of the partly hypoperfused brain. The CO_2 reactivity of the oligaemia was on the other hand only half of the control values of the neighbouring, normally perfused brain. Metabolic autoregulation, i.e. the regional increases of blood flow to physiological activity such as hand movements and listening, was markedly impaired in the hypoperfused regions, while the adjacent normally perfused tissue activated normally [28,30]. Between attacks, patients had normal blood flow regulation. The confinement of the regulation abnormalities to the hypoperfused parts of the brain indicated that local vasomotor function was at fault, closely related to the process of vasoconstriction and not the cerebral circulation as a whole.

Persistent cortical hypoperfusion during spontaneous classical migraine attacks, and normal perfusion pattern in common migraine

Another 11 patients with spontaneous attacks of classical migraine were studied two to three hours after onset of prodromes when their symptomatology was largely steady, consisting of weak neurological symptoms and headache. Eight of the patients displayed an asymmetrical flow pattern consisting of a unilateral region of hypoperfusion in the hemisphere appropriate to the present or previous focal neurological symptoms. Three patients exhibited a normal flow map. The tomographic approach to rCBF examination used in this study permitted us to localise the region of hypoperfusion to the cortex, while the subcortical structures showed a largely normal flow distribution (Figure 3). The hypoperfusion remained unchanged in repeated measurements of blood flow at 30 to 45 minute intervals for the subsequent one to three hours indicating a steady state of the cerebral perfusion. The patients were re-examined after ergotamine treatment or spontaneous recovery, when symptom-free. At this time blood flow had normalised in most patients, four to six hours after onset of attack. Migraine headache was not in any patient associated with hyperaemia [31].

In 12 patients with common migraine examined from seven to 20 hours after onset of the attack, no significant alterations of rCBF were seen. Taken together with the observation of normal blood flow in the initial phases of red-wine induced attacks in common migraine [32] we concluded that the common migraine attack was infrequently associated with intercranial perfusion changes [31].

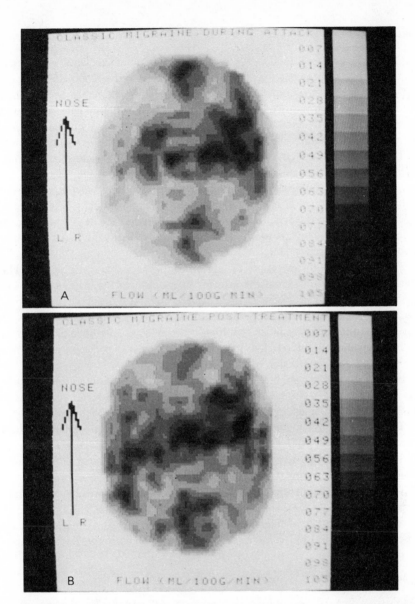

Figure 3. Tomographic cerebral blood flow study of patient with classical migraine. CBF tomogram of patient with classical migraine. This 24-year old woman with familial hemiplegic migraine arrived at the clinic after right scintillations, hemiparesis, and aphasia, and suffered at the time of rCBF study from right arm paraesthesias, left-sided headache, nausea, and photophobia. The tomogram 5cm above the orbitomeatal line shows reduced blood flow corresponding to the tomographic representation of left lateral temporal, parietal and frontal cortex (A). Between attacks, blood flow distribution was normal and symmetrical, except for the left insula which still showed some degree of hypoperfusion (B)

157

Conclusion

The compiled cerebral blood flow data in patients with induced and spontaneous classical migraine provides for a detailed description of the blood flow changes during the entire time course of the attack. 'Spreading oligaemia' accompanies the first one or two hours of the attack when the focal neurological symptoms develop and subside, and the headache ensues. The hypoperfused state persists for the following four to six hours until recovery to normal flow values occurs.

The following parallels can be drawn between the CBF changes of classical migraine and those of spreading depression of Leão: 'spreading oligaemia' of classical migraine starts in the posterior aspect of the brain which contains the highest density of neural elements, the density being maximal at the occipital pole. SD is most easily elicited in high density brains, and it is likely that a spontaneous SD in humans would begin in this region, and the rCBF reduction accordingly is secondary to a SD.

The velocity of propagation of 'spreading oligaemia' is 2–3mm/min. The hypoperfusion does not cross the primary sulci outlining the major macro- and microstructural changes of the cortical surface. SD likewise spreads at 2–5mm/min, and is stopped by abrupt architectonic changes of the cortex. The two phenomena thus behave similarly with regard to velocity and mode of evolution.

The reduction of blood flow in migraine is 20 to 25 per cent, comparable to the post-SD hypoperfusion of 25 to 30 per cent.

In both conditions abnormalities of blood flow regulation are restricted to the hypoperfused regions. The character of the regulation abnormalities is similar in the two conditions.

The blood flow reduction in migraine is cortical like the persistent, cortical hypoperfusion after SD. The hypoperfusion in the patients lasts for four to six hours. The post-SD hypoperfusion lasts for at least one hour, the perfusion changes at later stages are at the moment unknown.

The CBF studies therefore support the viewpoint that spreading depression is the most probable mechanism underlying classical migraine, and that SD may serve as an experimental migraine model. Conversely, we may regard classical migraine as an indication of how spreading depression can express itself in man.

Summary

Leão's spreading depression (SD) is a response of the cerebral cortex to noxious stimuli. Neuronal activity ceases completely, typically for a couple of minutes in regions a few millimetres across. The disturbance propagates through neural tissue at a rate of 2–5mm/min from the point of elicitation. In the post-SD period a reduced blood flow has been observed, and the reactivity of cerebral vessels to carbon dioxide is reduced by close to 50 per cent. The decrease in blood flow lasts for at least one hour and seems confined to the cortex.

In classical migraine the perfusion changes in a characteristic manner. Regional cerebral blood flow (rCBF) decreases at the beginning of the attack in the posterior part of the brain. The region of hypoperfusion progresses anteriorly at a rate of 2.2mm/min independent of the supply territories of the major arteries. The hypoperfusion does not cross the major cytoarchitectonic changes of the cortex and seems confined to the cortical tissues. The hypoperfusion outlasts the focal symptoms by several hours, thereby indicating the absence of a causal relationship. Hyperperfusion was not seen during development of unilateral pain.

The parallels between changes of blood flow in classical migraine and SD supports the view that SD occurs in migraine.

Acknowledgment

This work was in part supported by grants 12-1998, 12-3552, and 12-3836 from the Medical Research Council (Denmark), the Foundation for Experimental Research in Neurology, and Den lægevidenskabelige Forskningsfond for København, Faerøerne og Grønland. The author wishes to thank Ellen Munch, Vibeke Sejer and Annette Damgaard for expert technical assistance.

References

1 Gowers WR. *The Borderland of Epilepsy*. London: Churchill. 1907
2 Lashley KS. Patterns of cerebral integration indicated by the scotomas of migraine. *Arch Neurol Psychiatry 1941; 46:* 331–339
3 Leão AAP. Spreading depression of activity in cerebral cortex. *J Neurophysiol 1944; 7:* 359–390
4 Leão AAP, Morrison RS. Propagation of spreading cortical depression. *J Neurophysiol 1945; 8:* 33–45
5 Milner PM. Note on a possible correspondence between the scotomas of migraine and spreading depression of Leão. *Electroencephalogr Clin Neurophysiol 1958; 10:* 705
6 Dalessio DJ. *Wolff's Headache and Other Head Pain*. New York, Oxford: Oxford University Press. 1980
7 Hubschmann OR, Kornhauser D. Effect of subarachnoid hemorrhage on the extracellular microenvironment. *J Neurosurgery 1982; 56:* 216–221
8 Van Harreveld A, Stamm JS. Cortical responses to metrazol and sensory stimulation in the rabbit. *Electroencephalogr Clin Neurophysiol 1955; 7:* 363–370
9 Grafstein B. Mechanism of spreading cortical depression. *J Neurophysiol 1956; 19:* 154–171
10 Sugaya E, Takato M, Noda Y. Neuronal and glial activity during spreading depression in cerebral cortex of cat. *J Neurophysiol 1975; 38:* 822–841
11 Leão AAP. Further observations on the spreading depression of activity in the cerebral cortex. *J Neurophysiol 1947; 10:* 409–419
12 Hansen AJ, Zeuthen T. Changes of brain extracellular ions during spreading depression and ischemia in rats. *Acta Physiol Scand 1981; 113:* 437–445
13 Hansen AJ, Olsen CE. Brain extracellular space during spreading depression and ischemia. *Acta Physiol Scand 1980; 108:* 355–365
14 Bures J, Buresova O, Krivanek J. *The Mechanisms and Applications of Leão's Spreading Depression of Electroencephalographic Activity*. New York: Academic Press. 1974

15 Shinohara M, Dollinger B, Brown G et al. Cerebral glucose utilization: local changes during and after recovery from spreading cortical depression. *Science 1979; 203:* 188–190

16 Gjedde A, Hansen AJ, Quistorff B. Blood-brain glucose transfer in spreading depression. *J Neurochem 1981; 37:* 807–812

17 Mayevsky A, Zeuthen T, Chance B. Measurements of extracellular potassium, ECoG and pyridine nucleotide levels during cortical spreading depression in rats. *Brain Res 1974; 76:* 347–349

18 Krivanek J. Concerning the dynamics of the metabolic changes accompanying cortical spreading depression. *Physiol Bohemoslov 1962; 11:* 383–391

19 Carew TJ, Crow TJ, Petrinovich LF. Lack of coincidence between neural and behavioural manifestations of cortical spreading depression. *Science 1970; 169:* 1339–1341

20 Nicholson C, Kraig RP. The behaviour of extracellular ions during spreading depression. In Zeuthen T, ed. *The Application of Ion-selective Microelectrodes.* Amsterdam: Elsevier, North-Holland Biomedical Press. 1981: 217–238

21 Leão AAP. Pial circulation and spreading depression of activity in the cerebral cortex. *J Neurophysiol 1944; 7:* 391–396

22 Hansen AJ, Quistorff B, Gjedde A. Relationship between local changes in cortical blood flow and extracellular K^+ during spreading depression. *Acta Physiol Scand 1980; 109:* 1–6

23 Lauritzen M, Balslev Jørgensen M, Diemer NH et al. Persistent oligemia of rat cerebral cortex in the wake of spreading depression. *Ann Neurol 1982; 12:* 469–474

24 Lauritzen M. Cerebral blood flow regulation of rat brain after spreading depression. *J Cereb Blood Flow Metab 1983; 3:* S254–S255

25 Lauritzen M, Trojaborg W, Olesen J. EEG during attacks of common and classical migraine. *Cephalalgia 1981; 1:* 63–66

26 Sveindottir E, Larsen B, Rommer P, Lassen NA. A multidetector scintillation camera with 254 channels. *J Nucl Med 1977; 18:* 168–174

27 Stokely EM, Sveinsdottir E, Lassen NA, Rommer P. A single photon dynamic computer assisted tomograph (DCAT) for imaging brain function in multiple cross sections. *J Comput Assist Tomogr 1980; 4:* 230–240

28 Olesen J, Larsen B, Lauritzen M. Focal hyperemia followed by spreading oligemia and impaired activation of rCBF in classic migraine. *Ann Neurol 1981; 9:* 344–352

29 Lauritzen M, Skyhøj Olsen T, Lassen NA, Paulson OB. The changes of regional cerebral blood flow during the course of classical migraine attacks. *Ann Neurol 1983; 16:* 463–471

30 Lauritzen M, Skyhøj Olsen T, Lassen NA, Paulson OB. The regulation of regional cerebral blood flow during and between migraine attacks. *Ann Neurol 1983:* in press

31 Lauritzen M, Olesen J. Regional cerebral blood flow during migraine attacks by Xenon-133 inhalation and emission tomography. *Brain 1983:* submitted

32 Olesen J, Tfelt-Hansen P, Henriksen L, Larsen B. The common migraine attack may not be initiated by cerebral ischemia. *Lancet 1981; ii:* 438–440

33 Gjedde A, Hansen AJ, Siemkowicz E. Rapid simultaneous determination of regional cerebral blood flow and blood-brain glucose transfer in brain of rat. *Acta Physiol Scand 1980; 108:* 321–330

12

SPREADING CORTICAL DEPRESSION AND ANTIMIGRAINE DRUGS

A J Hansen, M Lauritzen, P Tfelt-Hansen

Introduction

Spreading depression of Leão (SD) represents a peculiar set of events, which can be elicited in most parts of the central nervous system, including the retina [1]. The elicitation requires some chemical, electrical or mechanical stimulation of the brain. The chief feature is, as the name implies, a transient reduction of electroencephalographical activity, spreading from the site of elicitation at a speed of approximately 3mm/min.

One feature of classical migraine is the prodromal phase, where either visual, sensory or motor symptoms develop, often in a mode which suggests that the mechanism is a disturbance of the brain, moving slowly in the cerebral cortex. The process causes a transient 'dysfunction' (Scotoma, when a visual cortex, paralysis in motorcortex or anaesthesia in sensory cortex) often preceded by enhanced function (fortification lines of visual cortex, twitching and paraesthesia of motor and sensory cortex). The involvement of a process in the cortex, consisting of a short excitatory and then followed by an inhibitory period was already, in 1941, suggested by Lashley [2], who, from studies of his own visual disturbances in classical migraine attacks, calculated that they were caused by a process moving at a speed of 3mm/min in the visual cortex. Spreading depression was first reported in 1944 by Leão [3], who soon after, without the knowledge of Lashley's work, connected spreading depression and migraine [4]. The connection was later rephrased by Milner [5].

Despite the obvious similarities between the prodromal phase in classical migraine and spreading depression, little research has been conducted on this line. One reason for this could be that spreading depression has been considered an event only occurring in the pathological damaged brain, especially in liss-encephalic animals. Spreading depression has, however, been demonstrated in the cerebral cortex in a number of animals [1, 6] whereas no electrophysiological evidence has so far been presented on its occurrence in cerebral cortex of man. However, in man, spreading depression has been demonstrated in the caudate nucleus and in hippocampus [7]. It remains of course to be established clearly that spreading depression is actually involved in the prodromal phase in migraine. The best study, hitherto, of this kind has been provided by Lauritzen and co-workers (see page 149). During studies of regional cerebral blood flow in man using the intracarotid Xenon injection technique a classical migraine attack was sometimes elicited in these patients. These resulted in a particular pattern of blood flow changes in the brain cortex. A state of low perfusion developed in the occipital pole and progressed anteriorly. In the invaded area, the blood vessels were unable to react to changes in $PaCO_2$. When similar flow studies were extended to spreading depression in a rat model, a similar flow depression as well as paralysis to changes in $PaCO_2$ were found.

The state of the art is such that much evidence, although circumstantial, links spreading depression with classical migraine, but little if any, which does not. This paper gives a brief description of the various changes occurring during spreading depression and the effect on some antimigrainous drugs on the event.

Spreading depression

Spreading depression has in the past been devoted to much research. Several reviews exist to which the reader is referred [1, 6, 8–10].

Definition of spreading depression

The following events must be considered as obligatory for a spreading depression in the brain:

1. Extinction of intrinsic (electroencephalographic activity) and evoked neuronal activity.

2. A rate of propagation in the order of 3mm/min.

3. A negative extracellular potential (so-called DC-potential) of at least 10mV when recorded with a micro-electrode against a remote electrode.

4. An increase in local extracellular K^+ concentration, $[K^+]_e$ to at least 20mM and decreases of $[Na^+]_e$, $[Cl^-]_e$ and $[Ca^{++}]_e$.

5. A refractory period of one to two minutes for the elicitation and propagation of another spreading depression.

The listed changes should be transient. If not the occurrence of anoxia/ischaemia or hypoglycaemia is likely.

Elicitation and propagation of spreading depression

In experimental animals, spreading depression is usually elicited by superfusion of the exposed cortex with solutions containing high (more than 150mM) KCl or local electrical stimulation, either AC or DC, or mechanical interferences (e.g. needle stab). They have in common that they will increase $[K^+]_e$. Other agents, such as excitatory amino acids, inhibitors of Na-K pump, agents interfering with glucose combustion (e.g. iodoacetate), local cooling and hydration or dehydration of the cortex can also elicit spreading depression. As mentioned earlier, spreading depression is easily elicited in small lissencephalic animals but with more difficulty in the bigger gyrencephalic animals. It is, however, possible to condition the brain by exposing it to any of the above mentioned agents, thereby lowering the threshold.

Three hypotheses have been forwarded for the development of spreading depression: they state that either potassium, glutamate or transmitters are the crucial substance for spreading depression. We shall devote ourselves to the

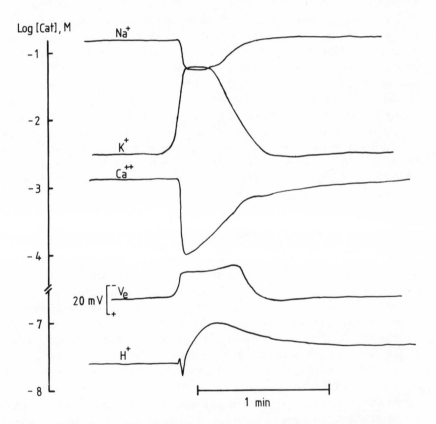

Figure 1. This shows the changes of extracellular cation activities and DC-potential (V_e) in rat cerebral cortex during a spreading depression. The concomitant changes of $[K^+]_e$, $[Na^+]_e$ and $[Ca^{++}]_e$ are mediated by increased ion permeability in the nerve membrane [11]. The prolonged increase of $[H^+]_e$ involves an enhanced glycolytic activity followed by accumulation of lactate [14]

163

transmitter hypothesis since it provides an explanation for most of the observed events [10]. It states that a local increase of $[K^+]_e$ leads to depolarisation of the pre-synaptic terminals thereby inducing release of transmitters, excitatory and inhibitory. The transmitter opens up ion channels with a diameter of approximately 0.7nm [11] in the post-synaptic membrane thereby allowing the ions to distribute according to their electrochemical potentials. This results in an increase of $[K^+]_e$ to about 60mM and a decrease of $[Na^+]_e$, $[Cl^-]_e$ and $[Ca^{++}]_e$ to 55, 75 and 0.1mM, respectively. This is similar to the changes observed in brain ischaemia [27]. The normal values of extracellular brain ion concentrations are (mM): K^+ 3.0, Na^+ 150, Cl^- 130 and Ca^{++} 1.3. The elicited increase of $[K^+]_e$ is transmitted by diffusion to surrounding nerve cells and the changes of events are repeated. Figure 1 shows the changes of extracellular ions in rat cerebral cortex during spreading depression.

The ensuing recovery of the extracellular ion milieu is an energy requiring process, which involves increase of blood flow [12] and local glucose metabolism [13]. There is a four-fold increase of local lactate concentration at the peak of the ionic changes [14]. This accumulation of lactate has an important bearing on the relationship between migraine and spreading depression since Skinhøj [15] showed an increased lactate concentration in CSF from patients during a migraine attack. It was attributed to hypoxia. Measurements of local PO_2 during spreading depression has in fact shown a decrease during the normalisation of the extracellular ion concentrations [16]. However, it could be that the pronounced stimulation effect mediated by the changed ion gradients on the Na-K^+ ATPase as well as the influx of Ca^{++} could stimulate the glycolysis so much that lactate was produced.

Substances which interfere with spreading depression

There have been few reports dealing with this matter. Spreading depression can be blocked or the threshold elevated by a variety of substances [1]. Among the more significant are divalent ions which antagonise Ca^{++} (Mg^{++}, Mn^{++} and Co^{++}), whereas TTX which blocks the Na-channels, involved in the action potential does not block spreading depression [17]. Other Na^+-channel blockers like cocaine and procaine have been claimed to arrest spreading depression [8].

The fact that inhalation of air mixtures with high CO_2 content arrest a spreading depression [18] has special interest for the link between spreading depression and migraine. Marcussen and Wolff [19] showed that a similar treatment relieves the early symptoms in migraine. The above mentioned substances can of course not be used in treatment of migraine due to the systemic effects and since the ionic species never will reach the brain extracellular fluid in sufficient quantity due to the presence of the blood-brain barrier.

The observation that the brain cortex is refractory for a period after elicitation or passage of a spreading depression shows that the brain in itself possesses an anti-spreading depression mechanism. It is likely that this effect is due to enhanced ion pumping induced by the transient increase of $[K^+]_e$ and $[Na^+]_i$. Koroleva and Bureš [20] showed that a spreading depression did not invade an epileptic focus established by topical application of penicillin or an area electrically stimulated. This effect lasted a few minutes after end of stimulation or epileptic activity. It is highly likely that the spreading depression propagation is arrested by enhanced K^+ clearance, thereby preventing $[K^+]_e$ reaching threshold levels.

Effects of antimigraine drugs on spreading depression

Only a single report has so far dealt with the subject. Wauquier et al [21] studied the effect of flunarizine, a prophylactic antimigraine drug, on spreading depression in rats. They found that the compound did not prevent spreading depression, but significantly reduced the DC-potential change and shortened the recovery time. We shall here communicate our own experiments dealing with this matter.

Drugs used were: flunarizine (a gift from Janssen), propranolol (a gift from ICI) and methysergide (a gift from Sandoz). The drugs were dissolved in a 1% solution of Tween 80 in distilled water. The concentrations were 2mg/ml of flunarizine, 2mg/ml of propranolol and 1mg/ml of methysergide. The drugs were administered per os via a gastric tube. Some rats had, every morning, 20mg/kg of flunarizine [22] and 10mg/kg of methysergide [23] for five days. Others had propranolol 20mg/kg twice a day [24] for four days and in the morning on the fifth day. Control rats were given 1ml Tween solution per 100g weight for five days. The experiments were performed on the fifth day.

Experimental procedure

The rats were initially anaesthetised with ether followed by pentobarbital (20mg/kg). The head was secured in a headholder and craniotomy performed on the left side. Elicitation of spreading depression was performed by needle-stab through the craniotomy in the frontal bone, with subsequent recording in the parietal cortex of tissue potential, using a single-barrelled micropipette filled with mock-CSF, and $[Ca^{++}]_e$ using double-barrelled Ca^{++}-sensitive micro-electrode. The electrodes were lowered 0.5mm below the cortical surface. The construction and use of the ion-selective electrodes has been described elsewhere [25]. Two spreading depressions were elicited and the rate of spread, the magnitude of the voltage shift and the induced $[Ca^{++}]_e$ changes determined. An example of a recording is shown in Figure 2.

The result of the study is presented in Table I. The study showed no influence of the various drugs on the change of events during spreading depression in this rat model.

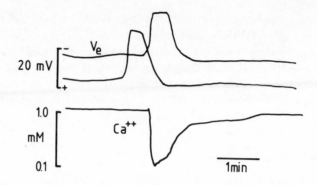

Figure 2. This shows the changes recorded in extracellular space of cerebral cortex during a spreading depression in a rat treated for five days with flunarizine. The spreading depression is elicited in the frontal cortex. The DC-potential is recorded anteriorly in the parietal cortex with a single-barrelled ion-selective microelectrode recording the changes of Ca^{++} as well

TABLE I. Effect of antimigraine drugs on cortical spreading depression

	Amplitude of V_e (mV)	Velocity of spreading depression (mm/min)	$[Ca^{++}]_e$ in spreading depression (mM)	
			Before	During
Control (n = 5)	25.0 ± 2.4	3.3 ± 0.7	1.34 ± 0.2	0.11 ± 0.01
Flunarizine (n = 6)	25.7 ± 5.4	3.7 ± 0.6	1.28 ± 0.2	0.10 ± 0.02
Methysergide (n = 5)	24.2 ± 3.8	3.5 ± 0.6	1.42 ± 0.2	0.13 ± 0.03
Propranolol (n = 4)	25.1 ± 2.6	3.9 ± 0.5	1.50 ± 0.3	0.18 ± 0.05

Values are means ± SD. Rats were treated for five days with per oral administration of the drugs. The doses are given in the text. Spreading depression was induced in the cerebral cortex by a needle stab in the frontal cortex. The change of the extracellular potential (V_e) and the extracellular calcium concentration ($[Ca^{++}]_e$) was measured by microelectrodes. The rats were spontaneously breathing and had arterial blood pH of ca. 7.40, pCO_2 of ca. 35mmHg and pO_2 of ca. 90mmHg. No significant differences in the blood values or the parameters recorded during spreading depression were observed among the groups.

Discussion

We have treated male Wistar rats, weighing 300g, with three antimigraine drugs. We chose to study the effect of two well-established, methysergide and propranolol and a new, flunarizine, prophylactic agents for migraine in this model. A drug

166

influencing spreading depression could theoretically do so by increasing the threshold for the elicintg, by modifying the mode of progression, or by arresting the process. A suitable natural agent for eliciting spreading depression is unknown and we therefore chose to elicit spreading depression by a needle stab and then monitor the rate of progression, the amplitude of the extracellular potential as well as the amplitude of the decrease of extracellular $[Ca^{++}]_e$. To simulate the clinical situation the effects of drugs were studied after chronic dosing for five days. The doses used for propranolol, methysergide and flunarizine were rather high but were well tolerated by the rats. The doses used for propranolol and flunarizine are known to have an effect on the central nervous system in rats whereas such information is lacking for methysergide.

The fact that we observed no effect of the drugs on spreading depression in this rat model does of course not exclude the possibility of spreading depression having any role in classical migraine. The rats may in fact be ill-suited for such a study since its lissencephalic cortex has a very high susceptibility for spreading depression. However, Wauquier et al [21] did find a decrease of the DC-potential in spreading depression in flunarizine treated rats. Gardner-Medwin [18] also using rats, showed that inhalation of gas-mixtures with a high content of CO_2 arrests spreading depression during its spread in the cortex. This was attributed to the dilatory effect of CO_2 on cerebral vessels, but its effect on pH in brain as well as its effect on glycolysis [26] could be important for spreading depression [13]. Further studies are certainly needed so that the CO_2 effect can be adequately explained.

The fact that we did not observe any effect on Ca^{++} movements during spreading depression nor during ischaemia in the flunarizine treated rats deserves attention. Our experiments were usually terminated by arresting the heart action by i.v. injection of saturated KCl whereafter we observed the well-known decrease of $[Ca^{++}]_e$ [27]. Flunarizine, although termed a drug with Ca^{++}-blocking properties, cannot be expected to block the Ca^{++} entry into cells during those two special events, since the movement is probably not mediated by ordinary Ca^{++} channels, but via the former mentioned unselective channels [11]. The fact that flunarizine was shown to diminish the Ca^{++} accumulation in nerve cells after hypoxia [28] must be due to some other action beside transport across the membrane.

Consideration for future studies

A more extensive knowledge of the cause of the start of spreading depression and its propagation in the brain cortex is crucial for understanding the effect of various drugs on spreading depression and for designing drugs which could possibly interfere with the process.

The theory that the $[K^+]_e$ has to surpass a threshold level (ca. 10mM) in brain cortex for the elicitation of spreading depression [10] deserves special attention. If one were to design a drug with an inhibitory effect on spreading depression, it should, accordingly, hinder the build-up of $[K^+]$ in the extra-cellular space – either by inhibition of the release of K^+ which occurs from the neurones or promoting the ensuing uptake, by glia and nerve cells [29]. There are a number of observations which suggest that this line of thinking could be fruitful. The theory that glial cells are involved in spreading depression comes from the observation that spreading depression is very easily elicited in small animals, where the neurone/glial index is higher than in bigger animals [30]. Compounds which condition or elicit spreading depression all tend to cause glial swelling. Van Harreveld and Stamm [31] treated rabbits with sub-conclusive doses of Metrazol, which also induces glial swelling [32]. They observed that light-flashes delivered to the eye, which otherwise failed to cause a spreading depression in the visual cortex now were capable of doing so. This could imply that interfering with one of the glial cell functions i.e. the K^+ buffer mechanism, facilitates the induction of spreading depression. There are special structural aspects of the visual cortex which have important bearing on the relationship between migraine and spreading depression. Attacks of classical migraine start most frequently in the visual cortex in the area corresponding to the macula. This part of the visual cortex is known to have a very high neuronal density [33]. Thus, this area is liable to have the highest increase of $[K^+]_e$ when stimulated. In relation to migraine it could be that some disturbance in the fluid metabolism, i.e. pre-menstrual water retention, caused swelling of glial cells thereby compromising K^+ buffer mechanisms. Adequate light stimuli could then increase $[K^+]_e$ to the necessary threshold for elicitation of spreading depression. For a more elaborate description of the glia-buffer mechanism in relation to migraine the reader is referred to [18]. The details given above also suggest that further studies on the effect of drugs on spreading depression should be dedicated to the effects on $[K^+]_e$ transient in brain especially those which are induced by afferent stimuli i.e. peripheral nerve stimulation or light stimulation to the retina.

Summary

There are obvious similarities between spreading depression and the prodromal phase of a classical migraine attack. Spreading depression is associated with a rise of extracellular K^+ concentration and may be elicited by manoeuvres which increase extracellular K^+ concentration to approximately 10mM. However, it is not established whether the extracellular rise of K^+ in itself is sufficient for the propagation of the spreading depression wave. We rather favour the idea that transmitters are crucial mediators in this respect.

Our group studied the effects of flunarizine, propranolol and methysergide in a rat model where spreading depression was elicited by mechanical stimulation. We could not find any influence of any of these drugs on the change of events during spreading depression, in contrast to others who found that flunarizine attenuated the electrical changes associated with a spreading depression wave in (another) rat model [21]. However, even if antimigraine drugs failed to prevent the spreading of spreading depression, this would not reject the hypothesis that spreading depression plays a role in classical migraine.

Further studies on the effect of antimigraine drugs on spreading depression should include an evaluation of their potential effect on potassium shifts in brain neurones, since potassium concentration has to surpass a threshold level in brain cortex in order to elicitate spreading depression.

References

1   Bures J, Buresova O, Krivanek J. *The Mechanisms and Applications of Leão's Spreading Depression of Electroencephalographic activity.* New York: Academic Press. 1974
2   Lashley KS. Patterns of cerebral integration indicated by the scotomas of migraine. *Arch Neurol Psychiatry 1941; 46:* 331–339
3   Leão AAP. Spreading depression of activity in cerebral cortex. *J Neurophysiol 1944; 7:* 359–390
4   Leão AAP, Morrison RS. Propagation of spreading cortical depression. *J Neurophysiol 1945; 8:* 33–45
5   Milner PM. Note on a possible correspondence between the scotomas of migraine and spreading depression of Leão. *Electroencephalogr Clin Neurophysiol 1958; 10:* 705
6   Marshall WH. Spreading cortical depression of Leão. *Physiol Rev 1959; 39:* 239–279
7   Sramka M, Brozek G, Bures J, Nadvornik P. Functional ablation by spreading depression: possible use in human stereotactic neurosurgery. *Appl Neurophysiol 1978; 40:* 48–61
8   Ochs S. The nature of spreading depression in neural networks. *Int Rev Neurobiol 1962; 4:* 1–69
9   Leão AAP. Spreading depression. In Penry JK, Purpura DP, Tower DB, Walter RD, Woodbury DM, eds. *Experimental Models of Epilepsy: A Manual for the Laboratory Worker.* New York: Raven Press. 1972: 173–196
10 Nicholson C, Kraig RP. The behaviour of extracellular ions during spreading depression. In Zeuthen T, ed. *The Application of Ion-selective Microelectrodes.* Amsterdam: Elsevier, North-Holland Biomedical Press. 1981: 217–238
11 Nicholson C, Phillips JM. Microelectrodes for novel anions and their application to some neurophysiological problems. In Lübbers DW, Acker H, Buck RP, Eisenman G, Kessler M, Simon W, eds. *Progress in Enzyme and Ion-selective Electrodes.* Berlin: Springer-Verlag. 1981
12 Hansen AJ, Quistorff B, Gjedde A. Relationship between local changes in cortical blood flow and extracellular K^+ during spreading depression. *Acta Physiol Scand 1980; 109:* 1–6
13 Gjedde A, Hansen AJ, Quistorff B. Blood-brain glucose transfer in spreading depression. *J Neurochem 1981; 37:* 807–812
14 Hansen AJ, Mutch WAC. Acid shift of brain interstitial pH during Leão's spreading depression. *J Physiol 1983.* In press
15 Skinhøj E. Hemodynamic studies within the brain during migraine. *Arch Neurol 1973; 29:* 95–98
16 Tsacopoulos M, Lehmenkühler A. A double-barreled Pt-microelectrode for simultaneous measurement of pO_2 and bioelectrical activity in excitable tissues. *Experientia 1977; 33:* 1337
17 Tobiasz C, Nicholson C. Tetrodotoxin resistant propagation and extracellular sodium changes during spreading depression in rat cerebellum. *Brain Res 1982; 241:* 329–333

18   Gardner-Medwin AR. Possible roles of vertebrate neuroglia in potassium dynamics, spreading depression and migraine. *J Exp Biol 1981; 85:* 111–127

19   Marcussen RM, Wolff HG. Effects of carbon dioxide-oxygen mixtures given during preheadache phase of the migraine attack. *Arch Neurol Psychiat 1950; 63:* 42–51

20   Koroleva VI, Bureš J. Blockade of cortical spreading depression in electrically and chemically stimulated areas of cerebral cortex in rats. *Electroencephal Clin Neurophysiol 1980; 48:* 1–15

21   Wauquier A, Ashton D, Clincke C, Van Reempts J. Pharmacological protection against brain hypoxia: The efficacy of flunarizine, a calcium entry blocker. In Rose FC, Amery WK, eds. *Cerebral Hypoxia in the Pathogenesis of Migraine.* London: Pitman. 1982: 139–154

22   Michiels M, Hendriks R, Knaeps F et al. *Absorption and Tissue Distribution of Flunarizine in Rats, Pigs and Dogs. Report from Janssen Pharmaceutic Research Laboratories, Beerse, Belgium.* 1982

23   Griffith RW, Grauwiler J, Hodel CH et al. Toxicological considerations. In Berde B, Schild HO, eds. *Ergot Alkaloids and Related Compounds. Handbook of Experimental Pharmacology Vol 49.* Berlin: Springer-Verlag. 1978: 805–851

24   Papanicolaou J, Vadja FJE, Summers RJ, Louis WJ. Role of adrenoreceptors in the anticonvulsant effect of propranolol on leptazol-induced convulsions in rats. *J Pharm Pharmacol 1982; 34:* 124–125

25   Hansen AJ. Extracellular potassium concentration in juvenile and adult rat brain cortex during anoxia. *Acta Physiol Scand 1977; 99:* 412–420

26   Siesjö BK. *Brain Energy Metabolism.* New York: John Wiley and Sons. 1978

27   Hansen AJ, Zeuthen T. Changes of brain extracellular ions during spreading depression and ischemia in rats. *Acta Physiol Scand 1981; 113:* 437–445

28   Van Reempts J, Borgers M. Morphological assessment of pharmacological brain protection. In Wauquier A, Borgers M, Amery WK, eds. *Protection of Tissues Against Hypoxia.* Amsterdam: Elsevier Biomedical Press. 1982: 263–274

29   Nicholson C. Dynamics of the brain cell microenvironment. *Neurosci Res Program Bull 1980; 18:* 177–322

30   Tower DB, Young OM. The activities of butyrylcholinesterase and carbonic anhydrase, the rate of anaerobic glycolysis, and the question of a constant density of glial cells in cerebral cortices of various mammalian species from mouse to whale. *J Neurochem 1973; 20:* 269–278

31   Van Harreveld A, Stamm JS. Cortical responses to metrazol and sensory stimulation in the rabbit. *Electroencephalogr Clin Neurophysiol 1955; 7:* 363–370

32   De Robertis E, Albericic M, De Lores Arnaiz RG. Astroglial swelling and phosphohydrolases in cerebral cortex of metrazol convulsant rats. *Brain Res 1969; 12:* 461–466

33   Bailey P, von Bonin G. *The Isocortex of Man.* Illinois: University of Illinois Press. 1951

13

POTENTIAL ROLE OF NEUROTRANSMITTER DEFICIENCY IN MIGRAINE: THERAPEUTIC IMPLICATIONS

F Sicuteri, M G Spillantini, A Panconesi, F Cangi

Introduction

In considering the mechanism of migraine and correlated headache, one cannot forget that even today the cause and effect relationship is not well defined. Attempted definitions (vascular, muscular, psychogenic, disnociceptive) can be accepted only as examples of working hypotheses: otherwise as with any dogmatic assumption, they can divert medical thinking. The unique disease classification is that of idiopathic headache (IH). Four particular aspects should be considered in supporting this conclusion:

1. IH sufferers can experience in 20–40 years of life, an impressive amount of pain, without any signs of damage to the particular regions (eye, temple, front, neck) affected by the severe pain. This is a unique example of human pathology where a repetitive (migraine) and/or chronic (daily headache) pain, does not result in an apparent anatomical lesion.

2. These pains frequently occur with other sensations, for example, dysesthesias or distortion of body image.

3. The pain usually parallels other facultative extra-pain vegetative phenomena, such as vomiting, horripilation, fever, orthostatic hypotension, vertigo or depression. Since these extra-pain phenomena are not dependent on, but rather independent of the pain itself (they in fact can emerge in some patients before the start of the ache) one can hypothesise that they derive from a common mechanism.

4. These peculiar pains are attenuated or interrupted by analgesic and non-analgesic drugs (ergotamine, methysergide, lisuride). This supports the conclusion that these non-analgesic drugs act on a peculiar mechanism of the pain.

Physiological and pathological (hallucinatory) pain

Pain is the physiological result of the activation of a highly specialised system. Only the circulatory system shares the wide distribution of the nociceptive system (NCS). Both the circulatory system and NCS are strictly controlled by emotions, differing in that the circulatory system is activated by emotions, not vice versa.

Nociception can be considered as a sixth sense, having the task of advertising to the consciousness, by means of a disagreeable sensation, damage to some particular parts of our body. All five conventional senses are susceptible to functional or organic damage: the results can be elementary or elaborated hallucinations, intended as perceptions without adequate stimulus. One can admit that even nociception can also be disrupted in its function, resulting in 'sine materia' pain sensation; therefore, this pain can be considered as a nociceptive hallucination (Table I). The mechanism impairing nociception can arise intermittently, chronically or as a mixture of both, provoking accessional, daily or mixed hallucinatory pains.

TABLE I. Intercorrelations between nociception (and dysnociception) and other autonomic functions (and dysfunctions)

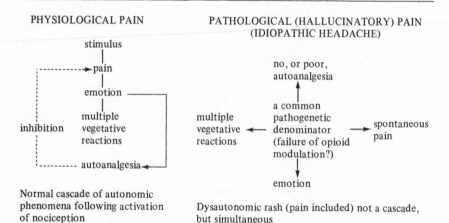

PHYSIOLOGICAL PAIN	PATHOLOGICAL (HALLUCINATORY) PAIN (IDIOPATHIC HEADACHE)
stimulus ↓ pain ↓ emotion ↓ inhibition — multiple vegetative reactions autoanalgesia	no, or poor, autoanalgesia ↑ a common multiple pathogenetic vegetative ← denominator → spontaneous reactions (failure of opioid pain modulation?) ↑ emotion
Normal cascade of autonomic phenomena following activation of nociception	Dysautonomic rash (pain included) not a cascade, but simultaneous

Multiple vegetative phenomena: a common denominator

Emotion triggers a constellation of vegetative reactions ending in the defense of the organism. This defense can take an active form (attack or escape) or a passive one (loss of consciousness and immobility simulating death). This manner of reacting to emotion varies in different animal species. In man it varies strongly, even within individuals. Pain constantly provokes emotion; the intensity of the emotion is dependent upon the reality, existence of pain and the personal emotional profile.

172

During pathological pain, for example migraine, are the vegetative phenomena a consequence (through the emotion: pain→emotion→vegetative reactions) or merely concomitant? In other words, are the vegetative phenomena, pain included, interdependent or interindependent? This is the fundamental question on which the speculation concerning the mechanism of these vegetative (nociceptive and extra-nociceptive) diseases, called headache, must revolve.

Two considerations are of importance in this dilemma:

1. Intense vegetative phenomena (for instance vomiting over a long period of time i.e. sea sickness, or variable circulatory changes, for instance sauna or sexual intercourse, or sports) are not pain provoking in non-headache sufferers. Even extreme vasodilatation, induced by vasodilatator (but per se not pain producing) drugs, are not painful.

2. Vegetative phenomena can precede pain in a migraine attack (aura with yawning, somnolence, emesis, nausea, vertigo, horripilation and shivering). Therefore, we must assume that a migraine attack is a multiple vegetative storm. Such a dysautonomic rash emerges clinically with a chronological succession, repetitive intraindividually, but not interindividually. It seems unlikely that many different mechanisms simultaneously impair such a mosaic of autonomic functions. It is instead credible that there exists an 'unicum movens', involving multiple functions, each controlled by various (noradrenergic, cholinergic, dopaminergic, etc) aminic transmitters. In this sense, the demonstration that the dysautonomia concerns other regions of body, apart from that of the head, is relevant in supporting the possibility of a common systemic denominator.

The 'empty neurone' as background of the autonomic storm of migraine

The vegetative storm of migraine attack, is characterised by an acute hyperfunction of multiple and different autonomic neuroeffector junctions. Vasoconstriction followed by vasodilatation with nasal and conjunctival congestion, lacrimation, nasal obstruction, vomiting, horripilation and fever, oliguria followed by poly-uria and hypernociception can be listed as the most common symptoms. It is of interest that this acute vegetative storm is reproducible through suitable pharmacological manipulations. The clinical phenomena are usually evoked by drugs which modify the secretion of the transmitters into the synaptic cleft or which act on the pre- or the post-synaptic receptors. The most salient examples from investigations are as follows:

'Empty adrenergic neurone' of the iris (ipsilateral to pain) in cluster headache patients: patent and silent Horner syndrome

In cluster headache (CH) patients, without visible Horner syndrome, the bilateral conjunctival instillation of tyramine, a noradrenaline releaser, provokes long-lasting (1−2 hours) anisocoria, due to poor mydriasis of the pupil ipsilateral to the pain. The bilateral instillation of phenylephrine, an α-adrenoceptor agonist, provokes an isocoric mydriasis [1]. The results of these two tests (phenylephrine, tyramine) are compatible with the assumption that there is a diminished quantity, or poor secretion, or excessive re-uptake of NA in the sympathetic neurones. In other words, a Horner syndrome is constantly present manifesting itself spontaneously [2] or latently, but pharmacologically unmaskable [3]. The tyramine anisocoria is present even in periods free from cluster attack, even many months after the last attack. In an eight year old child, the tyramine test was positive after third attack of the first cluster, suggesting that the 'empty neurone' condition precedes the clinical manifestations and is not a consequence of the vegetative storm of repetitive attacks. In our laboratory it has been observed that a latent Horner syndrome, unmaskable with bilateral conjunctival instillation of tyramine, is present even in asymptomatic children of patients suffering from CH. Normal children and adults, when tested with tyramine, exhibit an isocoric mydriasis. In the majority of asymptomatic children the tyramine anisocoria is ipsilateral to that of the father. Then the asymmetry of the sympathergic innervation could serve as a genetic marker in this peculiar pain disease.

Asymmetry of the vegetative system can be detected in other autonomic functions such as in profuse sweating [4], in circulation [5] and finally in the heart [6]. The most exciting question is if the asymmetry is irrelevant to the mechanism of the clinical phenomena or if this imbalance between right and left autonomic innervation in specific areas, can be expressed in clinical terms.

Syncopal migraine: dramatic dopamine hyperreactivity

Some migraine patients, usually non-epileptic females, experience a loss of consciousness for several minutes during some migrainous attacks. If a tablet of bromocriptine (2.5mg), a powerful and long-lasting dopamine agonist, is given to the patients in a migrainous free-period after lying in a supine position for one hour, then, when asked to stand the patient frequently faints: within a few seconds or minutes of standing there is a fall of systolic and diastolic pressure without compensatory tachycardia. Domperidone (a dopamine antagonist, unable to cross blood brain barrier) prevents or reverses the effect of bromocriptine, confirming both the peripheral and the dopaminergic nature of this phenomenon (Figure 1).

This dramatic effect of bromocriptine in syncopal migraine could be due to: 1) an excess of sensitivity of dopamine receptors (dopamine hypersensitivity) located on the sympathetic ending of the neuro-vascular and neuro-cardiac junction, resulting in an inhibition of noradrenaline synaptic secretion at the moment of the orthostasis; 2) an 'empty neurone' of the sympathetic neuro-vascular junction, with normal dopamine receptoral sensitivity: instead of the partial inhibition of NA release by bromocriptine, there is a total inhibition

174

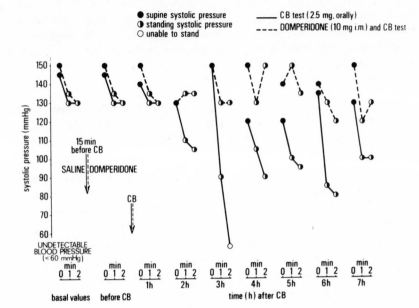

Figure 1. Domperidone antagonism on bromocriptine (CB)-induced hypotension in a migraineur (M.S. ♀ 32 years). While saline solution did not abolish the hypotensive reaction to bromocriptine, after domperidone, bromocriptine-induced hypotension did not take place. (From Sicuteri F et al. *Advances in Neurology 33.* New York: Raven Press. 1982)

due to poor storage of NA. The effects are impressive, especially at the moment of request for increased secretion of NA for the postural change. The inhibition from bromocriptine of NA secretion is proved by the fact that the physiological increase of plasma NA concentration at the moment of orthostasis [7] is reduced or absent when the subject has received the dopamine agonist.

Apomorphine headache

It has never been possible to exactly reproduce pharmacologically an attack in migraine sufferers. Nitroglycerin, reserpine, histamine, histamine liberator, tyramine can trigger some of the more salient phenomena (pain, nausea and vomiting) of the spontaneous attack. The sufferers affirm that the induced crisis is recognisable from the spontaneous one. For instance, the pre-critical phenomena (as yawning, lacrimation, nasal occlusion, somnolence, horripilation, anhedonia) are not reproduced by these migraine precipitating agents.

The only drug which mimics, with high fidelity, the migraine attack is apomorphine. When given by various routes (sublingual, muscular, subcutaneous, venous) in doses which are unable to provoke any reaction (or slight somnolence and nausea) in normal subjects, the migraine sufferers will feel those sensations

175

identical in quality and order, which they feel during the spontaneous crisis. The apomorphine attack lasts approximately 12–36 hours, similar to the spontaneous one. The apomorphine headache is of theoretical interest mainly for four reasons:

1. Strict similarity with pain and extra-pain phenomena of IH;

2. Since it is a quasi pure dopaminomimetic agent, it offers a possible explanation for headache provoking (acutely) and improving (chronically) capacity of ergot derivatives, such as ergotamine, methysergide, lisuride (all dopaminomimetics);

3. The fact that domperidone administration in apomorphine treated subjects, partially or completely antagonises nausea, vomiting, shivering, orthostatic hypotension but not (or poorly) pain, suggests that this pain is central in nature;

4. The repetition of the same dose induces tolerance, with gradual disappearance of the apomorphine evoked phenomena: the tolerance not rapidly (tachyphylactic), but slowly arises suggesting a gradual modification of number and/or function of the dopamine receptors.

Poor opioid modulation suggests new trends in migraine therapy

Since vegeto-affective disorders are multiple, encompassing different aminergic and peptidergic transmitters, they appear to be dependent on an impairment of a unique system, common to relative affected functions. As mentioned above, the pattern of impairment affecting different neurones is mainly that of 'empty neurone': a scarce neuronal release (apparently due to a poor intraneuronal availability of transmitter) and a compensatory superreactivity to the transmitter of the effector cell (Figure 2). This common pathological condition could be due to a defect in modulator mechanism. Three factors indicate the opioid system as the main factor in such a hypomodulation:

1. Histochemical preparations, show that opioids are located in 'personal' interneurones which are in contact with the ending of different neurones; alternatively opioids cohabit with classical transmitters in the same neurones [8];

2. Pharmacological stimulation of the opioid receptors mainly result in an inhibition of the activity of other (aminergic, peptidergic) neuronal functions [9, 10];

3. The behavioural, vegetative phenomena emerge during withdrawal in opiate tolerant animals as well as in human heroin addicts. The similarity of the cascade of clinical manifestations in abstinence and migraine has been previously suggested [11]. Here, simply, one would stress that abstinence in man is, unfortunately, the most adequate pattern of topographic and functional

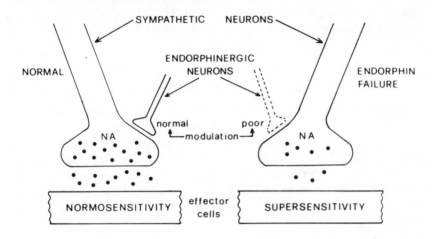

Figure 2. *Left:* an opioid interneurone impacts a sympathetic neurone, and modulates the release of NA. *Right:* a deficient opioid modulation can provoke a chronic incontinence of neuronal NA, with exhaustion in transmitter: consequently the effector cell acquires a compensatory superreactivity. (From Sicuteri F et al. *Int J Clin Pharm Res 1981; 1*)

strategy of opioid (mainly μ type) receptors. Some differences between abstinence and migraine can be easily explained, when the type of interested opioid receptors and neurones, and their topography (systemic in addiction, regional and frequently lateral in migraine) are accounted for. The evidence of opioid hypomodulation in migraine is somewhat indirect. It mainly concerns the reduced amount of β-endorphin in both CSF and plasma, the poor action (and rapid tolerance) of the opiates in migraine-pain, the scarce effectiveness of acupuncture on pain and β-endorphin plasma concentration, and finally the loss of the capacity to serotonin tachyphylaxis in migraine sufferers.

Reduced concentrations of opioids

These are detected initially in the CSF of migraine and cluster headache sufferers [12] and successively in their plasma [13]. An interesting finding is that during a migraine attack the plasma β-endorphins tends to decrease, in spite of the dramatic stress of pain and vegetative disorders. Similar stresses provoke, in both animal and normal man, an increase of humoral endogenous opioids. Even acupuncture, which in normal subjects provokes an increase of plasma opioid concentrations [14], is without effect in these patients [15]. The fact that the enkephalin, which in peripheral blood seems to be mainly generated by the adrenal glands, increases in plasma during an attack, supports the implication

177

that β-endorphin is mainly located in brain stem and in the anterior lobe of the pituitary. The major question is if this deficiency in β-endorphin is a consequence (that is an exhaustion) of repetitive stress of the attack, or if it is an upstream defect in the neuronal transmission, due to a reduced synthesis, neuronal incontinence, or an excess of the enzymatic degradation.

Loss of the 5-hydroxytryptamine tachyphylaxis (TPX)

5-hydroxytryptamine (5-HT) provokes a spasm in the dorsal hand vein in man in vivo [16]. This effect is rapidly tachyphylactic. 5-HT-TPX is a usual phenomenon in muscular tissue of different species of animals, both in vitro [17–20] and in vivo [21]. Indirect evidence suggests that 5-HT-TPX is due to an exhaustion of the neuronal noradrenaline, since the 5-HT spasm is mainly indirect, being due in part to the release of NA from a stimulation of pre-synaptic 5-HT receptors [18–20]. Confirming the 5-HT-TPX in man, two additional aspects have been observed:

1. A 5-HT fatigued vein, following a local inoculation of naloxone (a quasi pure opioid antagonist), promptly re-acquires sensitivity to 5-HT (Figure 3). This

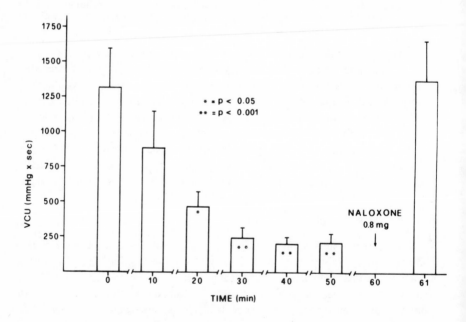

Figure 3. In animal as in normal man a 5-HT-TPX is present in vivo, when dorsal hand vein is utilised (computerised venotest): since 5-HT-TPX is naloxone revertible it seems to correlate with a progressive excitation of local opioid apparatus (14 cases, 8♂, 6♀: 28–53 years). (From Sicuteri F et al. *Clin Neuropharmacol 1983*. In press)

178

suggests that 5-HT-TPX is not due (or only in part) to a mere depletion of NA, but rather to an excitation of the local opioid apparatus. In this sense TPX is not a passive but rather an active phenomenon, i.e. a progressive activation of a modulator system. Even in vitro, animal investigations show a revival by naloxone in fatigued organs [22, 23].

2. It also has been observed that vasoconstrictor peptides such as angiotensin and vasopressin are not able to provoke a spasm in the dorsal hand vein in vivo at clinical doses. Neuropeptides such as bradykinin and tachykinins (eledoisin and physalemin) and angiotensin, do not display spasmogenic activity, with one exception: somatostatin (SS) vigorously spasms the vein even in doses which do not affect systemic circulation. The SS venospasm is rapidly and constantly tachyphylactic in nature; the SS-TPX is long-lasting, approximately an hour. Almost all biologically active peptides (substance P, angiotensin) constantly produce in animals TPX through an unclear mechanism. In 50 per cent of subjects tested with SS (computerised venotest),

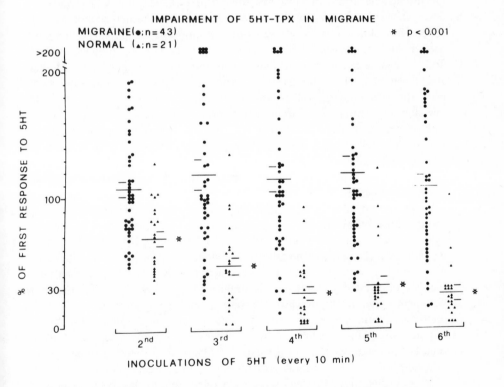

Figure 4. IH sufferers (•) do not display vein 5-HT-TPX when compared with subjects personally and familiarly exempt from IH. This could be due to a deficiency of the local opioid apparatus. (From Sicuteri et al. *Cephalalgia 1983*. In press)

179

naloxone partially restores the sensitivity to SS, suggesting some implications of opioid apparatus even in SS-TPX.

Tyramine spasms the hand dorsal vein tachyphylactically. Naloxone is able to partially and inconsistantly, but significantly, reverse the tyramine TPX, stressing again the putative opioid mechanism in the phenomenon of fatigue.

It is interesting to note that 5-HT and tyramine (but not SS) TPX is partially or totally absent in migraine sufferers (Figure 4) supporting the hypothesis of some impairment (metabolic and/or receptoral in nature) in the local opioid apparatus. In conclusion, TPX is apparently opioid dependent. The loss of TPX could be a new tool in the explorations of both painful and non-painful autonomic diseases.

Migraine therapy: a clinical pharmacological chiaroscuro

Modern pharmacological and pathophysiological assumptions do not agree with various past dogmatic interpretations concerning the mechanism of action of antimigraine drugs. For example some drugs, LSD-25 in non-hallucinogenic doses, methysergide and pizotifen, were suggested for the prophylaxis of migraine [24]. Their action was correlated to their main properties displayed in animal studies, i.e. antagonising 5-HT. Currently evidence is being found that these drugs, when tested in man at clinical concentrations are agonists rather than antagonists of 5-HT (Figure 5). In high (non-clinical) doses they display even in man, the well known 5-HT antagonism. Therefore, if 5HT is relevant to the migraine mechanism, these agents act as pro-, rather than anti-5-HT [25, 26].

Ergotamine displays in clinical (i.e. not venospastic) concentrations, an important 5-HT potentiation [27]. Since 5-HT, together with endogenous opioids, dopamine and others, serves as transmitter in the antinociceptive system, the 5-HT potentiations could play a role in the specific antimigraine analgesic properties of these drugs. It has been shown that IH sufferers are sometimes tremendously hyperreactive to dopaminomimetic agents including apomorphine, bromocriptine and other ergot derivatives [28]. Their exaggerated reactivity can be acutely moderated or totally inhibited by haloperidol, domperidone, metoclopramide and other dopamine antagonists. Then, as an alternative interpretation, the ergot derivatives could act partially or not at all as pure 5-HT agonists or antagonists, but as dopaminomimetics [29, 30]. The long-term treatment could act by desensitising some dopamine receptors, probably those pre-synaptic, thereby correcting the derangement of the dopamine hyper-responsivity. This possibility is supported by the copious increase (10 to 20 times) of tolerance to the painful, emetic and hypotensive effects of apomorphine, following chronic (2 to 4 months) treatment with increasing doses of this drug.

If, according to a pathological rationale, one wishes to classify the pharmacological agents capable of correcting the main imbalance of IH (pain plus other vegetative phenomena, and dopamine hyperreactivity), one could classify the antimigraine drugs as follows:

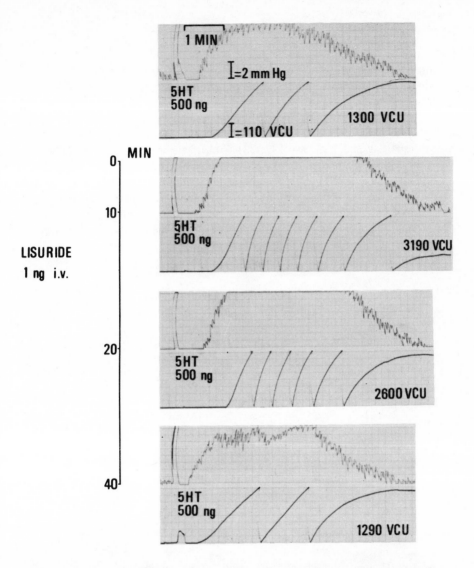

Figure 5. An example of 5-HT potentiation from serotoninomimetic drugs: lisuride (5-HT antagonist when tested in high doses) in clinical doses potentiates very small amount of 5-HT. (From Del Bianco PL et al. *Advances in Neurology 33*. New York: Raven Press. 1982)

1. Those which principally correct a putative deficiency of analgesic promoting transmitters (endorphins, 5-HT and dopamine);

2. Those which correct the superreactivity to some transmitters, mainly to dopamine.

Drugs (or manoeuvres) tending to correct the putative deficiency of the transmitters on the antinociceptive system

Antienkephalinase   Since it is not possible to increase the synthesis or the storage of endogenous opioids, attempts are made at the possibility of lowering their enzymatic inactivation. We are testing three types of antienkephalinases as therapeutic agents [31]. The inhibitor of ACE (angiotensin converting enzyme) potentiates the analgesic promoting effects of morphine and enkephalins possibly by inhibiting enkephalinase [32, 33]. Enkephalinase is an enzyme which has been recently characterised [34] in animal brain, as well as in plasma and in CSF of man [35–37]. Surprisingly, captopril (since apparently this drug does not cross the blood brain barrier) is able to inhibit enkephalinase both in plasma and in CSF (Figure 6). Captopril significantly improves the clinical course of common migraine and particularly the headache associated with arterial hypertension.

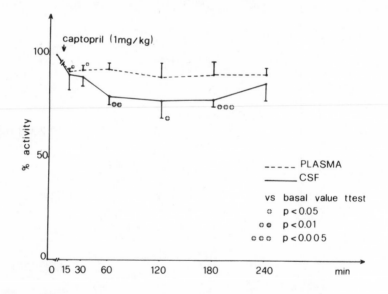

Figure 6. Captopril, which displays therapeutic efficacy in migraine is even able to inhibit in man (plasma and CSF) enkephalinase. (From Spillantini MG et al. In press)

D-phenylalanine, another enkephalinase inhibitor which displays an analgesic promoting effect on different painful conditions [38] has not been sufficiently tested in migraine.

Thiorphan is a powerful antienkephalinase agent [39] : even in man it strongly inhibits, in plasma in vivo, and in CSF in vitro, the enkephalin destroying enzyme (Figures 7 and 8). This supports the hypothesis that if it crosses the blood

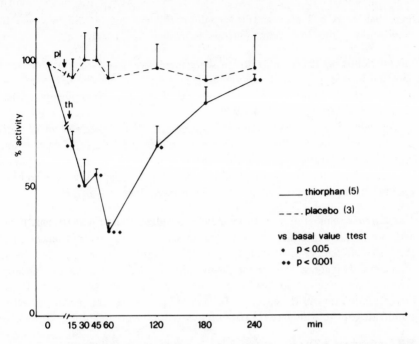

Figure 7. Inhibition in man in vivo (self-experiment) of plasma enkephalinase by thiorphan; enkephalinase activity was evaluated by a spectrophotofluorimetric method in plasma after i.v. thiorphan administration (3mg/kg)

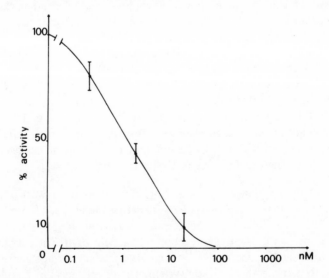

Figure 8. Inhibition in vitro of enkephalinase in human CSF by thiorphan. (From Spillantini MG et al. *J Neurochem*. In press)

183

brain barrier it will also be able to inhibit this enzyme in CSF in 'vivo'. Its therapeutic validity in migraine must be defined.

Insulin Following insulin injection, a sharp increase of β-endorphin is constantly observed in man [4]. The insulin-induced hyperendorphinaemia is possibly due to its increased release from the pituitary gland, activated by adrenaline, which in turn is released by the hypoglycaemia.

The daily use of small progressive doses in fasting subjects is an efficient therapy, probably due to an increased synthesis and release of endogenous opioid in the pituitary and in the brain stem. During insulinic 'microshock' the patients exhibit an enhanced pain threshold and a major tolerance to headache producing agent such as nitroglycerin or histamine.

Acupuncture Sometimes this therapeutic manoeuvre improves IH, but in the majority of cases it is ineffective or counteractive. According to a recent study [15] the efficiency of acupuncture in IH sufferers can be explained by its incapacity to increase the plasma β-endorphin level. The absence or transitory effect of acupuncture in headache is in agreement with the theory of poor opioid modulation in IH sufferers. In fact, in both animal and man acupuncture should attempt to stimulate the secretion by opioid neurones [41].

5-HT precursors The content of 5-HT in the antinociceptive system (intended as an analgesic transmitter) is increased in animals by administering l-tryptophan or l-5-hydroxytryptophan (5-HTP) [42].

The 5-HTP benefit (more evident in children) could depend on the increased brain concentration of 5-HT (intended as one of the analgesic promoting transmitters of the antinociceptive system).

In 'hyperreactive children' 5-HTP is considered an efficient modulator of the excess of unco-ordinated activity, resulting in difficulty in intellectual concentration. Frequently migrainous children are hyperreactive, and 5-HTP treatment is able to improve both conditions.

Finally, the rationale of therapy with precursors depends on the observation of its spontaneous increase in plasma (as free fractions) as well as in the CSF of headache sufferers, which could be interpreted as a type of positive feed-back, activated by an increased request of 5-HT during pain [43, 44].

Placebo This is a typical active human drug. It does not work in animals in standard conditions. Placebo acts by stimulating the emotion, correlated to the concept of a new drug. The spontaneous analgesia induced by painful sensation could be due to the emotional reaction to the pain itself. The consideration, of fundamental significance, is that even emotions, which do not depend on pain, are able to activate the analgesic system. The effectiveness of placebo in IH is directly proportional to placebo-emotion, and inversely to the existence of the impairment of the antinociceptive system.

Theoretical assumption of dopamine desensitisation is based on three facts: a) the superreactivity of IH sufferers to dopaminomimetics (sometimes in impressive levels: see bromocriptine test in syncopal migraine); b) the dopaminomimetic activity of all ergot derivatives and various (apomorphine, levodopa) drugs displaying some therapeutic usefulness in migraine; c) the approximate proportion between the entity of clinical results and reduction of dopamine hyperreactivity following long-term treatment with dopaminomimetic agents.

However when the concept of desensitisation is applied, some practical aspects remain to be explained. For example, the mechanism of the frequent rebound of the clinical phenomena (a type of specific abstinence with a burst of violent attacks) is seen following the withdrawal, from long-lasting treatment with methysergide, ergotamine, but never with lisuride, apomorphine and levodopa.

Another puzzling fact concerns the therapeutic effects of dopamine antagonists, which are sometimes rapid and excellent.

Haloperidol, even in small doses (long-term treatment) should be an excellent antimigrainous drug. Unfortunately it frequently provokes (20% of adults, 40% of teenagers) a picture of typical reversible depression, following one to three month treatment-free period.

Domperidone is active in migraine attacks [45]. It is efficacious even when administered for many months in reducing the fainting seen in syncopal migraine as well as attenuating the intensity and frequency of the attacks. Perhaps the contrast between strict pharmacological mechanisms (agonism and antagonism) varies according to multifactorial conditions, including affinity, which is different for pre- and post-synaptic receptors. Other examples suggest the reconsideration of the therapeutic mechanism of antimigraine drugs.

Ergotamine, but not other powerful vasoconstrictor agents, acts through vasoconstriction. Platelet anti-aggregation drugs are considered beneficial, because of the increased platelet aggregation during migraine attack. Beta-blockers are useful because of potentiation of the spontaneous vasoconstriction as a consequence of the β-receptor inhibition, with consequent emergence of α-receptor activity. Unfortunately pure α-receptor stimulants are not active in migraine.

Flunarizine is an excellent antimigraine drug. Its action is obscure (calcium antagonism? modulator of vascular tone?). However, one must consider the increase of appetite and body weight, which are 'quasi specific' central side-effects of the majority of antimigraine drugs. One final example is the interpretation of the therapeutic mechanism of clonidine. Clonidine acts as an obstacle to vasoconstriction which is a necessary step, according to the migraine vascular theory, for the successive painful vasodilatation. However clonidine is even an efficacious drug for attenuating the clinical phenomena seen in acute abstinence in opiate addicts [46]. The migraine attack has been compared to an acute opiate abstinence [11]. Clonidine displays also an analgesic activity at the central level [47].

Summary

The pharmacological manipulation of those painful autonomic disorders, traditionally known as migraine, is one of the most efficient operative tools in understanding their nature. The emerging characteristic of the idiopathic headache (IH) is the lability of nociception as well as of other satellite vegetative functions. In confronting the IH mechanism, the scientist has at his disposal scarce or absent anatomical lesions, a few chemical disorders and multiple peculiar repeatable pharmacological reactions. Apomorphine, and various other dopaminomimetics, when given acutely, are capable of evoking in IH sufferers pain and extra-pain phenomena which is indistinguishable from that of the spontaneous attack. When these agents, ergot derivatives included, are administered chronically (months), the dopamine hyperreactivity and spontaneous manifestations appear to be gradually reduced. This suggests that the basic therapeutic mechanism of ergot derivatives could be identified in a dopamine desensitisation. A second promising trend is the possibility of directly modulating the nociception by reinforcing the autoanalgesia (apparently deteriorated in IH) by drugs (5-HT precursors, antienkephalinase agents) and/or manoeuvres (placebo, special positive emotions, acupuncture). Finally, medications or manoeuvres able to control several aggravating factors (scalp muscle contraction, arterial pulsation, venous congestion) attenuate the complaints of IH sufferers.

Acknowledgments

We are greatly indebted to Mr J O'Donnel for the revision of the English text.
This work was supported by the National Research Council (CNR-Rome), Gruppo Finalizzato 'Chimica Fine e Secondaria'.

References

1   Fanciullacci M. Iris adrenergic impairment in idiopathic headache. *Headache 1979 19:* 8–13
2   Horton BT, McLear AR, McCraig W. A new syndrome of vascular headache: result of treatment with histamine: preliminary report. *Proc Clin 1939; 14:* 257
3   Fanciullacci M, Pietrini U, Gatto G et al. Latent dysautonomic pupillary lateralization in cluster headache. A pupillometric study. *Cephalalgia 1982; 2:* 135–144
4   Sjaastad O. Evaporimetry in the cluster headache syndrome. In Sjaastad O, Russel D, eds. *Proc of the Scandinavian Migraine Society, Rǿros Meeting, Sandoz informasjon 1981; Suppl 1:* 41–42
5   Kudrow L. Thermographic a doppler flow asymmetry in cluster headache. *Headache 1979; 19:* 204–208

186

6   Morace G, Boccuni M, Pietrini U et al. Possible lateralization of the cardiac sympathetic function in cluster headache. *G Ital Cardiol 1982; 12:* 799–804

7   Ziegler MG, Lake CR, Kopin IJ. The sympathetic-nervous-system defect in primary orthostatic hypotension. *N Engl J Med 1977; 296:* 293–297

8   Hokfelt T, Johansson O, Ljungdahl A et al. Peptidergic neurones. *Nature 1980; 284:* 515–521

9   Trendelenburg U. The action of morphine on the superior cervical ganglion and on the nictitating membrane. *Br J Pharmacol Chem 1957: 12:* 79–85

10   Handerson G, Hughes J, Kosterlitz HW. A new example of a morphine-sensitive neuro-effector junction: adrenergic transmission in the mouse vas deferens. *Br J Pharmacol 1972; 46:* 764–766

11   Sicuteri F. Headache as the most common disease of the antinociceptive system: analogies with morphine abstinence. In Bonica JJ, Liebeskind JC, Albe-Fessard DG, eds. *Advances in Pain Research and Therapy 3.* New York: Raven Press. 1979: 359–365

12   Sicuteri F, Anselmi B, Curradi C et al. Morphine-like factors in CSF of headache patients. In Costa E, Trabucchi M, eds. *Advances in Biochemical Psychopharmacology. The Endorphines 18.* New York: Raven Press. 1978; 363–366

13   Baldi E, Salmon S, Anselmi B et al. Intermittent hypoendorphinaemia in migraine attack. *Cephalalgia 1982; 2:* 77–81

14   Clement-Jones V, Tomlin S, Rees LH et al. Increased β-endorphin but not met-enkephalin levels in human cerebrospinal fluid after acupuncture for recurrent pain. *Lancet 1980; ii:* 946–948

15   Facchinetti F, Nappi G, Savoldi F, Genazzani AR. Primary headache: reduced circulating β-lipotropin and β-endorphin levels with impaired reactivity to acupuncture. *Cephalalgia 1981; 1:* 195–201

16   Del Bianco PL, Sicuteri F. Computerized venospasm: a method for exploring the neurovascular junction in man. *J Pharmacol Methods 1978; 1:* 329–340

17   Innes IR. An action of 5-hydroxytryptamine on adrenaline receptors. *Br J Pharmacol 1962; 19:* 427–441

18   Pluchino S. Direct and indirect effects of 5-hydroxytryptamine and tyramine on cat smooth muscle. *Naunyn Schm Arch Pharmacol 1972; 272:* 189–224

19   Fozard IR, Mwaluko GMP. Mechanism of the indirect sympathomimetic effect of 5-hydroxytryptamine on the isolated heart of the rabbit. *Br J Pharmacol 1976; 57:* 115–125

20   Collis MG, Vanhoutte PM. Tachyphylaxis to 5-hydroxytryptamine in perfused kidneys from spontaneously hypertensive and normotensive rats. *J Cardiovasc Pharmacol 1981; 3:* 229–235

21   Spira PJ, Mylecharane EJ, Lance JW. The effect of humoral agents and antimigraine drugs on the cranial circulation of the monkey. *Res Clin Stud Headache 1976; 4:* 37–75

22   Van Nueten JM, Janssen PAJ, Fontaine J. Unexpected reversal effects of naloxone on the guinea pig ileum. *Life Sciences 1976; 18:* 803–810

23   Puig MM, Gascon P, Musacchio J. Electrically induced opiate-like inhibition of the guinea-pig ileum: cross tolerance to morphine. *J Pharmacol Exp Ther 1978; 206:* 289–302

24   Sicuteri F. Prophylactic treatment of migraine by means of lysergic acid derivatives. *Triangle 1963; 6:* 116–125

25   Aellig WH. Agonists and antagonists of 5-hydroxytryptamine on venomotor receptors. In Critchley M, Friedman AP, Gorini S, Sicuteri F eds. *Advances in Neurology 33.* New York: Raven Press. 1982: 321–324

26   Muller-Schweinitzer E, Fanchamps A. Effects of arterial receptors of ergot derivatives used in migraine. In Critchley M, Friedman AP, Gorini S, Sicuteri F, eds. *Advances in Neurology 33.* New York: Raven Press. 1982: 343–356

27   Fanciullacci M, Franchi G, Sicuteri F. Ergotamine and methysergide as serotonin partial agonists in migraine. *Headache 1976; 16:* 226–231

28 Boccuni M, Fanciullacci M, Michelacci S, Sicuteri F. Impairment of postural reflex in migraine: possible role of dopamine receptors. In Corsini GU, Gessa GL, eds. *Apomorphine and other Dopaminomimetics 2.* New York: Raven Press. 1981: 267–273

29 Sicuteri F, Fanciullacci M. Dopamine as agonist in opiate and endogenous opioid (migraine) abstinence. In Calne DB, Horowski R, McDonald RJ, Wuttke W, eds. *Lisuride and Other Dopamine Agonists.* New York: Raven Press. 1983: 481–488

30 Schachter M, Bedard P, Debono AG et al. Role of D-1 and D-2 receptors. *Nature 1980; 286:* 157–159

31 Fanciullacci M, Michelacci S, Baldi E. Analgesizing activity of captopril in migraine: a clinical pharmacological approach. In Ehrenpreis SP, Sicuteri F, eds. *Proc International Workshop: Degradation of Opioid Peptides and its Relevance in Human Pathology, Capri (Italy) 1982.* New York: Raven Press. In press

32 Stine SM, Yang HY, Costa E. Inhibition of in situ metabolism of ^{3}H(met^5)-enkephalin and potentiation of (met^5)-enkephalin analgesia by captopril. *Brain Res 1980; 188:* 295–299

33 Igic RP, Gafford JT, Erdos EG. Effect of captopril on proteins and peptide hormones. *Biochem Pharmacol 1981; 30:* 683–685

34 Schwartz JC, Malfroy B, De La Baume S. Biological inactivation of enkephalins and the role of enkephalin-dipeptidyl carboxipeptidase ('enkephalinase'). *Life Sci 1981; 29:* 1715–1740

35 Llorens C, Malfroy B, Schwartz et al. Enkephalin dipeptidyl carboxipeptidase (enkephalinase) activity. Selective radioassay, properties and regional distribution in human brain. *J Neurochem 1982; 39:* 1081–1089

36 Erdos EG, Johnson AR, Bayden NT. Hydrolysis of enkephalin by culture of endothelial cells and by purified peptidil peptidase. *Biochem Pharmacol 1978; 27:* 843–848

37 Spillantini MG, Malfroy B, Schwartz JC. Characterization of enkephalinase in human plasma, CSF and amniotic fluid by a spectrophotofluorimetric method. *J Neurochem 1983.* In press

38 Ehrenpreis SR, Balagot RC, Myles S, Advocate-Comaty EJ. Further studies on the analgesic activity of D-phenylalanine in mice and humans. In Way EL ed. *Endogenous and Exogenous Opiate Agonists and Antagonists.* New York: Pergamon. 1980: 379–382

39 Roques BP, Fournie-Zaluski MC, Soroca E et al. The enkephalinase inhibitor thiorphan shows antinociceptive activity in mice. *Nature 1980; 288:* 286–288

40 Nakao K, Nakai Y, Jingarni H et al. Substantial rise of plasma beta-endorphin levels after insulin-induced hypoglicemia in human subjects. *J Clin Endocrinol Metab 1979; 49:* 838–841

41 Abbate D, Santamaria A, Brambilla A et al. Beta-endorphin and electro-acupuncture. *Lancet 1980; i:* 1309

42 Tenen SS. The effects of p-chlorophenylalanine, a serotonin depletor, on avoidance, acquisition, pain sensitivity and related behaviour in the rat. *Psychopharmacology 1967; 10:* 204–219

43 Anselmi B, Baldi E, Casacci F, Salmon S. Endogenous opioids in cerebrospinal fluid and blood in idiopathic headache sufferers. *Headache 1980; 20:* 294–299

44 Salmon S, Bonciani M, Fanciullacci M et al. A putative 5HT central feed-back in migraine and cluster headache attacks. In Critchely M, Friedman AP, Gorini S, Sicuteri F, eds. *Advances in Neurology 33.* New York: Raven Press. 1982: 265–274

45 Amery WK, Waelkens J. Prevention of the last chance: an alternative pharmacological treatment of migraine. *Headache 1983; 23:* 37–38

46 Gold ME, Redmond DC, Kleber HD. Clonidine blocks acute opiate withdrawal symptoms. *Lancet 1978; ii:* 599–601

47 Paalzow L. Analgesia produced by clonidine in mice and rats. *J Pharm Pharmacol 1974; 26:* 361–363

Part II

CLINICAL PHARMACOLOGY

14

MARKERS OF THE MIGRAINE TERRAIN

F Clifford Rose

The main problem that bedevils the therapy of migraine is its precise definition. In order to separate it from the many other varieties of headache, a number of clinical characteristics have been used e.g. its throbbing (pulsating) quality, unilaterality, gastrointestinal symptoms such as anorexia, nausea and vomiting, prodromal syndromes, photophobia and phonophobia, family history, as well as response to drugs such as ergotamine. None of these is pathognomonic. The more of these features that are present, the more likely is the diagnosis of migraine to be widely accepted.

It is because of this clinical uncertainty that the search for more specific markers continues, whether biochemical, electrophysiological or haematological.

Biochemical

Serotonin

Serotonin is the neurotransmitter most often invoked as playing a significant part in the migraine attack. It was the work with reserpine-induced headaches that first gave emphasis to the part that serotonin (5-hydroxytryptamine, 5-HT) plays, since reserpine releases 5-HT, the dense storage granules in platelets disappearing. Given to migraineurs, reserpine produces, five hours later, migraine which is relieved by intravenous 5-HT or its precursor 5-hydroxytryptophan (5-HTP). The rise in urinary levels of its breakdown product, 5-hydroxyindole-acetic acid (5-HIAA), during the migraine attack was found first by Sicuteri in 1961 [1] but is not a consistent finding and it may be that the excretion of free serotonin in urine is of more significance.

Whilst it is generally accepted that plasma 5-HT decreases during an attack, there is no clear relationship between this fall and the headache, (it may indeed be raised during an attack), nor is there any alteration in tryptophan, its precursor. Nearly all of the 5-HT in blood is carried in the platelets but the precise nature of its releasing factor is still unknown. Its exact metabolism is still not fully understood since only some of it is excreted in urine either as 5-HT or 5-HIAA. Although serotonin has been of interest and a stimulus to research, it is unlikely to be a useful routine marker for identifying migraine.

Free fatty acids (FFA)

The factor that releases serotonin from platelets has a MW of less than 50,000 – so it is probably not a protein, FFA (e.g. stearic, linoleic, palmitic and oleic acids) could qualify, particularly as they release serotonin in vitro. Total plasma FFA rises during a migraine attack, the order of magnitude varying with the different acids e.g. 95 per cent for oleic and 36 per cent for stearic. Linoleic acid shows the highest rise (137.5%) and since it is the precursor of prostaglandins it was thought to be significant [2] but, because of work in our own laboratory on prostacyclin infusion, we doubt whether a prostaglandin is the platelet releasing factor [3].

Also in our laboratory we found that adrenaline and noradrenaline (NA) infusions produced a rise of FFA, but these catecholamines are weak releasers of serotonin [4].

Catecholamines

Stress is probably the commonest trigger factor for migraine and since it stimulates the central noradrenergic pathway, catecholamines have been investigated in migraine. The cell bodies of noradrenergic neurones to cerebral vessels are either in the superior cervical ganglia or brain-stem nuclei, chiefly the locus coeruleus. These neurones are more extensively found in the carotid arterial tree than in the vertebral system. Contractile responses are mediated by alpha-adrenoceptors and vasodilatation by beta-adrenoceptors. There is a rapid degradation of NA by monoamine oxidase (MAO) (and catechol-O-methyltransferase) so that the low MAO could cause vasodilation.

Plasma noradrenaline is raised three hours before early morning migraine, and then falls, this being most marked one to two hours before the maximum headache. An increase of urinary vanyl mandelic acid (VMA) has been found, but not always confirmed, in migraine attacks, and noradrenaline infusion relieves migrainous headache. Between attacks, dopamine B hydroxylase, an enzyme active in the synthesis of noradrenaline, is raised.

Adrenergic function varies between the two sexes and in the female at different stages of the menstrual cycle [5].

Acetylcholine

Because of the presumed involvement of the autonomic nervous system in migraine, acetylcholine in CSF has been estimated and some, but not all, cases

192

show a marked rise.

If potent parasympathetic agents are given e.g. methacholine 20mg s.c., this does not produce headache in migraineurs, but acetylcholine given during a migraine attack can abort it. Acetylcholine dilates cerebral arteries experimentally but other findings indicate that the relationship may not be straightforward and it may act by modifying NA release.

Dopamine

Because some of the clinical features of migraine (gastrointestinal and vaso-constrictor) are similar to the effects of dopamine and its agonists, it has been suggested that migraine could be due to dopamine hypersensitivity; it is far-fetched to compare the photophobia and phonophobia of migraine with the visual and auditory hallucinations of L-dopa medication.

There is little doubt that dopamine receptors are involved in vomiting, which was the commonest side-effect when L-dopa was given. Similarly, dopamine receptors are found in areas of the brain involved with pain perception, affect and blood pressure; these receptors have an approximately four fold increase of sensitivity at the height of a migraine attack and pharmacological responses to antagonists are marked.

Bès et al [6] have suggested that dopamine hypersensitivity could be used as a diagnostic marker for migraine. They gave an intravenous infusion 0.1mg/kg of piribedil, a dopamine agonist, to twenty migraineurs and ten controls. Piribedil crosses the blood-brain barrier and has less peripheral effect than apomorphine.

There was no change in cerebral blood flow in the normals but in migraineurs there was a nearly 20 per cent increase with a more than 30 per cent decrease in blood pressure which was absent in controls. Most controls could take a dose 0.2mg/kg piribedil for half an hour before nausea and vomiting ensued but most migraineurs developed nausea after 15 minutes of 0.1mg/kg; the infusion had to be stopped in 18 of the migraineurs because of nausea but not in the controls. Domperidone was given to five of the migraineurs and the piribedil repeated. Domperidone suppressed the nausea and fall in blood pressure but did not affect the cerebral blood flow.

Others [7] had also shown a hypotensive reaction in migraineurs to a dopa-mine agonist, bromocriptine.

It has been suggested that dopamine blockade given at the first warning can prevent migraine attacks [8].

Adenosine triphosphate, nucleosides and nucleotides

Nearly 20 years ago, it was found that some autonomic nerves were neither cholinergic nor adrenergic. It was suggested that adenosine triphosphate (ATP) was the neurotransmitter. Both adenosine and ATP produce cerebral vasodilation, but the latter is 10 to 100 times more potent and can cross the blood-brain barrier.

Whatever the cause of the prodromal vasospasm, this produces ischaemia, hypoxia and reactive hyperaemia. Burnstock [9] has recently argued that ATP and its metabolites (ADP, AMP and adenosine) are the mediators for this.

Adenine nucleotide in platelets is higher in migraine patients and rises still further during attacks. ATP interferes with platelet aggregation which we know is altered during the migraine attack. A very potent vasodilator, as are its metabolites, ATP produces pain if applied to blisters or cutaneous afferent nerve fibres. ATP also stimulates prostaglandin synthesis and interferes with platelet aggregation. Aspirin is effective in migraine, and may be acting, not as a prostaglandin synthetase inhibitor, but as an adenosine antagonist. This thesis may not be compatible with the fact that Persantin (dipyridamole), a compound known to inhibit adenosine uptake aggravates migraine, but this may be due to its direct vasodilating effect.

Tyramine

In 1965 it was reported that patients on monoamine oxidase inhibitors developed violent headaches and hypertension on taking cheese. The offending amine was found to be tyramine and because of this Hanington [10] postulated that a similar effect might explain dietary migraine. One hundred milligrammes of tyramine given to such patients [11] produced 78 per cent positive response for headache whereas lactose capsules produced only a six per cent response. When double-blinded the effect was by no means as easily demonstrable [12,13] and could not be confirmed [14].

Tyramine is metabolised by MAO A and B but only the B form is found in platelets. We confirmed the transitory decrease in platelet MAO during, but not between attacks [15] and that there seemed no difference between dietary and non dietary migraine.

The tyramine pressor response test

The patient lies down for at least half an hour and when the blood pressure (BP) is steady for at least 10 minutes an intravenous injection of tyramine is given. Intravenous tyramine produces a transient rise of blood pressure by releasing stores of catecholamines. The initial dose is 0.5mg and increased until the systolic BP is increased by 30mmHg, the dose of tyramine needed being recorded. Less tyramine is needed to raise the blood pressure in migraine patients than in controls [16] but this has not been confirmed [17] although a significant proportion of patients with dietary migraine developed a headache after tyramine whether given orally or intravenously. The headache, unlike that following

194

prostacyclin administration [3], was typical of migraine. Since it is not related to the pressor effects and develops after a period, it is unlikely to be due to catecholamine release. Still indoramine, an alpha-adrenoceptor blocker, prevents to some extent post-tyramine headache.

Monoamine oxidase (MAO)

Monoamine oxidase (MAO) catalyses oxidative deamination of biologically active monoamines. The human platelet contains only MAO B [18], an enzyme that has among its substrate preferences phenylethylamine, 'trace amines', and *tele-* methylhistamine [18].

Whilst several authors found that mean platelet MAO activity in migraine patients between attacks is significantly less than that of controls [15], others dispute this finding.

Platelet MAO

A migrainous population has a wider scatter in values than controls [18]. Whilst low platelet MAO levels occur in psychiatric patients, the decrease in migraine is a transitory one. The level is usually stable for any individual but can vary transiently in normals, for example, after exercise [4]. In female patients, the mean MAO activity was not significantly different from controls. Mean values in males with classical migraine and with tension headache were significantly lower than those of controls (p <0.01). Although some decrease in activity was present in males with common migraine the difference was not statistically significant.

We found that mean platelet MAO activity between attacks in males with classical migraine, with tension headache and with cluster headache was significantly lower than that of a control group [19]. We were unable to show such a reduction with common migraine despite the fact that patients belonging to this group from an earlier study still had low values on retesting. Maleness had not previously been recorded as a significant contributory factor to low MAO activity in migraine, although in control populations it has frequently been observed that females have higher mean activity than males.

If these are ruled out, the central question is whether platelet MAO defects reflect an abnormal platelet population or an abnormality of the enzyme itself. Platelets from migrainous patients aggregate more readily, even when studied outside an attack and a number of accompanying changes have been noted during attacks including release of 5-hydroxytryptamine and B-thromboglobulin [20], as well as a decrease in specific MAO activity, but we do not know whether these changes are specific to migraine. In studies of platelet function in migraine, care needs to be taken to ensure a representative yield of platelets but it may be that low platelet enzyme activity reflects a similar change throughout the body, and is a predisposing factor to headache.

Another major class of dietary chemicals is the phenols, which are widely distributed in foods, including cocoa, alcoholic drinks, milk products, tinned orange juice and coffee. Most analyses of phenols have been qualitative rather than quantitative, so that the exact concentration of them is unknown but we have been measuring phenolsulphotransferase (PST) in relationship to dietary migraine. PST catalyses the addition of sulphate to a wide range of phenols, a metabolic transformation that inactivates them and facilitates excretion.

PST exists in two forms, P and M which have a different distribution and substrate specificity. The activity of both is highest in the intestine, presumably because their function is to inactivate dietary phenols. PST M acts predominantly on monoamine phenols such as tyramine, dopamine and noradrenaline, while PST P acts on phenol itself, p-cresol, other synthetic phenols such as o-methoxyphenol and resorcinol, and probably many others. Both forms of PST are present in human platelets, which is the source of the enzyme used for clinical studies [21].

In studying platelet PST P and M activity in migraine there was a small mean reduction in PST M group, but it did not reach statistical significance, so that this was not the explanation of the observation, made ten years ago, of a defect of tyramine conjugation in dietary migraine. The patients with dietary migraine showed a highly significant decrease in PST P compared with the non-dietary groups ($p<0.01$) and controls ($p<0.02$).

These results could provide a marker and even a possible mechanism for dietary migraine. Patients could have a relative inability to detoxicate certain dietary phenols, allowing them to pass into the circulation in relatively high concentration, to initiate the migraine cascade. If our experience with platelet MAO activity in headache patients provides a precedent, it indicates the need to examine a large population before meaningful and reproducible results can be obtained. Mean differences between groups are probably relatively small and superimposed upon within-group heterogeneity. Even if small, it does not mean that they are unimportant. Predisposition to migraine is multifactorial and there is a need to identify the many contributory factors of which diminished PST P activity may be one.

Electrophysiological studies

Although visual evoked potentials (VEP) are in standard use for the confirmation of pathological lesions in the optic pathway, they are also abnormal in neurotransmitter deficiencies e.g. Parkinsonism [22] and migraine [23–25]. The latter workers studied migraineurs between attacks using a checkerboard stimulus and found that, compared to controls, the latency of the major positive wave was greater and the amplitude larger. Patients with left sided headaches had greater amplitudes.

Gawel et al [26] used unpatterned flash responses at six increasing intensities. They found that the Nizo peak had a substantially larger amplitude in migraineurs. The delayed latency of N 120 peak was most marked at the brighter intensities.

These findings suggest an alteration in migraine patients of sensory input modulation. The levels of neurotransmitters have been found to be greater in the left hemisphere than in the right, viz thalamic noradrenaline [27] and hemispheric choline acetyl transferase [28].

Vestibular abnormalities

There is a large literature on the association of headache and vertigo. The first report was by Escat in 1904 when he presented a paper on 'migraine otique' at the 7th International Congress of Otology in Bordeaux [29].

Barre [30] thought that headache as well as vertigo could be due to 'cervical arthritis' and cervical or cervicogenic migraine has been repeatedly reported in the continental literature [31]. The association is characteristic of basilar artery migraine, first delineated by Bickerstaff in 1961 [32].

The main pathogenetic hypotheses have been either of a common vascular aetiology or a common neurotransmitter disorder. Autonomic dysfunction of the pupil has been found on the ipsilateral side in Ménière's disease, as evidenced by the response to mecholyl [33].

Similar drug approaches have been made to both Ménière's disease and migraine and Skinhoi [34] suggested that the two disorders are interconvertible. Dursteler [35] found 57 per cent of his series of 30 per cent migraine patients had ENG abnormalities while in another series it was 79 per cent [36], a figure that a more recent study on 20 headache patients has confirmed [37]. Guidetti et al [38] studied 53 unrelated headache patients including 25 with common and 12 with classic migraine. In this series 51 of the 53 patients (96%) had ENG abnormalities. The chief criticism of this study is that there were no age-matched controls. Behan and Carlin [39] reported a series of 32 cases of benign recurrent vertigo who responded to antimigraine therapy e.g. pizotifen or propranolol, even though less than a third complained of headache.

Ansink reported in 1983 at the Scandinavian Migraine Association meeting in Helsinki that of 30 migraine patients (22 common, 8 classical) 27 had an abnormal ENG with scored tests but found that their presence was not predictive of their response to flunarizine, nor was there any relationship between the severity of the ENG abnormalities and the frequency of the migraine attacks.

For these reasons, it is unlikely that vestibular tests will be proved clinically useful as a marker for migraine.

Pupillometry

The pupil is an invaluable aid in many clinical diagnoses. Pharmacologically using its size as an indicator, it can be used to measure the effects of drugs on the neuromuscular apparatus which has both adrenergic, and cholinergic nerve supply. Being both a non-invasive and reproducible technique, it is eminently acceptable [40]. The average pupillary diameter in migraineurs is no different from normal controls. Age matching is important because the pupil becomes smaller with ageing. There is a mild degree of anisocoria in 17 per cent of the normal population. A Horner's syndrome due to sympathetic paralysis is well recognised in cluster headaches, but is far less common in migraine.

Using photography, the pupil diameter can be accurately measured with standardised techniques [41]. Electronic pupillometry using television cameras can also be used [41].

Although different types of drugs produce different reactions in headache patients, they do not distinguish between different types of headache syndromes and are unlikely to be useful as a marker for migraine.

Herman [42] instilled five per cent cocaine into the eyes of 16 patients with migraine, both classical and common and four patients with cluster. Pupillography demonstrated anisocoria in 65 per cent of his series before, and 90 per cent after, cocaine instillation. A normal reaction is at least a 30 per cent dilatation of the pupil with cocaine. Less than this suggests sympathetico-deficiency and was found in 15 of his 20 patients. He found also that the anisocoria increased following cocaine instillation.

Although cocaine does not distinguish between a pre- and post-ganglionic lesion, the work of the Florence group with adrenaline and noradrenaline indicates that the pupillary abnormality is post-ganglionic.

Although in cluster headache, the miosis is on the side of the pain, in migraine where the headaches are unilateral, the smaller pupil may occur on either side, suggesting that any sympathetic deficiency is bilateral [42].

Venotests

Because of differences with animal pharmacology, it is scientifically preferable, where possible, to study the actions of drugs in humans. The dorsal veins of the hand are eminently suitable for studies of drugs acting on veins because they are subcutaneous and easily visible [43].

In 1964, Sicuteri and his colleagues [44] introduced a technique, the veno-constriction test, where the pressure in the dorsal venous test was measured using a pressure transducer. With the subject supine, a needle is inserted into a vein and effects of drugs acting locally and producing constriction can be measured before and after their introduction; this technique was later computerised. The area under the pressure-time curve is a measure of venoconstriction.

An alternative technique is the measurement of venous diameter at constant pressure. With the patient supine the arm is placed on a rigid support sloping up at an angle of 30° so that the superficial veins are completely empty [45]. A stereomicroscope is focused on the summit of a suitable vein and refocused after

after a sphygomanometer cuff around the upper arm is inflated to 45mmHg; the difference in readings is a measure of the change in venous diameter [46]. Based on the same principle, compliance can also be measured [47] by using a linear variable differential transformer placed directly over the back of the hand using a small tripod, with the light metal core in the central hole of the transformer placed over the vein summit. The alteration of voltage in the outer coils is proportional to the venous diameter directly.

Again, although venotesting is of much pharmacological and research interest, it is unlikely to prove to be a routine test for migraine.

Summary

Since migraine cannot always irrefutably be diagnosed from clinical features, more specific markers have been sought.

Firstly, biochemical: plasma levels of serotonin, free fatty acids and noradrenaline have been measured, as has acetylcholine in CSF, the response to potent cholinomimetics, dopamine hypersensitivity, tyramine provocation as well as MAO, adenine nucleotide and phenolsuphotransferase activity in platelets. Secondly, there are electrophysiological markers, such as abnormal visual evoked potentials, but these are non-specific.

Finally, vestibular tests, pupillometry and venotesting have been useful as research tools but are unlikely to provide useful routine markers for migraine.

The search should continue since a biochemical marker may have been found for cluster headache.

References

1 Sicuteri F, Testi A, Anselmi B. Biochemical investigations in headache: increase in hydroxyindoleocetic acid exertion during migraine attacks. *Arch Allergy Appl Immunol 1961; 19:* 55
2 Anthony M. Role of individual free fatty acids in migraine. *Res Clin Stud Headache 1978; 6:* 110–116
3 Peatfield RC, Gawel MJ, Rose FC. The effect of infused postacyclin in migraine and cluster headache. *Headache 1981; 21:* 190–195
4 Gawel MJ, Glover V, Burkett M et al. The specific activity of platelet monoamine oxidase varies with platelet count during severe exercise and noradrenaline infusion. *Psychopharmacology 1981; 72:* 275–277
5 Ghose K, Turner P. The menstrual cycle and the tyramine pressor response test. *Br J Clin Pharm 1977; 4:* 500–502
6 Bès A, Géraud G, Güell A, Arne-Bès MC. Hypersensibilite dopaminergique dans la migraine: un test diagnostique? *La Nouvelle Presse Medical 1982; IIm:* 1475–1478
7 Fanciullacci M. This volume
8 Amery WK, Waelkens J. Dopamine blockade at the prodromal warning prevents migraine. In Rose FC, ed. *Progress in Migraine Research 2.* London: Pitman. 1984
9 Burnstock G. Nervous control of cerebral blood vessels: a new hypothesis for the mechanisms underlying migraine. In Rose FC, Zilkba KJ, eds. *Progress in Migraine Research 1.* London: Pitman. 1981: 17–32

10 Hanington E. Preliminary report on tyramine headache. *Br Med J 1967; 2:* 550–551
11 Hanington E, Horn M, Wilkinson M. Further observations on the effect of tyramine. In Cochrane AL, ed. *Background to Migraine.* London: Heinemann. 1970: 113–119
12 Moffett A, Swash M, Scott DF. Effect of tyramine in migraine, a double-blind study. *J Neurol Neurosurg Psychiat 1972; 35:* 496–499
13 Ryan RE. A clinical study of tyramine as an aetiological factor in migraine. *Headache 1974; 14:* 43–48
14 Ziegler DK, Stewart R. Failure of tyramine to induce migraine. *Neurology 1977; 27:* 725–726
15 Glover V, Sandler M, Grant E et al. Transitory decrease in platelet monoamine oxidase activity during migraine attacks. *Lancet 1977; i:* 391–393
16 Ghose K, Cappen A, Carroll D. Intravenous tyramine response in migraine before and during treatment with indoramine. *Br Med J 1977; 1:* 1191–1193
17 Sandler M, Peatfield R, Glover V, Littlewood J. Tyramine response and platelet monoamine oxidase and platelet monoamine oxidase activity in migraine. In Clifford Rose F, ed. *Advances in Migraine Research and Therapy.* New York: Raven Press. 1982
18 Glover V, Littlewood J, Sandler M et al. Why is platelet monoamine oxidase activity low in some headache patients? In Clifford Rose F, ed. *Advances in Migraine Research and Therapy.* New York: Raven Press. 1982
19 Glover V, Peatfield RC, Zammit-Pace R et al. Platelet monoamine oxidase activity and headache. *J Neurol Neurosurg Psychiat 1981; 14:* 786–790
20 Gawel M, Burkitt M, Rose FC. The platelet release reaction during migraine attacks. *Headache 1979; 19:* 323–327
21 Glover V, Littlewood JT, Sandler M et al. Dietary migraine: looking beyond tyramine. In Clifford Rose F, ed. *Progress in Migraine Research 2.* London: Pitman. 1984
22 Gawel M, Das P, Vincent S, Rose FC. Visual and auditory evoked potentials in Parkinson's disease. *J Neurol Neurosurg Psychiatry 1981; 44:* 227–232
23 Kennard C, Gawel M, Rudolph N de M, Rose FC. Visual evoked potentials in migraine subjects. *Res Clin Stud Headache 1978; 6:* 73–80
24 Nyrke T, Lang AH. Spectral analysis of visual potentials evoked by sine wave modulated light in migraine. *EEG and Clin Neurophys 1982; 53:* 436–442
25 Simon RH, Zimmerman AW, Tasman A, Hale MS. Spectral analysis of photic stimulation in migraine. *EEG and Clin Neurophys 1982; 53:* 270–276
26 Gawel M, Connolly JF, Rose FC. Migraine patients exhibit abnormalities in the visual evoked potential. In Clifford Rose F, ed. *Advances in Migraine Research and Therapy.* New York: Raven Press. 1982
27 Oke A, Mefford I, Adams RM. Lateralisation of norepinephrine in human thalamus. *Science 1978; 200:* 1411–1413
28 Amaducci L, Sorbi S, Bracio L et al. Right and left differences of cholinergic system in the human temporal areas. *Excerpta Medica Int Congr Ser 1981; 548*
29 Escat H. De la migraine otique. In *7th Congres Internationale d'Otologie.* Bordeaux: Gounouilhou. 1904
30 Barre JA. Sur un syndrome sympatique cervical postereur et sa cause frequente, larthrite cervicale. *Rev Neurol 1926; 55:* 1246–1248
31 Bärtschi-Rochaix W. *Migraine Cervicale.* Bern: Huber. 1949
32 Bickerstaff ER. Basilar artery migraine. *Lancet 1961; i:* 15–17
33 Uemura T, Hoh M, Kikuchi N. Autonomic dysfunction on the affected side in Ménière's disease. *Acta Otolaryngol 1980; 89:* 109–117
34 Skinhøj F. Migraine converted into Ménière's disease. In *Headache.* Florence: New Vistas Biomedical Press. 1977: 9–12
35 Dursteler MR. Migraine und vestibularapparat. *J Neurol 1975; 210:* 253–269
36 Rafaelli E, Monan AD. Migraine and the limbic system. *Headache 1975; 15:* 69–78
37 Kuritzky A, Toglia KJ, Thomas D. Vestibular function in migraine. *Headache 1981; 21:* 110–112
38 Guidetti G, Bergamini G, Pini LA. Neuro-otological abnormalities in headache sufferers. In Clifford Rose F, ed. *Progress in Migraine Research 2.* London: Pitman 1984

39   Behan PO, Carlin J. Benign recurrent vertigo. In Clifford Rose F, ed. *Advances in Migraine Research and Therapy*. New York: Raven Press. 1982

40   Turner P. The human pupil as a model for clinical pharmacological investigations. *J R Coll Physicians London 1975; 9:* 165–172

41   Fanciullacci M, Pietrini K, Boccuni M. Disruption of iris adrenergic transmission as an index of poor endorphin modulation in headache. In Critchley M, Friedman AP, Gorini S, Sicuteri F, eds. *Headache: Physiopathological and Clinical Concepts*. New York: Raven Press. 1982

42   Herman P. The pupil and headaches. *Headache 1983; 23:* 102–105

43   Nachev C, Collier JG, Robinson BF. Simplified method for measuring compliance of superficial veins. *Cardiovasc Res 1971; 5:* 147–156

44   Sicuteri F, Del Bianco PL, Fanciullacci M, Franchi G. Il test, della venocostiizione per la misura della sensibilita alla 5-idiossitriptamina ed alla catecholamine nell. *Boll Soc Italy Biol Spe 1964; 40:* 1148–1150

45   Aellig WH. Use of a linear variable differential transformer to measure compliance of human hand veins in situ. *Br J Clin Pharmacol 1979; 8:* 395 (Abstr)

46   Aellig WH. A new technique for recording compliance of human hand veins. *Br J Clin Pharmacol 1981; 11:* 233–243

47   Aellig WH. Agonists and antagonists of 5-hydroxytryptamine on venomotor receptors. In Critchley M, Friedman AP, Gorini S, Sicuteri F, eds. *Headache: Physiological and Clinical Concepts*. New York: Raven Press. 1982

15

ANTIMIGRAINE DRUGS AND DOPAMINE HYPERSENSITIVITY

A Bès, B Comet, Ph Dupui, A Guell, M C Arne-Bès, G Géraud

Considering the role of neurotransmitters and particularly monoamines in migraine pathogenesis, serotonin has had and doubtlessly retains a preponderant role. However, the place of dopamine has increased in the last few years, mainly under the influence of F Sicuteri's work and concepts [1,2]. More recently, our group has obtained results apparently supporting the concept of dopaminergic hypersensitivity (DAHS) in migraine patients [3]. This interesting, and much discussed theory may have practical consequences, prompting a deeper study of drugs working on the dopaminergic system in migraine. It will be seen that this venture has promise, but numerous doubts persist, and certain paradoxes remain to be explained.

Dopaminergic hypersensitivity in migraine patients

F Sicuteri has gathered a certain number of arguments indicating a probable dopaminergic hypersensitivity (DAHS) in migraine patients, making him call dopamine 'the second protagonist', after serotonin, in headache patients.

We can cite (a) a much more marked emetic action of apomorphine given intramuscularly in idiopathic headache (IH) patients compared with non-cephalalgic control subjects [1]; (b) the same very marked action of L-dopa in the same headache patients [4]; (c) on the contrary, the improvement of headaches by small doses of haloperidol, this neuroleptic blocking post-synaptic receptors [5]; (d) the marked hypotensive action of bromocriptine in migraine patients after only one oral dose [6]; and (e) the interesting results of an objective method, venospasm measurement.

The computerised venotest shows the striking hypersensitivity to dopamine (from 20 to 30 times) and even more to serotonin, during a migraine attack. Therefore there are many arguments in support of the DAHS concept in migraine patients.

202

In these conditions, we have studied the action of dopaminergic agonist on cerebral circulation, in order to verify if this DAHS existed on the level of the cerebral arterioles. Actually, although the point of impact is worth discussing, the initial idea was the hypothesis of a probably greater sensitivity of the cerebral arterioles in migraine patients to dopamine, than that which has been demonstrated in vitro for other amines [7].

ACTION ON THE CEREBRAL BLOOD FLOW

The dopaminergic agonist chosen was piribedil, because it crosses the blood-brain barrier. McCulloch [8] showed that giving a 0.2mg/kg dose of piribedil to monkeys caused an increase of cerebral blood flow (CBF) reaching 40 per cent. Guell [9] verified the increase of CBF (22%) in man under 0.2mg/kg of drug. We then established that in control subjects without headache the perfusion of 0.1mg/kg of piribedil did not cause a significant increase of CBF in 30 minutes. Figure 1 shows on the left the results obtained with 10 control subjects; it can be seen that there has been no CBF increase except a moderate one in one subject [10].

On the contrary, the same dose of piribedil causes a significant increase of CBF in migraine patients, as observed in 18 out of 20 of the examined subjects. This increase attains an average of over 18 per cent, and the extremes go from 10 per cent to 39 per cent.

The migraine subjects examined were chosen because of their characteristic aetiology, they had all the usual cardinal signs of common migraine, and they had high scores in the established scale, between 12 and 14 with a maximum of 14.

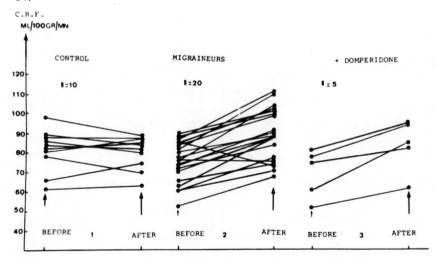

Figure 1

Therefore piribedil, a dopaminergic agonist crossing the blood-brain barrier, caused a definite increase in CBF in migraine patients at a dose that has no effect on cerebral flow in non-cephalalgic control subjects. It would seem that we may conclude that the migraine patients showed a DAHS on the cerebral or cerebrovascular level.

PERIPHERAL ACTION

It is also worth studying the peripheral effects of the dopaminergic agonist perfusion in question. A 0.2mg/kg dose of piribedil, infused over 30 minutes, causes nausea in non-migraine subjects between the 20th and 30th minute, sometimes with vomiting. The 0.1mg/kg dose causes little or no upset in control subjects, the dose can be given in totality, sometimes with slight nausea at the end. The same 0.1mg/kg dose is much less well tolerated by migraine patients: nausea can be felt towards the 10th minute, and if the perfusion continues, vomiting may cause it to be interrupted. Decreased blood pressure and other important vegetative signs were seen: in the 20 characterised migraine subjects examined, the

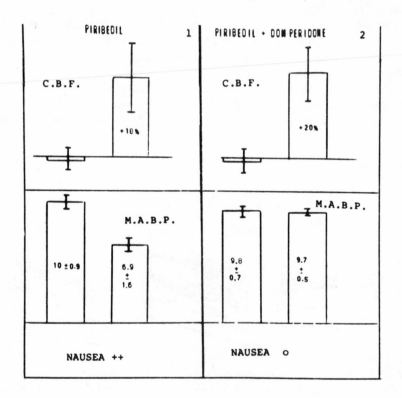

Figure 2

204

average value of MABP passed from 10 to 6.9cmHg, i.e. a 32 per cent decrease. No migraine subject retained the normal values of blood pressure during the test. These results are displayed in Figure 2, on the left. The decrease in blood pressure would have been greater if the test had been continued beyond the first sign of intolerance, but the perfusion was interrupted as soon as this happened.

The dopaminergic hypersensitivity is therefore not limited to cerebral blood flow. The 'peripheral' signs, nausea or vomiting, and decreased blood pressure, have led us to propose a piribedil test in order to examine those headache subjects difficult to classify, and for whom there is the question as to whether they are migraine sufferers or not. The demonstration of dopaminergic hypersensitivity in those patients i.e. the more or less quick appearance of nausea and the tendency to decrease in blood pressure, would lead us to consider them probable cases of migraine. Conversely, a negative test would lead us to consider psychogenic headache or something other than migraine. Our clinical experience on 150 subjects has been published elsewhere [11].

It was interesting in these conditions to study the action of dopaminergic antagonists in migraine patients, with the hypothesis that the correction of dopaminergic hypersensitivity during a migraine attack would also relieve the symptoms whose dopaminergic nature is probable, and perhaps have an influence on the pain syndrome itself.

The antidopaminergic drugs in migraine patients

Domperidone

This is a powerful dopaminergic antagonist which blocks dopaminergic receptors at the periphery, but which, at the doses used, has little or no penetration across the blood-brain barrier. On the other hand, it acts on the chemoreceptors of the vomiting centre, in the postrema area, which is not protected by the blood-brain barrier. Its use has been proposed in order to permit a better tolerance of dopaminergic agonists in the treatment of Parkinson's disease [12].

a) Giving a 20mg per os dose of domperidone before the piribedil test does not seem to modify the response observed at the cerebral blood flow level: in five subjects examined, an average CBF increase of 20 per cent was observed under these conditions (Figures 1 and 2, on the right). On the other hand, the characteristic migraine patients, examined under this protection, showed no nausea, nor any blood pressure decrease. It can be seen on Figure 2 that the blood pressure at cessation of perfusion has remained comparable.

Other authors [13] have observed that giving domperidone does not prevent the episodes of orthostatic hypotension connected with bromocriptine, and have tried to conclude from this fact that the hypotension provoked by the dopaminergic agonists were of central origin. Our results do not indicate this, but rather lead us to prefer a peripheral origin of the hypotension connected with dopaminergic agonists.

b) We studied the effects of domperidone injected intravenously in 10 volunteer typical migraine sufferers 15 minutes before the perfusion of piribedil. This was a randomised double-blind cross-over study, with either 8mg of domperidone or of a placebo.

As far as gastrointestinal effects were concerned, six subjects out of 10 were well protected by domperidone, whereas they had nausea or vomiting with the placebo two subjects were not protected by the domperidone. It must be remarked that this kind of double-blind experiment is sometimes difficult to interpret, especially in the cases where a first test has caused very marked upset, and a conditioning.

As far as effects on blood pressure are concerned, Figure 3 shows a characteristic protective effect by domperidone with regard to the decreased blood pressure caused by the piribedil test administered without protection.

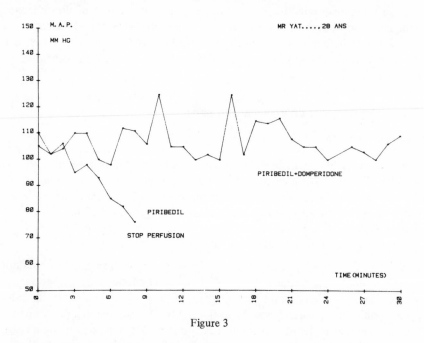

Figure 3

However, during this study we did not observe sufficient cases of clear arterial hypotension in the group with placebo to permit establishing a statistically significant result in favour of domperidone.

Figure 4 shows the protective effect of domperidone which reduces the upset due to the dopaminergic hypersensitivity of migraine patients: a score has been established, taking into account all the problems precipitated by the

206

dopaminergic agonist, i.e. nausea and vomiting, hypotension, while also taking into account their speed of appearance.

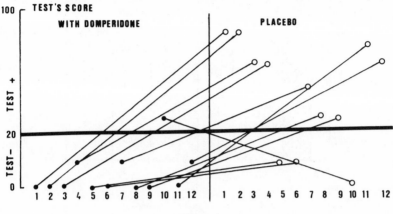

Figure 4

c) Does domperidone have a place in the clinic? Of course it can help in treating attacks by efficiently eliminating the disorders connected to dopaminergic hypersensitivity, especially nausea and vomiting. But can more be asked of it, and is it capable of halting an attack? There is still little clinical evidence. One study [14] shows that domperidone given intravenously during an attack efficiently eliminates nausea and vomiting. Another conducted double-blind study with placebo [15,16] with 19 subjects having complete migraine, domperidone given with the appearance of the first symptoms prevents the attack in 66 per cent of cases, against five per cent for the placebo. The last step will consist of studying the possibility of chronic treatment with this drug.

Substituted benzamide

We have used another dopaminergic antagonist, a substituted benzamide, which is mainly a D2 antagonist. It protects very efficiently against the emetic effects of apomorphine, the drug reaching easily the vomiting centres of area postrema. It increases plasma prolactin, as much as sulpiride does.

The drug was given in a 100mg dose one and a half hours before the piribedil test. The subjects examined were characteristic migraine patients. This trial was not a double-blind study, but in order to avoid a conditioning due to the unpleasant effects of the first positive test, : protection by the active drug was systematically given at the first test, and a placebo before the second test. This trial design seems to us to be appropriate for certain types of study using migraine patients.

Figure 5 shows the results on blood pressure. It will be noted that in all cases,

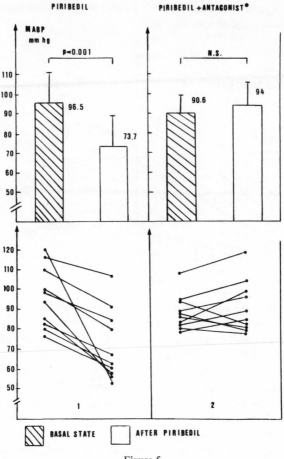

Figure 5

a fall in blood pressure has been avoided, and that a certain number of subjects even showed a discrete tendency towards increased blood pressure, a fact difficult to interpret at the moment.

Figure 6 shows the effect of prevention of nausea or vomiting. It can be noted that the dopaminergic agonist piribedil given alone to these hypersensitive patients, quickly causes nausea, from the second to the 10th minute, and the perfusion has usually to be interrupted between the fifth and the 17th minute. On the other hand, in the 10 subjects protected by the benzamide derivative, the perfusion could be continued for 30 minutes in all cases, and no nausea appeared, and especially no arterial hypotension.

Figure 7 shows the clear difference in score according to whether the subjects were protected by the antagonist or not. All protected subjects had a negative test, and all subjects without antagonist had a positive test. We stress that the

208

score takes into account the totality of signs of dopaminergic hypersensitivity and their time of appearance.

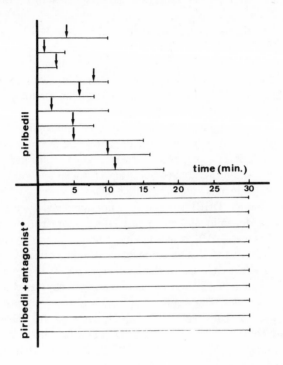

Figure 6

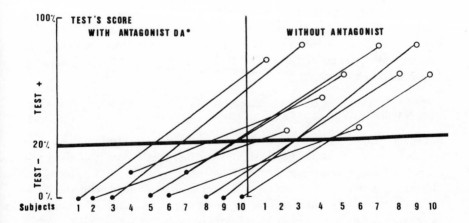

Figure 7

These are well known for their dopaminergic antagonism of D1 or D2 receptors, or globally.

Haloperidol is an antagonist on the level of D1 and D2. Sicuteri points out [1] that it reduces venospasm in idiopathic headache patients, and that it improves them clinically, but it causes in them a high incidence of depression. Lechin [17] proposes using haloperidol in association with sulpiride and pro-pranolol, in order to effect a complex blocking of the monoaminergic systems, but gives primary importance to dopaminergic blocking.

Sulpiride alone, an antagonist of D2 receptors, appeared to be more potent in blocking post rather than pre-synaptic dopaminergic receptors [18].

Metoclopramide is an antagonist of the pre-synaptic dopaminergic receptors [18]. This action should result in a releasing of dopamine without blockade of post-synaptic dopaminergic receptors following low doses.

Dihydroergotamine (DHE) is classically a noradrenergic agonist, more recently shown to have a dopaminergic antagonist effect, more particularly on the D2 receptors, and Horowski [19] makes the hypothesis that the favourable effect of DHE on migraine is due to this dopaminergic antagonist effect.

Our personal experience has for several years led us to prescribe combined DHE/haloperidol at a small dose (0.75 to 1mg per day) as chronic treatment of intractable migraines. The results seem positive to us, but must be verified by a double-blind study. The mechanism may appear doubtful, since DHE is at the same time antagonist D1 and antagonist D2. This last effect is also shown by haloperidol, which would therefore be synergistic with DHE in the chronic treatment of migraine.

We have shown several attempts at treating migraine by products which reduce dopaminergic hypersensitivity. It is somewhat paradoxical to see that dopa-minergic agonists have also been used to this end: bromocriptine has been shown favourably in preventing the occurrence of menstrual migraines [20]. Lisuride would seem to have a favourable effect [21]. However, it does not modify, at the doses used, the amount of prolactin and the active mechanism is therefore independent of it.

General remarks

A certain number of facts have contributed to giving a significant place to dopamine in the physiopathogenesis of migraine. DAHS on the cerebral and peripheral levels, seems established, and may make up an important element of the 'migraine terrain'. It is logical to expect an improvement with the dopa-minergic antagonists that reduce hypersensitivity. Actually, dopaminergic antagonists eliminate certain awkward symptoms during the attack, even may check the attack and perhaps also constitute a preventive chronic treatment.

But the extraordinary complexity of migraine pathogenesis, and the number of points of impact of therapeutics, cannot be forgotten. Even with monoamines, we are dealing with multiple hypersensitivities, with serotonin of course, but also with noradrenaline, as well as tryptamine, etc.

Finally, the blocking of hypersensitive receptors is perhaps not the only therapeutic way. We can imagine giving agonist substances in chronic treatment, in minimal doses and over a period of time, thus re-establishing a sufficient quantity of mediators in the synaptic gap, and eliminating post-synaptic hypersensitivity. Perhaps in this way we may understand the efficacy of dopaminergic agonists, bromocriptine, lisuride, noradrenergic (DHE), and serotoninergic (pretonin) in the chronic treatment of the disorder. Therefore we propose classifying drugs into those which mask hypersensitivity, of the neuroleptic type, and those which correct it, the dopaminergic agonists.

The development of dopaminergic hypersensitivity in one subject is, at best, one of the most interesting factors. Probably it is not always of the same importance. Numerous experimental facts have already revealed to what extent the responses of migraine patients vary to different stimulations, notably by the neuromediators, according to whether the subject is having an attack or is in a period of quietude. Longitudinal studies of hypersensitivity are of the greatest interest. On the other hand, the more we have manageable tests at our disposal, the more we can appreciate the modification of hypersensitivity attributable to one drug, and in consequence, define efficacy more objectively.

Summary

Migraineurs seem to have a dopaminergic hypersensitivity. This phenomenon was studied using the dopaminergic agonist piribedil. Given to such patients at a dose (0.1mg/kg) which had no effect in control subjects, it not only increased cerebral blood flow (CBF) but it also induced peripheral effects.

Various antidopaminergic drugs have been tested in an attempt to correct the dopaminergic hypersensitivity. The peripheral dopamine blocker domperidone did not prevent an increase of CBF but seemed to protect against induced nausea, vomiting and blood pressure decrease. Domperidone has been found by others to be useful in the treatment of migraine patients. A centrally acting substituted benzamide did similarly antagonise the emetic and hypotensive effects of piribedil. The clinical usefulness of a series of other drugs (haloperidol, sulpiride, metoclopramide, DHE) in migraine may also be related to their dopamine blocking properties. Paradoxically, some dopamine agonists (bromocriptine) have also given favourable results.

Clearly, much has still to be learned about dopaminergic hypersensitivity in migraineurs. Longitudinal studies of this hypersensitivity may be of the greatest interest in this respect.

References

1 Sicuteri F, Fanciullacci M, Del Bene E. Dopaminergic system and migraine. *Joint Meeting of the Italian and Scandinavian Headache Societies.* Florence. 1976: 41–42
2 Sicuteri F. Migraine, a central biochemical dysnociception. *Headache 1976; 16:* 145–159
3 Bès A, Géraud G, Guell A, Arne-Bès MC. Hypersensibilite dopaminergique dans la migraine: un test diagnostique? *La Nouvelle Presse Medicale 1982; 11,19:* 1475–1478
4 Fanciullacci M, Franchi G, Sicuteri F. Ergotamine and methysergide as serotonine partial agonist. *Headache 1976; 16:* 226–231
5 Sicuteri F. Dopamine, the second putative protagonist in headache. *Headache 1977; 17:* 129–131
6 Fanciullacci M, Michelacci S, Curradi C, Sicuteri F. Hyper-responsiveness of migraine patients to the hypotensive action of bromocriptine. *Headache 1980; 20:* 99–102
7 Del Bianco PL, Franchi G, Anselmi B, Sicuteri F. Monoamine sensitivity of smooth muscle in vivo in nociception disorders. *Adv Neurol 1982; 33:* 391–398
8 McCulloch J, Edvinsson L. Cerebral circulatory and metabolic effects of piribedil. *Eur J Pharmacol 1980; 66:* 327–337
9 Guell A, Géraud G, Jauzac P et al. Effects of a dopaminergic agonist (piribedil) on cerebral blood flow in man. *J Cereb Blood Flow Metabol 1982; 2:* 255–257
10 Bès A, Guell A, Victor G et al. Effects of a dopaminergic agonist on CBF in migraine patients. In Heistad DH, Marcus ML, eds. *CBF: Effects of Nerves and Neurotransmitters.* New York: Elsevier Biomedical. 1982: 163–168
11 Géraud G, Bès A, Courtade M et al. Interet du test au piribedil dans le diagnostic de migraine. A propos de 150 cas. *Rev Neurol (Paris) 1983; 139:* 215–218
12 Agid Y, Pollak P, Bonnet AM et al. Bromocriptine associated with a peripheral dopamine blocking agent in the treatment of Parkinson's disease. *Lancet 1979; i:* 570–572
13 Quinn N, Illas A, Lhermitte F, Agid Y. Bromocriptine in Parkinson's disease. A study of cardiovascular effects. *J Neurol Neurosurg Psych 1981; 44:* 426–429
14 Friedman AP. Migraine. *Med Clin North Am 1978; 62:* 481–494
15 Waelkens J. Domperidone in the prevention of complete classical migraine. *Br Med J 1982; 284:* 144
16 Amery WK, Waelkens J. Prevention of the last chance: an alternative pharmacologic treatment of migraine. *Headache 1983; 23:* 37–38
17 Lechin F, Van Der Dijs B, Lechin E et al. The dopaminergic and noradrenergic blockades: a new treatment for headache. *Headache 1978; 18:* 69–74
18 Alander T, Anden NE, Grabowska-Anden M. Metoclopramide and sulpiride as selective blocking agents of pre and postsynaptic dopamine receptors. *Naunyn Schmiedeberg's Arch Pharmacol 1980; 312:* 145–150
19 Horowski R. Some aspects of the dopaminergic action of ergot derivatives and their role in the treatment of migraine. *Adv Neurol 1982; 33:* 325–334
20 Hockaday JM, Peet KMS, Hockaday TDR. Bromocriptine in migraine. *Headache 1976; 16:* 109–114
21 Dorow R, Horowski JM, Lusse KH, Graf KJ. Differences between acute and chronic effects of the potent dopaminergic agonist lisuride. *Sixth International Congress of Endocrinology,* Melbourne. Canberra: Union Offset Co. 1980: Abstract 873

16

MIGRAINE, ANTIMIGRAINE DRUGS AND TYRAMINE PRESSOR TEST

K Ghose

Effect of dietary tyramine in migraine

The association between migraine attacks and foods/drinks containing tyramine was first demonstrated by Hanington in a placebo controlled study [1]. Oral tyramine precipitated migraine attacks in patients with a history of dietary migraine [1]. Although some investigators were unable to confirm this observation [2], tyramine's role in the pathogenesis of migraine remained under consideration. Intravenous tyramine injection has been reported to induce attacks in migraine patients [3], and accentuation of the pre-existing electroencephalographic abnormalities in patients suffering from dietary migraine and migraine with epilepsy was observed following oral tyramine administration [4]. Harper and co-workers postulated a defect in the blood brain barrier of migraine patients, particularly those in whom an item of diet may trigger on an attack [5]. This defect is likely to make the cerebral circulation vulnerable to variations in circulatory levels of vasoactive substances [5]. Defective conjugation of tyramine due to an enzyme deficiency in some migraine patients has also been reported [6,7]. This would increase the duration of tyramine's pharmacological effect following oral ingestion. Dietary tyramine, therefore, probably plays a significant part in the genesis of migraine attacks in a subgroup of patients.

Role of endogenous tyramine in migraine

In addition to defective sulphate conjugation, migraine patients were observed to have low platelet monoamine oxidase (MAO) level [8,9]. Furthermore, a transitory decrease in platelet MAO activity during migraine attacks has also been reported [10]. The main metabolic pathways of tyramine are oxidative deamination and β-hydroxylation by the enzymes MAO and dopamine β-hydroxylase

(DBH) respectively [11]. Any decrease in the activity of MAO is likely to prolong tyramine's tissue half-life. In addition, with the possible deficiency of other catabolic routes, the conversion of tyramine to octopamine by the enzyme DBH would become more significant. Octopamine has the properties of a neurotransmitter in many invertebrates and in mammals, it appears to be a co-transmitter with NA [12]. Therefore, both endogenous tyramine and its metabolite octopamine, a putative neurotransmitter, could be responsible in producing migraine attacks in susceptible subjects. Increased circulating NA and tyramine during migraine attacks have been postulated [13]. Harper et al suggested that the blood brain barrier could be intact in non-dietary migraine patients, but release of monoamines (and prostaglandins) from the brain itself could account for the migraine attacks [5]. Tyramine, in addition to NA, releases other vasoactive substances such as 5-hydroxytryptamine (5-HT) [14] and increases the biosynthesis of prostaglandins [15]. In animal experiments, the concentration of striatal tyramine has been reported to be increased by drugs which reduce dopamine turnover, such as apomorphine and piribedil [16].

Possible mechanism(s) of tyramine-induced migraine

Tyramine is an indirectly acting sympathomimetic amine and produces its pharmacological effect by releasing intraneuronal NA [17]. The studies on the cardiovascular effects of tyramine in animals indicated that both cardiac (ionotropic) and peripheral vasoconstrictor responses of tyramine are involved in the systemic pressor effects [18]. Although transient increase in blood pressure (BP) was observed within one to three minutes of an intravenous injection of tyramine, the patients experienced migraine attacks usually between one to 36 hours after an injection [3]. This time lag raises the possibility of tyramine's indirect effect (other than mediated via NA) in the pathogenesis of migraine. As mentioned above, tyramine is rapidly metabolised by the enzymes MAO and DBH. A defective sulphate conjugation and low platelet MAO activity were observed in some patients [6,9]. Therefore, in these patients, the majority of tyramine is likely to be converted by DBH to octopamine, a putative neuro-transmitter. Unlike tyramine, octopamine tends to remain in the tissue for longer periods [12]. Its vasoconstrictor effect is similar to NA and may act alone or as a co-transmitter with the latter. The conversion of tyramine to octopamine can be blocked (or reduced) by disulfiram, a drug which inhibits the enzyme DBH [19] and increases adrenergic activity in man [20]. In a double blind crossover study, the incidence of migraine, and in particular post-tyramine attacks, were observed to be more during treatment with 400mg disulfiram daily for six days than during placebo treatment [21]. It is, there-fore, unlikely that octopamine plays any major role in the pathogenesis of migraine.

214

ASSESSMENTS

Tyramine as a pharmacological probe

In view of tyramine's possible role in the pathogenesis of migraine attacks, it is of paramount importance that this amine's pharmacological effect is studied in patients suffering from migraine. However, methodological problems limit such investigations in humans and only the peripheral effect has been studied in man [22]. Tyramine has a very short tissue and pharmacodynamic half life. NA (like other monoamines) is also rapidly metabolised by the enzyme catechol-O-methyl transferase (COMT) outside the cell and the mitochondrial MAO inside the cell [23]. However, the majority of the released NA is taken up actively by the nerve terminals to the storage site, as shown in Figure 1 [24]. Tyramine is also taken up actively by the same membrane pump which reaccumulates intraneuronal NA to the storage site (Figure 1). Therefore, tyramine's pharmacological effects will depend on (1) its uptake by the nerve terminals; (2) intraneuronal store of NA and its release to the synaptic cleft; (3) sensitivity of the

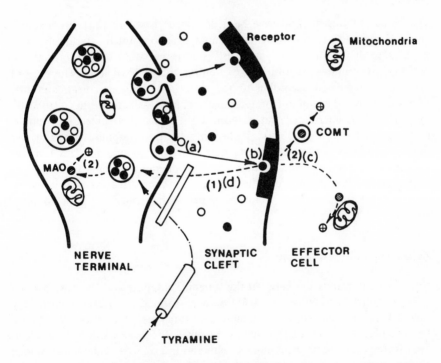

Figure 1. Schematic diagram of nerve terminal illustrating mechanism of tyramine's pharmacological action. (1) Uptake of tyramine by the nerve terminal, (a) release of NA, (b) interaction with the receptors. (2) (c) Extra neuronal metabolism. (2) Intraneuronal inactivation. (1) (d) Reuptake of released NA

215

α-adrenergic receptors, and (4) the activity of the various enzymes responsible for their metabolism [22,23]. In view of that, the effect of exogenously administered tyramine in migraine patients should be interpreted with caution and preferably be compared with drug free healthy control subjects matched for age and sex.

Tyramine has several pharmacological effects of which pressor response to intravenous injection, mydriasis following conjunctival instillation and local venoconstrictor effect during slow intravenous infusion were studied in man by the author [25]. The pressor response test was observed to produce reproducible and reliable information regarding a subject's peripheral adrenergic activity, and no significant morbidity was observed [22]. This method was used to study (1) the adrenergic activity of patients suffering from migraine; (2) the relationship between the migraine attacks and tyramine, and (3) the peripheral adrenergic interactions of various antimigraine drugs in man.

Determination of tyramine pressor test

The details of this method have been described elsewhere [25]. Briefly, tyramine is injected as short bolus intravenous injection, usually starting from an initial dose of 0.25mg. The systolic BP is measured at 30 second intervals for at least five minutes or until the BP returns to the basal level. The dose of tyramine is increased according to the systolic BP response. From the dose response curve, the amount of tyramine required to increase the systolic BP by 30mmHg is determined and is taken as an index of a subject's peripheral adrenergic activity [22]. Figure 2 illustrates the dose response curves in two migraine patients before and during treatment with indoramin. This test was performed in normal healthy volunteers and migraine patients in a series of investigations. Permission from the local ethical committee for each investigation and informed consent from the patients were obtained prior to these studies.

Tyramine pressor test in controls

No significant correlation between the tyramine response and age was observed [22], although an increase in MAO activity with age has been reported by others [26]. Female controls required less tyramine to increase systolic BP by 30mmHg than the male controls, matched for age as shown in Table I. That is, female subjects were more sensitive to intravenous tyramine. In animal studies, increased hepatic MAO activity in female rats following testosterone administration [27], and reduced MAO activity in male rats after castration [28] were reported. These observations in animals suggest the influence of sex hormones in adrenergic activity.

216

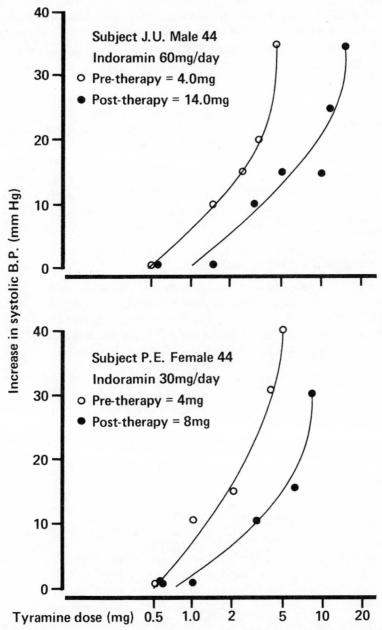

Figure 2. Tyramine dose pressor response curves in two migraine patients. The amount of tyramine required to increase the systolic BP by 30mmHg was (= tyramine sensitivity) determined from these curves. The shifts of the dose response curves to right indicate increased tyramine requirement, or decreased tyramine sensitivity during indoramin therapy

TABLE I. Tyramine pressor test in control subjects and migraine patients

	n	Age (years) Mean	SEM	Tyramine (mg) Mean	SEM
Male					
Controls	13	41.5	3.2	6.62	0.54
Patients	11	38.4	4.2	4.13†	0.47
Female					
Controls	23	37.1	2.9	5.22*	0.29
Patients	30	36.4	1.8	3.60†	0.34
All					
Controls	36	39.4	2.8	5.89	0.44
Patients	31	37.1	1.9	3.84†	0.23

* compared to male $p < 0.05$
† compared to controls $p < 0.05$

Tyramine pressor test and menstrual cycle

In order to study the effect of sex hormones on tyramine sensitivity, tyramine pressor test was performed at weekly intervals for four weeks in five premenopausal healthy drug-free subjects [29]. They required less tyramine during the premenstrual and menstrual periods (weeks four and one respectively) as compared to the mid cycle period (week three). This is illustrated in Figure 3. All

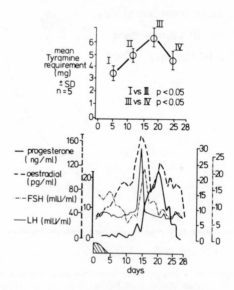

Figure 3. The relationship of tyramine sensitivity with menstrual cycle and female sex hormones (taken from Searle's diagnostic chart). Reproduced from *Br J Clin Pharmac* [29] by kind permission of the editor and co-author

218

the four females sex hormones are at peak during mid cycle (week three) as shown in Figure 3 (taken from Searle's diagnostic chart). Hence, it is difficult to comment which of these four hormones, if any, is responsible for this altered tyramine sensitivity. In a further double blind crossover study, tyramine sensitivity was determined in three postmenopausal patients with affective disorder. These patients were receiving prophylactic lithium therapy and their affective state was normal at the time of this study. They were selected randomly to receive either conjugated oestrogen (premarin) tablets (daily dose of 1.25mg) or matched placebo tablets first, and each treatment period lasted for six weeks (unpublished observation). The patients required more tyramine, that is, they were less sensitive to tyramine during oestrogen therapy. Variations in autonomic responsiveness during the different phases of the menstrual cycle have been considered in the past [30]. This investigation, although studied only in three subjects, indicates oestrogen's possible effect on the adrenergic system.

Tyramine pressor test in drug-free migraine patients

This was studied as a part of a double blind placebo controlled crossover study where the efficacy of a selective α-adrenergic receptor blocking drug in migraine was evaluated. Each treatment period lasted for four weeks and the pressor response test was performed on the 28th day of each phase. No other medication was prescribed. The results obtained during the drug-free period were compared with a group of drug-free healthy normal subjects, matched for age and sex, as shown in Table I. Both male and female patients suffering from migraine required less tyramine to increase the systolic BP by 30mmHg than the control subjects. In other words, migraine patients appear to be more sensitive to intravenous tyramine.

There could be several explanations. Firstly, consideration should be given to the possibility of an increased uptake of tyramine by the nerve terminals (Figure 1). Although no data are available regarding tyramine's uptake in migraine patients, several studies have demonstrated a reduced uptake of 5-HT by platelets in patients within a five day period after a migraine attack [31,32]. No difference between the control subjects and the migraine patients during the attack-free period, however, was observed by them. It is difficult to comment on whether a similar defect in tyramine's uptake by membrane pump exists in migraine sufferers. In any event, reduced uptake will decrease tyramine sensitivity. Therefore, increased uptake is unlikely to be a possible explanation.

Secondly, increased circulating NA and tyramine during a migraine attack has been postulated in the past [13]. Hsu et al measured the plasma NA concentrations in migraine patients suffering from night attacks [33]. Plasma NA levels were observed to be significantly higher in the three hour period preceding a migraine attack, not only in the corresponding period when the same subject did not wake with migraine, but also in the similar three hour period in those waking without migraine. It is possible that there is increased release of NA following tyramine injection in migraine patients.

Thirdly, α-adrenergic receptors may be supersensitive in migraine patients [34,35], although direct evidence in support of this hypothesis is sparse.

Fourthly, since there is decreased platelet MAO activity in patients with migraine [7–9], the pharmacological effect of tyramine (and NA) will be prolonged or increased and the subjects will be more sensitive to tyramine.

Intravenous tyramine pressor sensitivity has also been studied by Sandler et al who were unable to observe any difference between the migraine patients and control subjects [36]. Tyramine is well known for its tachyphylactic property [37], and the amount of tyramine, during determination of a dose response curve should be prudently increased [22]. This could account for differences in observations between two investigators. Besides, tyramine sensitivity is known to be influenced by several drugs [25]. In Sandler et al's study, all prophylactic medication was discontinued only for 24 hours prior to the test, and it has also remained unclear whether any other medication for acute migraine attack was allowed on the day of the test [36].

Tyramine pressor test and migraine attacks

The association between tyramine and migraine attacks was studied by using tyramine pressor test [3]. The patients were asked to keep a record of their migraine attacks for 36 hours after a tyramine pressor response test. None of these patients experienced migraine attacks immediately after the injection and there appeared to be a time lag of between one and 36 hours. Migraine attacks, therefore, were divided into four grades. Grade 0 represented no attack within 36 hours of injection; Grades I and II indicated attacks during 25 to 36 hours and 13 to 24 hours respectively; Grade III comprised attacks occurring within 12 hours of injection. Forty-six per cent of patients experienced headache within 36 hours of injection [3]. In a further study, post-tyramine headache was observed to correlate with the total amount of tyramine injected [38]. However, no association was found between the occurrence of post-tyramine migraine and a history of dietary or premenstrual migraine. Similar incidence of post-tyramine migraine attacks was observed by other investigators [36].

Post-tyramine migraine and disulfiram

It is postulated that the delayed onset of post-tyramine headache is due to tyramine's indirect action and is probably related to one of its metabolites, such as octopamine. In order to study octopamine's role in the pathogenesis of migraine, a double blind crossover study was carried out in which eight patients with classical migraine received 400mg of disulfiram (an inhibitor of DBH) daily for six days or matched placebo tablets first. The alternative medication was given after a two weeks washout period. Tyramine pressor response test was performed on the sixth day of each treatment period. The patients experienced post-tyramine headache during both phases as shown in Figure 4 and Table II. Furthermore, the severity of post-tyramine migraine index correlated with the total amount of tyramine injected during both placebo (r=53) and disulfiram (r=73) treatments (Figure 4) [38]. Since the conversion of tyramine to octopamine was suppressed by inhibiting the enzyme DBH, it is highly unlikely that octopamine plays any significant role in the pathogenesis of migraine.

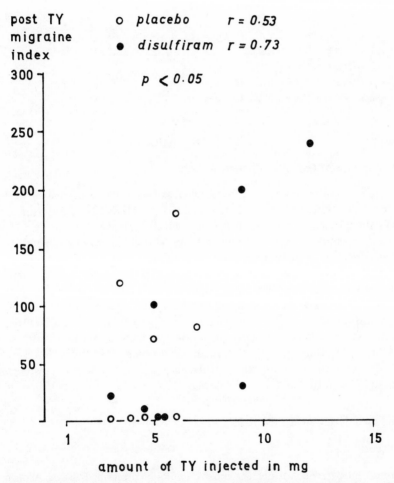

Figure 4. Correlation between post-tyramine migraine index and the total amount of tyramine injected to determine tyramine sensitivity during placebo/disulfiram medication. Post-tyramine migraine index = severity of attack (4 point scale) x duration in hours x grade [3,38]

TABLE II. Tyramine pressor test and post-tyramine migraine attacks

Group	n	Incidence		*Grade			Reference
		n	%	III	II	I	
Placebo	13	6	46	5	2	–	[3]
Indoramin	13	1	8	–	–	1	
Placebo	4	3	75	2	1	–	[38]
Propranolol	4	1	25	–	1	–	
Placebo	8	5	63	5	–	–	[38]
Disulfiram	8	6	75	4	1	1	

* Grade III = attacks within 12 hours
  Grade II = attacks between 13–24 hours
  Grade I = attacks between 25–36 hours

EFFECT OF DRUGS

Tyramine pressor test and antimigraine drugs

If migraine attacks are related to sudden excessive transient release of NA and/or supersensitivity of the adrenergic receptors [13,33–35,39], this condition should ideally be treated by drugs which antagonise adrenergic activity in man. Tyramine pressor response test can be used to assess a subject's peripheral adrenergic activity and its interactions with drugs [22]. In addition, as discussed above, intravenous tyramine injections can precipitate a migraine attack in a susceptible subject [3,36,38]. Tyramine pressor sensitivity test, therefore, can be used as a pharmacological challenge before and during a prophylactic drug therapy in migraine patients in order to evaluate its efficacy [3,38]. At present, several drugs claimed to possess antimigraine effects are available [40]. Unfortunately, information regarding these drugs' interactions with tyramine, both in animals and humans, is rather deficient. This is summarised in Table III and discussed below.

Drugs used during an acute attack

Analgesics

Aspirin and paracetamol are the most commonly prescribed drugs. Aspirin is known to possess antiplatelet agglutination properties, and probably also has prophylactic activity in migraine [41]. In the therapeutic dose, they probably do not interact with tyramine.

222

TABLE III. Summary of the interactions between antimigraine drugs and tyramine (Ty)

Drug	Interaction/comment	Source
Aspirin	Possibly no interaction	Postulation
Metoclopramide	? weak α-adrenoceptor blocking effect	Postulation
Domperidone	Probably decreases Ty sensitivity	Postulation
Methysergide	Effect on several autocoids	Ref 48
	Possibly will interact	Postulation
Clonidine	α-adrenoceptor blockers	
Indoramin	Decreases Ty sensitivity (indoramin)	Ref 3
	Reduction in post-Ty migraine	Ref 3
Propranolol	No interaction observed	Ref 38
	Reduction in post-Ty migraine	Ref 38
Pizotifen	Structural similarity to tricyclic antidepressants	Ref 52
	Probably decreases Ty sensitivity	Postulation
Amitriptyline	Decreases Ty sensitivity	Ref 22
Lithium salts	No interaction	
	(Increases amine uptake and blocks α-receptors)	Refs 22,54
Flunarizine	Inhibits vasoconstriction	Ref 56
	Probably decreases Ty sensitivity	Postulation

Dopamine antagonists

These drugs, such as metoclopramide, were initially prescribed to reduce nausea [42,43], but are now known to enhance the absorption and effectiveness of oral aspirin [43]. Domperidone, another dopamine antagonist, in addition to controlling nausea and vomiting during an acute attack [44], is also observed to have a prophylactic effect in classical migraine [45]. Most drugs in this group possess weak α-adrenergic receptor blocking activity and hence are likely to alter tyramine sensitivity [22]. Domperidone has been shown to have no significant effect on peripheral β-adrenoceptors [46], but its effect on α-adrenoceptors remains unclear.

Ergotamine/dihydroergotamine

Drugs in this group are also prescribed for both acute attacks and prophylaxis. The influence of various ergot alkaloids on venous tone in man has been studied [47]. Their venoconstrictor effect was considered to be mainly due to α-adrenoceptor stimulation. Hence, these drugs are likely to potentiate tyramine's pressor effect.

223

Drugs used in prophylaxis

Methysergide

It is now prescribed less frequently in view of the risk of retroperitoneal and intrathoracic fibrosis. Methysergide was initially considered to be a 5-HT antagonist, but the mechanism of its antimigraine activity has remained unclear. It interacts with a variety of autocoids [48], and is likely to interact with tyramine.

α-adrenoceptor blockers

The beneficial effect of clonidine, an α-adrenoceptor blocker, in the prophylaxis of migraine is established [49]. This drug possesses a number of pharmacological effects on the adrenergic system and is likely to decrease tyramine sensitivity. This has been demonstrated in relation to another selective α-adrenoceptor blocking drug, indoramin. Not only a dose related decreased tyramine sensitivity was observed during indoramin therapy, but also the incidence of post-tyramine headache was reduced from 46 per cent to eight per cent during this treatment [3].

β-adrenoceptor blockers

These are considered to be effective prophylactic drugs [50,51]. Although propranolol produced no significant effect on tyramine pressor sensitivity, the incidence of post-tyramine migraine was significantly reduced during this treatment [38].

Pizotifen

It is a 5-HT receptor blocker and observed to be effective in migraine prophylaxis [52]. Pizotifen, structurally, is a tricyclic compound similar to cyproheptadine and tricyclic antidepressant drugs, and shares many common pharmacological properties with them. It probably possesses α-adrenoceptor blocking and uptake blocking activities and is likely to decrease tyramine sensitivity. However, no experimental data is available to confirm this interaction.

Tricyclic antidepressants

Amitriptyline has been reported to be beneficial in reducing the frequency and severity of migraine attacks [53]. Other drugs in this group will probably be equally effective (or ineffective). These drugs have several effects on the adrenergic system and have been shown to decrease tyramine sensitivity in man [25].

224

Lithium salts

This drug's efficacy in cluster headache is now established but its beneficial effect in the prophylaxis of other types of migraine remains doubtful (personal observation). Lithium possesses a weak α-adrenoceptor blocking activity, but no significant change in tyramine sensitivity has been observed [22,53]. Lithium therapy is known to be associated with increased platelet monoamine uptake [54]. This increased amine uptake is probably responsible for normal tyramine response in the presence of α-adrenergic blockade during lithium therapy.

Flunarizine

It is considered to be an effective antimigrainous drug [55]. Flunarizine selectively inhibits vasoconstriction by decreasing the cell membrane permeability for calcium ions and probably will influence the tyramine sensitivity.

Drugs inducing migraine attacks

Phenelzine

This drug has been reported to be beneficial in migraine patients [56]. It is an MAO inhibitor and obviously increases sympathetic activity. Pharmacologically, putative antimigraine activity of any MAO inhibitor drug is difficult to reconcile with the autonomic theory of migraine. These drugs are known to produce hypertensive crisis and other complications following ingestion of food containing tyramine and, therefore, should be avoided in migraine patients.

Disulfiram

This is an inhibitor of DBH and increases the adrenergic activity in man [20] and indeed has been shown to increase the incidence of migraine attacks during disulfiram medication [38]. Although no significant change in tyramine sensitivity was observed, the post-tyramine headaches were increased during this therapy (Table II).

Oral contraceptives

Increased frequency and severity of migraine attacks are known to occur in patients receiving oral contraceptives with high progesterone content. The attacks appeared to be less in combination preparations with relatively larger doses of oestrogen [57]. In an unpublished study, oestrogen therapy was observed to be associated with decreased tyramine sensitivity.

Summary and concluding discussion

Increased autonomic activity is considered to be an aetiological factor in the genesis of migraine attack [39]. Although some investigators were unable to demonstrate any relationship between the migraine attacks and tyramine, there appears to be an association between them [1,3,21,36]. Tyramine releases intraneuronal NA, and increased circulating NA during migraine attacks has been reported by a group of investigators [33]. Furthermore, low platelet MAO activity [9] indicates an increase or prolongation of the pharmacological effects of NA and tyramine. Octopamine does not seem to play any significant role in the pathogenesis of migraine [38].

Tyramine pressor response test is a reliable technique for assessing peripheral adrenergic activity in man [22]. Migraine patients were more sensitive to this test as compared to the matched drug-free controls [3]. This indicates increased adrenergic activity. Similar observations were made in depressed patients [58]. An association between migraine and depression has been postulated [59], but there is as yet no conclusive evidence of a direct relationship between these two conditions.

Female subjects (both controls and patients) were observed to be more sensitive to tyramine pressor test [3], and this sensitivity appears to be greater during the premenstrual and menstrual periods [29]. Migraine attacks are known to be more frequent and severe during perimenstrual periods in some patients. These observations indicate the influence of female sex hormones on migraine attacks. Migraine attacks usually start at puberty, and the patients may feel better during pregnancy [40]. Oral contraceptives are known to increase the severity and frequency of migraine attacks [40,57]. Although high oestrogen content pills have been considered to increase migraine attacks by some, the incidence appears to be more with combination preparations containing higher progesterone contents and to be less in progestogenic pills containing higher doses of oestrogen [57]. Endometrial MAO activity after ovulation or during oral contraceptive administration has been reported to be increased [57,60]. This will lead into decreased tyramine sensitivity, as has been observed during week three (Figure 3) of a menstrual cycle [29], and during oral oestrogen therapy (unpublished personal observation). It is possible oestrogen decreases adrenergic activity in man.

Tyramine pressor test can be used to assess adrenergic interactions of drugs in man [22]. Furthermore, this test can also be used as a pharmacological challenge to evaluate efficacy of an antimigraine drug [3,38]. The incidence of post-tyramine migraine was observed to be reduced from 46 per cent to eight per cent and from 75 per cent to 25 per cent during treatment with a selective α-adrenergic blocking (indoramin) and a β-adrenoceptor blocking (propranolol) drug respectively. Since it is difficult to assess severity of migraine objectively [51], a pharmacological challenge like tyramine pressor test, undoubtedly will provide valuable information regarding a drug's efficacy in migraine.

References

1   Hanington E. Preliminary report on tyramine headache. *Br Med J 1967; 1:* 550–551
2   Ryan RE. A clinical study of tyramine as an etiological factor in migraine. *Headache 1974; 14:* 43–48
3   Ghose K, Coppen A, Carroll D. Intravenous tyramine response in migraine before and during treatment with indoramin. *Br Med J 1977; 1:* 1191–1193
4   Scott DF, Moffett A, Swash M. Observations on the relation of migraine and epilepsy. An electroencephalographic, psychological and clinical study using oral tyramine. *Epilepsia 1972; 13:* 365–375
5   Harper AM, MacKenzie ET, McCulloch J, Pickard JD. Migraine and the blood brain barrier. *Lancet 1977; i:* 1034–1036
6   Youdim MBH, Bonham Carter S, Sandler M et al. Conjugation defect in tyramine sensitive migraine. *Nature 1971; 230:* 127–128
7   Smith I, Kellow AH, Mullen PE, Hanington E. Dietary migraine and tyramine metabolism. *Nature 1971; 230:* 246–248
8   Sandler M, Youdim MBH, Hanington E. A phenylethylamine oxidising defect in migraine. *Nature 1974; 250:* 335–337
9   Glover V, Littlewood J, Sandler M et al. Why is platelet monoamine oxidase activity low in some headache patients? In Rose FC, ed. *Advances in Migraine Research and Therapy.* New York: Raven Press. 1982: 127–132
10 Glover V, Sandler M, Grant E et al. Transitory decrease in platelet monoamine oxidase activity during migraine attacks. *Lancet 1977; i:* 391–393
11 Carlsson A, Waldeck B. Beta-hydroxylation of tyramine in vivo. *Acta Pharmacol et Toxicol (Kobenhaven) 1963; 20:* 371–374
12 Axelard J, Saavedra JM. Octopamine. *Nature 1977; 265:* 501–504
13 Espin Herrero J, Bracia Marino C. Aspectos pathogenicos de la jaqueca. *Med Esp 1974; 71:* 65–77
14 Trendelenburg U. Classification of sympathomimetic amines. In Blaschko H, Muscholl E, eds. *Catecholamines Handb exp Pharmac 1972; 33:* 336–362
15 Collier HOJ, McDonald-Gibson HJ, Saeed SA. Stimulation of prostaglandin biosynthesis by capsaicin, ethanol and tyramine. *Lancet 1975; i:* 702
16 Juorio AV. Drug induced changes in the formation, storage and metabolism of tyramine in the mouse. *Br J Pharmac 1979; 66:* 377–384
17 Burn JH, Rand MJ. The action of sympathomimetic amines in animals treated with reserpine. *J Physol (Lond) 1958; 144:* 314–316
18 Harakal C, Sevy RW, Rusy BF. Haemodynamic effect of tyramine. *J Pharmac Exp Therap 1964; 144:* 89–96
19 Haley TJ. Disulfiram (tetraethylthioperoxydicarbonic diamide): a reappraisal of its toxicity and therapeutic application. *Drug Metabolism Reviews 1979; 9:* 319–335
20 Rogers WK, Benowitz NL, Wilson KM, Abbott JA. Effect of disulfiram on adrenergic function. *Clin Pharmacol Therap 1979; 25:* 469–477
21 Ghose K, Carroll JD. *Migraine and Monoamines: Disulfiram as Pharmacological Probe. Proceedings of Scandinavian Migraine Society.* Rφros, Norway. 1981: May 31 – June 2
22 Ghose K. Assessment of peripheral adrenergic activity and its interaction with drugs in man. *Europ J Clin Pharmacol 1980; 17:* 233–238
23 Kopin IJ, Gordon EK. Metabolism of administered and drug-released norepinephrine – 7-H3 in rat. *J Pharmac Exp Therap 1963; 140:* 207–216
24 Whitby LG, Axelrod J, Weil-Malherbe H. The fate of H3-norepinephrine in animals. *J Pharmac Exp Therap 1961; 132:* 193–201
25 Ghose K. Biochemical assessment of antidepressive drugs. *Br J Clin Pharmac 1980; 10:* 539–550
26 Robinson DS, Davis JM, Nies A et al. Relation of sex and aging to monoamine oxidase activity of human brain, plasma and platelets. *Arch Gen Psychiat 1971; 24:* 536–539

27   Wurtman RJ, Axelrod J. Sex steroids, cardiac ^{3}H-norepinephrine and tissue mono-amine oxidase levels in the rat. *Biochem Pharmac 1963; 12:* 1417–1419
28   Gaziri LCJ, Ladosky W. Monoamine oxidase variation during sexual differentiation. *Neuroendocrinology 1973; 12:* 249–256
29   Ghose K, Turner P. The menstrual cycle and the tyramine pressor response test. *Br J Clin Pharmac 1977; 4:* 500–502
30   Little BC, Zahn TP. Changes in mood and autonomic functioning during the menstrual cycle. *Psychobiology 1974; 2:* 579–590
31   Coppen A, Swade C, Wood K, Carroll JD. Platelet 5HT accumulation and migraine. *Lancet 1979; ii:* 914
32   Malmgreen R, Olsson P, Tornling G, Unge G. Migraine: a platelet disorder. *Lancet 1979; ii:* 1198
33   Hsu LKG, Crisp AH, Kalucy RS et al. Early morning migraine. Nocturnal plasma levels of catecholamines, tryptophan, glucose and free fatty acids, and sleep encepha-lographs. *Lancet 1977; i:* 447–450
34   Sicuteri F. Vasoneuroactive substances and their implication in vascular pain. *Research and Clinical Studies in Headache 1967; 1:* 6–10
35   Bès A, Guell A, Victor G et al. Effects of a dopaminergic agonist (piribedil) on CBF in migraine patients. *J Cerebral Blood Flow and Metabolism 1981; 1:* S519–S520
36   Sandler M, Peatfield R, Glover V, Littlewood J. Tyramine response and platelet monoamine oxidase activity in migraine. In Rose FC, ed. *Advances in Migraine Research and Therapy.* New York: Raven Press. 1982: 133–138
37   Day MD, Rand MJ. Tachyphylaxis in some sympathomimetic amines in relation to monoamine oxidase. *Br J Pharmac 1963; 21:* 84–96
38   Ghose K, Carroll JD. The role of tyramine and dopamine in the pathogenesis of migraine: disulfiram as pharmacological probe. In preparation
39   Johnson ES. A basis for migraine therapy – the autonomic theory reappraised. *Postgrad Med J 1978; 54:* 231–242
40   Management of migraine. *Drug and Therapeutics Bulletin 1981; 19:* 69–72
41   Deshmukh SV, Meyer JS. Cyclic changes in platelet dynamics and the pathogenesis and prophylaxis of migraine. *Headache 1977; 17:* 101–108
42   Tfelt-Hansen P, Olesen J, Aebelholt-Krabbe A et al. A double blind study of meto-clopramide in the treatment of migraine attacks. *J Neurol Neurosurg Psychiat 1980; 43:* 369–371
43   Wainscott G, Kaspi T, Volans GN. The influence of thiethylpenazine on the absorption of effervescent aspirin in migraine. *Br J Clin Pharmac 1976; 3:* 1015–1021
44   Jacques N, Lambrecht A, Schiettekatte L, Waelkens J. Treatment of nausea and vomiting during migraine attacks with intravenous domperidone. *Postgrad Med J 1979; 55 (Suppl 1):* 51–54
45   Waelkens J. Domperidone in the prevention of complete classical migraine. *Br Med J 1982; 284:* 944
46   Brogden RN, Carmine AA, Heel RC et al. Domperidone: a review. *Drugs 1982; 24:* 360–400
47   Aellig WH. Studies on the venoconstrictor effect of ergot compounds on man. *Triangle 1975; 14:* 39–46
48   Douglas WW. Autocoids. In Goodman LS, Gilman A, eds. *The Pharmacological Basis of Therapeutics, Fifth Edition.* New York: Macmillan Publishing Co Inc. 1975: 589–629
49   Shafar J, Tallett ER, Knowlson PA. Evaluation of clonidine in prophylaxis of migraine. Double-blind trial and follow-up. *Lancet 1972; i:* 403–407
50   Stensrud P, Sjaastad O. Comparative trial of tenormin (Atenolol) and Inderal (pro-pranolol) in migraine. *Headache 1980; 20:* 204–207
51   Weerasuriya K, Patel L, Turner P. α-adrenoceptor blockade and migraine. *Cephalagia 1982; 2:* 33–45
52   Lawrence ER, Hossain M, Littlestone W. Sanomigran for migraine prophylaxis; controlled multicentral trial in general practice. *Headache 1977; 17:* 109–112

53   Fann WE, Davis JM, Janowsky DS et al. Effect of antidepressant and antimanic drugs on amine uptake in man. *J Nerv Ment Dis 1974; 158:* 361–368

54   Murphy DL, Colburn RW, Davis JM, Bunney WE. Stimulation by lithium of mono-amine uptake in human platelets. *Life Sci 1969; 8:* 1187–1193

55   Amery WK, Wauquier A, Van Nueten JM et al. The antimigrainous pharmacology of flunarizine (R14950), a calcium antagonist. *Drugs Exptl Clin Res 1981; 7:* 1–10

56   Anthony M, Lance JW. Monoamine inhibition in the treatment of migraine. *Headache 1969; 21:* 263–268

57   Grant ECG. The influence of hormones on headache and mood in women. *Hemicrania 1975; 6:* 2–10

58   Ghose K, Turner P, Coppen A. Intravenous tyramine pressor response in depression. *Lancet 1975; i:* 1317–1318

59   Cough JR, Ziegler DK, Hassanien RS. Evaluation of the relationship between migraine headache and depression. *Headache 1975; 15:* 41–50

60   Southgate J, Grant ECG, Pollard W et al. Cyclic variations in endometrial monoamine oxidase: correlation of histochemical and quantitative biochemical assays. *Biochem Pharmac 1968; 17:* 721–723

229

17

ANTIMIGRAINE DRUGS AND VESTIBULAR FUNCTION

W J Oosterveld, L I Caers

Introduction

Migraine and vertigo seem to have close ties. Neurologists have long recognised that migraine may start with vertigo or dizziness, and several studies have shown an association between the two [1,2]. In addition, several recent reports have described the presence of vestibular dysfunction in migraine sufferers, vestibular disturbances being more frequent in such patients than in healthy subjects [3,4]. Most migraineurs actually appear to show abnormalities in their vestibular function [5–8]. Furthermore, a lot of migraine sufferers have been very susceptible to motion sickness in childhood [9]. Conversely, a substantial fraction of migraine patients reportedly develop vertigo later in their life [10]. The ties between migraine and vertigo are not perfect, however, since EEG readings are usually normal in patients with vestibular disorders, whereas they are often abnormal in migraineurs. Finally, mention should be made of Hungerford's observation that, besides labyrinthine changes, ischaemia of the upper bulbar centres may also occur in migrainous subjects [11]. In addition, headache may occur in patients with vestibular problems and the relationship between headache and vertigo in patients suffering from Ménière's disease vertebro-basilar insufficiency and vertigo of childhood has already been emphasised in this context [5].

Cluster headaches and vertigo may even have closer ties. Attacks of vertigo frequently occur in so-called cluster fashion, in 'benign positional vertigo' as well as in typical and in atypical Ménière's disease [10]. Many authors have pointed to the striking similarities between the time pattern shown by the headache attacks in cluster patients and that shown by the vertigo in both benign positional vertigo and Ménière's disease. Even the duration of the remissions, which may last for months or years in Ménière's disease, are reminiscent of that found in cluster headache. Furthermore, the age groups of patients affected by Ménière's disease and those of cluster headache sufferers are quite similar [12,13].

In addition, both conditions are characterised by unilateral involvement. Gilbert [12] assumes the presence of similar mechanisms of vasodilatation in both diseases, involving the region of the orbit in one case and the region of the inner ear in the other case. Vasodilatation in cluster headache produces pain and excessive secretions in the involved areas, whereas in Ménière's disease the excessive secretion results in the assumed state of 'endolymphatic hydrops'. Both conditions are a process of a recurrent paroxysmal focal dilatation.

Although vestibular abnormalities have been well documented in migraineurs, the relationship between migraine, cluster headache and vertigo remain poorly understood. Guidetti et al have recently stated that vestibular function tests could become important in the monitoring of drug treatment in headache sufferers [14]. It would seem, therefore, that time has come to start reviewing what is known about the vestibular activity of antimigraine drugs. That, then is the purpose of this paper.

SURVEY

Drugs for the abortive treatment of a migraine attack

Although ergotamine tartrate is probably the oldest drug used in the treatment of migraine, little is known up to now about its potential vestibular activity. Its pharmacological profile is very complex, however, both at the level of the CNS and at that of different smooth muscle cells [15]. It could thus well influence the processing of vestibular impulses. In two cases with benign recurrent vertigo, ergotamine in the treatment of an attack did not modify the characteristics of the attacks [16]. To our knowledge, no other reports have been published on the use of ergotamine in the treatment of vertigo attacks. This may be somewhat surprising in view of the similarity between Ménière's disease and cluster headache.

Drugs used in the prophylactic treatment of migraine

Drugs interfering with serotonergic receptors (Table I)

According to the results of Genco et al [17], serotonin receptor antagonism by methergoline, and to a lesser extent also by cyproheptadine, significantly decreases caloric nystagmus. This was shown in two groups of four normal volunteers treated orally with 8mg/day methergoline and 12mg/day cyproheptadine during four and five days respectively. Cyproheptadine, however, has both antihistamine and antiserotonin properties making this drug less reliable to evaluate the role of the serotonergic system on the labyrinth. Methergoline has been described to be effective in the prophylactic treatment of migraine,

231

TABLE I. Drugs interfering with serotonergic receptors and the labyrinthine system or vertigo

| Agent | Subjects | Findings | | Remarks | Ref. |
		ENG	Vertigo		
Methergoline	4 human volunteers (8mg/day over 4 days)	Duration ↓ Amplitude ↓	–	–	[16]
Cyproheptadine	4 human volunteers (12mg/day over 5 days)	Duration ↓ Amplitude ↓ in 2/4 men	–	Antihistamine component	[16]
Pizotifen	32 patients with recurrent vertigo 1mg t.i.d.	–	Complete relief in 23 patients Partial benefit in 3 patients	Antihistamine component	[18]
Methysergide	–	–	–	Dizziness as side effect	[17]

especially in children. In adults, it is less effective and poorly tolerated [18].

Other antiserotonin drugs like pizotifen and methysergide are widely used in the prophylaxis of migraine. The results with methergoline, discussed above, may suggest an inhibitory effect of such agents on an evoked nystagmus. Pizotifen also has an antihistaminic activity which is at least as pronounced as its antiserotonin effect.

Benham and Carlin [19] reported on 32 patients complaining of true vertigo as a main symptom of their migraine attacks. These patients were treated with pizotifen, 1mg, three times daily for six months to three years. Twenty-three patients had complete relief of the vertigo attacks and three obtained good to moderate benefit. In addition, difficulty in hearing during the attacks, as reported by two patients, was completely abolished by this treatment. Ten of 19 patients tested, were found to have vestibular abnormalities consisting of spontaneous nystagmus, positional nystagmus and abnormalities on caloric testing. In one patient, there was complete canal paresis. Follow-up vestibular testing was not performed.

Similar experiences with methysergide have not been reported. Possibly, this drug is not often prescribed for such patients since it may provoke dizziness itself.

Drugs interfering with the sympathetic nervous system

Clonidine is a central α-adrenergic agonist which reduces the peripheral vascular response to both vasoconstrictor and vasodilator substances. Its antimigraine

232

efficacy is well recognised [18]. Clonidine has been described by Vesternauge et al [20] to reduce the caloric response to a 30°C stimulus and to reduce the response to rotational stimulation in five healthy young volunteers orally treated with 0.3mg in a double-blind placebo-controlled trial. These authors attributed this effect to a rather doubtful 'unspecific' central sedation. Genco et al [17] reported a significant decrease of the duration, frequency and amplitude of a caloric evoked nystagmus, 15 minutes after the i.v. administration of 0.15mg clonidine.

Dizziness has been reported as a side effect of clonidine, but this is not necessarily due to an effect on the vestibular system, since it might as well be caused by orthostatic hypotension.

Beta-receptor antagonists

In some countries, propranolol has become a popular antimigraine drug. Apart from some individual cases, no information is available on the influence of this drug or of other β-blockers on the vestibular system or on vertigo.

In the patient population of Benham and Carlin [19], two patients with the poorly defined diagnosis 'recurrent vertigo', not responding to pizotifen, were successfully treated with propranolol, 40mg three times daily.

Calcium entry blockers

Calcium entry blockers are now under intensive investigation in the prophylactic treatment of migraine. Double-blind studies have been published for flunarizine, nimodipine, nifedipine and verapamil. Nifedipine and verapamil are calcium entry blockers used in cardiology and studies of these drugs in the prophylaxis of migraine are scarce [21, 22]. Recently, Gelmers [23] published a first study reporting the efficacy of nimodipine in migraine. Several studies on the prophylactic efficacy of flunarizine in migraine have been performed (for review, see [24]).

Except for flunarizine, there is hardly any information available on the effect of these drugs on the vestibular system or on vertigo. Hofferberth and Strelow (personal communication) [25] compared the labyrinthine effect of verapamil, nimodipine and flunarizine in rabbits. The frequency, the speed of the slow nystagmus component as well as the amplitude of the rotary induced nystagmus and the nystagmus after rotation, were inhibited by all three agents.

In eight of 10 patients with vertigo, due to vertebrobasilar insufficiency, treated with 40mg nimodipine, both the frequency and the speed of the slow nystagmus component were reduced. The total amplitude of the nystagmus, however, was increased.

We have investigated flunarizine rather extensively both with regard to its vestibular depressant action [26] and to its therapeutic action against vertigo [27, 28]. Flunarizine has been shown to be effective in various types of vertigo (for review, see [29]).

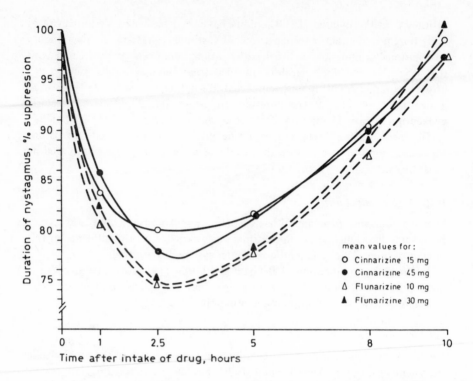

Figure 1. Course of vestibular depression by two dosages of cinnarizine and flunarizine with respect to time (human volunteers). From Oosterveld [26] with kind permission of S Karger AG, Basel

Flunarizine has a pronounced depressant action on the duration of the nystagmus in rabbits and in man (Figure 1). In humans, maximal depression occurs 2.5 hours after the intake of the drug (10mg) and this effect is associated with a decrease in the peak velocity of the slow nystagmus phase.

Why calcium entry blockers interfere with the labyrinthine system remains uncertain but it is known that calcium shifts play an important role within the vestibular system.

Drugs interfering with dopaminergic receptors

Several authors have ascribed an important role to dopamine in the pathogenesis of a migraine attack [30, 31]. Moreover, it has recently been shown [32] that a high dose of domperidone, a peripheral dopamine antagonist, can prevent a migraine attack if taken at the early appearance of premonitory signs, preceding the headache attack by six to 48 hours.

No significant effects of the dopamine agonists piribedil and bromocriptine and of the dopamine antagonist pimozide were found on the evoked nystagmus

234

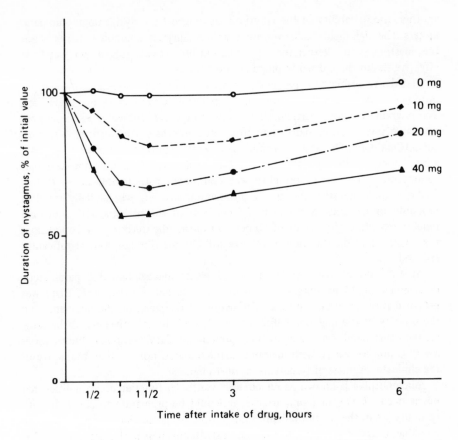

Figure 2.   Vestibular depression obtained in human volunteers with different doses of domperidone. From Oosterveld [33] with kind permission of S Karger AG, Basel

in human volunteers [17]. In our laboratory, however, a dose-dependent reduction of the duration of a rotation induced nystagmus in rabbits was shown after the administration of domperidone and results in human volunteers were similar (Figure 2) [33]. In contrast to flunarizine, the peak velocity of the slow nystagmus component was not influenced.

In addition, our (open) experience indicates that domperidone, administered by suppositories, 60mg four times daily, is effective in cutting off attacks of Ménière's disease, and this is my drug of choice nowadays.

Discussion and conclusions

This overview suggests that all agents, used in the prophylaxis of migraine and on which some vestibular research has been done, do reduce, in one way or another, the irritability of the labyrinth, as judged from nystagmographic parameters. The high incidence of vestibular abnormalities in migraine patients, raises the question as to whether there is a relationship between this property and the effectiveness of these drugs in migraine prophylaxis.

In order to evaluate the possible clinical significance of vestibular abnormalities in migraineurs, we started a study in co-operation with two migraine specialists. The migraine patients, participating in this study, were subjected to a complete vestibular investigation, before and after three months of treatment with flunarizine, 10mg daily. Our interim results, as recently reported by Ansink et al [34], are as follows: of 30 migraine patients, 27 were found to have at least one vestibular abnormality and this abnormality was considered pathological in 24 (80%).

After three months, the drug's antimigraine efficacy was globally rated as probably or certainly effective in 77 per cent of the patients with a median reduction of attack frequency of 50 per cent during the third month. In addition, the severity and the duration of attacks still coming through, were significantly reduced.

At the end of the treatment period electronystagmographic parameters, determined in 23 patients, had remained unchanged. Furthermore, there was no correlation between the total ENG-scores at the start, on the one hand, and the severity of the migraine before the study and the effectiveness of the drug, on the other hand. According to these preliminary data, vestibular abnormalities are thus not correlated with migraine characteristics, nor are they predictive of the clinical usefulness of flunarizine against migraine.

Since nothing is known about possible vestibular function abnormalities that might occur *during* migraine attacks, it would be premature to conclude with certainty that the vestibulodepressant action of prophylactic drugs, used in migraine, bears no relevance to their clinical effectiveness in this disease.

Information on the vestibular action of most antimigraine drugs is limited. The existing material, however, indicates that those antimigraine drugs which have been investigated in this respect, do seem to have a more or less pronounced depressant activity on the vestibular system. With the growing evidence of vestibular abnormalities in migraine patients, the possible role of the vestibular system in migraine, and as a consequence, the role of a vestibular depressant activity of antimigraine agents would seem to deserve further evaluation. Our preliminary study was a first step in this direction, but further research is warranted to clarify whether the vestibular abnormalities are a mere epiphenomenon or, to the contrary, play a genuine role in the pathogenesis of a migraine attack.

Summary

Migraine and cluster headache have close ties with vertigo. Migraine may start with vertigo or may manifest as vertigo, and a high incidence of vestibular abnormalities have been reported in migraine patients. An overview is given of what is known about the vestibular or the anti-vertigo activity of antimigraine drugs. Information is scarce, but all prophylactic drugs, that have been studied in this respect, seem to have a depressant effect on the labyrinth. Among these drugs are serotonin-antagonists, drugs interfering with sympathetic nervous system tonus, calcium entry blockers and dopamine antagonists. In preliminary findings no correlation was found between vestibular abnormalities and migraine characteristics, neither were such abnormalities predictive of the clinical usefulness of flunarizine, a drug used in migraine prophylaxis. At this very moment no judgement can be given whether the vestibular abnormalities are a mere epiphenomenon or, on the contrary, play an important role in the pathogenesis of a migraine attack.

References

1   Bickerstaff ER. Basilar artery migraine. *Lancet 1961; i:* 15−17
2   Fenichel GM. Migraine as a cause of benign paroxysmal vertigo of childhood. *J Paediatr 1967; 71:* 114−115
3   Dürsteler MR. Migraine und Vestibularapparat. *J Neurol 1975; 210:* 253−269
4   McCann J. Migraines may manifest as vertigo. *JAMA 1982; 247:* 956−957
5   Galetti G, Guidetti G, Bergamini G et al. La sofferenza dell'apparato vestibolare nel paziente cefalalgico. Considerazioni a proposito di osservaxioni ENG in 53 casi. *Acta Otorhinol Ital 1982; 2:* 245−263
6   Ansink BJJ, Danby M, Oosterveld WJ, Schimsheimer W. In press
7   Kuritzky A, Toglia UK, Thomas D. Vestibular function in migraine. *Headache 1981; 5:* 110−112
8   Fedorova ML. Vestibulares syndrom by migraine. *Klin Med (Mosk) 1970; 48:* 70−76
9   Pearce J. General review of some aetiological factors in migraine. In Cumings JN, ed. *Background to Migraine.* New York: Springer Verlag. 1971: 1−7
10   Behan PO, Carlin J. Benign recurrent vertigo. *Adv Migraine Res and Ther 1982; 49−55*
11   Hungerford GD, Du Boulay GH, Zilkha KJ. Computerized axial tomography in patients with severe migraine. *J Neurol Neurosurg Psychiatry 1976; 39:* 990−995
12   Gilbert GJ. Cluster headache and cluster vertigo. *Headache 1970; 9:* 195−200
13   Oosterveld WJ. Paroxysmal vertigo with and without cochlear symptoms. *Acta Otolaryngol 1983; 95:* 391−393
14   Guidetti G, Bergamini G, Pini LA. Neuro-otological abnormalities in headache sufferers. *Proceedings Symposium of the Migraine Trust (London) 1982*
15   Ral TW, Schliefer LS. Oxytocin, prostaglandins, ergot alkaloids and other agents. In Goodman, Gilman, eds. *The Pharmacological Basis of Therapeutics.* New York: MacMillan Publishing Co. 1980: 935−950
16   Moretti G, Manzoni G, Caffarra P, Parma M. "Benign recurrent vertigo" and its connection with migraine. *Headache 1980; 20:* 344−346
17   Genco S, Puca F, Specchio L et al. Nistagmo evocato nell'uomo: analisi farmacologica di alcuni neurotransmettitori. *Riunione di primavera di Ferrara, Maggio 1976:* 353−357
18   Diamond S, Medina JL. Review article: current thoughts on migraine. *Headache 1980; 20:* 208−212
19   Behan PO, Carlin J. Benign recurrent vertigo. In Rose FC, ed. *Advances in Migraine Research and Therapy.* New York: Raven Press. 1982: 49−54
20   Vesternauge S, Mansson A, Bande-Petersen F et al. Vestibular effects of water immersion and clonidine. *Physiologist 1981; 24 (Suppl):* S87−S88

21   Kahan A, Weber S Amor B et al. Nifedipine in the treatment of migraine in patients with Raynaud's phenomenon. *N Engl J Med 1983; 308:* 1102–1103

22   Solomon GD, Steel JG, Spaccavento LJ. Migraine prophylaxis with verapamil. A preliminary report. *Headache 1983; 23:* 139

23   Gelmers HJ. Nimodipine, a new calcium antagonist, in the prophylactic treatment of migraine. *Headache 1983; 23:* 106–109

24   Amery WK. Flunarizine, a calcium channel blocker: a new prophylactic drug in migraine. *Headache 1983; 23:* 70–74

25   Hofferberth B. Calcium entry blockers in the therapy of dizziness. *Angiology meeting Brussels-Antwerp, May 1982*

26   Oosterveld WJ. Vestibular pharmacology of flunarizine compared to that of cinnarizine. *ORL 1974; 36:* 157–164

27   Oosterveld WJ. Pilot evaluation of flunarizine (R 14950) in vertigo. A double-blind trial. *Can J Otolaryngol 1974; 3:* 284–290

28   Oosterveld WJ. Flunarizine in vertigo. A double-blind placebo-controlled cross-over evaluation of a constant-dose schedule. *ORL 1982; 44:* 72–80

29   Wouters L, Amery W, Towse G. Flunarizine in the treatment of vertigo. *J Laryngol Otol 1983; 97:* 697–704

30   Fanciullacci M, Michelacci S, Curradi C, Sicuteri F. Hyperresponsiveness of migraine patients to the hypertensive action of bromocriptine. *Headache 1980; 20:* 99–102

31   Bès A, Géraud G, Güell A, Arne-Bès MC. Hypersensibilité dopaminergique dans la migraine: un test diagnostique? *Nouv Presse Méd 1982; 11:* 1475–1478

32   Waelkens J. Domperidone in the prevention of complete classical migraine. *Br Med J 1982; 284:* 944

33   Oosterveld WJ. Vestibular pharmacology of domperidone in rabbits and man. *ORL 1981; 43:* 175–180

34   Ansink BJJ, Danby M, Oosterveld WJ, Schimsheimer W. The influence of the calcium entry blocker flunarizine on migraine and on the vestibular system in migraine patients. *12th Scandinavian Migraine Society Meeting, Hanasaari, June 1983*

18

PUPIL AND VEIN AS DETECTORS OF NEURONAL MECHANISMS OF ANTIMIGRAINE DRUGS

M Fanciullacci, M Boccuni, U Pietrini, G Gatto

Recent studies agree with the hypothesis that migraine is 'in primis' essentially a disease of the nervous system [1], mainly involving monoaminergic and peptidergic neurotransmission which regulate pain sensitivity and other functions affected by a migrainous attack [2–4]. However, the map and sequence of the neurotransmission disorder in the central and peripheral nervous system remains unknown. Apart from these pathogenetic mechanisms of migraine it remains a fact that a great number of pharmacological agents capable of improving migraine exert their fundamental pharmacological action at the neuroreceptor level.

Despite the great progress in the last decade in understanding their pharmacological properties through animal experiments, much remains unknown about the analgesic action of these drugs in migraine headache. The availability of simple and valid methods for studying their actions on the neuroeffector junction directly in vivo in man, may contribute to an understanding of the neuronal mechanism of the drugs used in migraine.

It is the purpose of this paper to summarise our findings regarding the effect of some antimigraine drugs on migrainous iris and hand vein, two neuromuscular junctions, which can currently be explored with appropriate techniques.

Patients

All experiments were carried out on hospitalised patients suffering from migraine, complaining of four to six disabling attacks per month. All subjects had been drug-free for seven days prior to the investigations. The purpose and procedure of the investigations were fully explained to all subjects and their consent was obtained. The patients were tested during headache-free periods or when they complained of only a moderate headache.

Pupillometric experiments

Electronic and photographic pupillometry

With an original pupillographic technique, previously fully described elsewhere [5], pupil diameter could be measured accurately, rapidly and with a good reproducibility. Briefly, the apparatus consisted of a television (TV) camera (with infra-red tube) equipped with a special optical apparatus that allowed for proper magnification of the subject's eye, a digital interface between the TV camera and microprocessor, and a TV monitor that gave visual control during examination of the pupil. A particular TV raster line crossed the pupil in correspondence to the transverse diameter. This line was measured by a microcomputer and the signal was recorded by a writing apparatus. The TV camera was mounted on a sliding rule, which rapidly permitted eye focus.

Photographic technique was obtained with a Polaroid close-up '5-Land Camera'. Brackets were situated on both sides of the lens in order to obtain an equal focal distance between the objective and the patient's eyes. These brackets were opaque, thus reducing the corneal highlight provoked by the annular flasher. A macrophoto of both pupils in the ratio of 1:1 were taken and pupil diameters were measured directly on the photographs by using a magnifying optic dispositive.

Ergotamine abuse and withdrawal

By electronic pupillographic technique the influence of ergotamine abuse on pupillary sympathetic function was studied in migrainous patients. The test was carried out by instilling in the right conjunctival sac one drop of tyramine, a norepinephrine (NE) releaser, and two days later one drop of phenylephrine, a direct α-adrenoceptor agonist.

Migrainous patients taking 0.125–2mg of ergotamine daily from 4–20 years were tested. The control group was migrainous patients treated only with mild analgesics. Ergotamine abusers were tested again a week after the abrupt withdrawal from ergotamine medication. The entire group experienced a rebound headache from ergotamine discontinuation.

When compared to migrainous patients not using ergotamine, all ergotamine abusers showed a marked mydriatic response to tyramine. On the contrary, responsiveness to phenylephrine was similar in both groups (Figure 1).

Seven days after ergotamine discontinuation, tyramine-induced mydriasis was markedly reduced while pupillary response to phenylephrine remained unchanged (Figure 2).

Flunarizine investigations

These investigations were carried out by using the photographic technique instead of the electronic pupillographic technique as the study was performed in a section

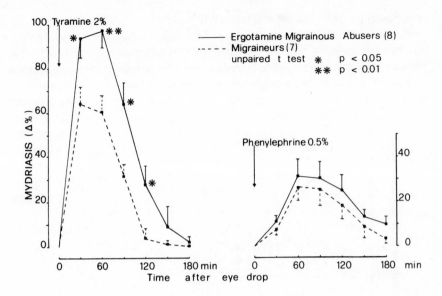

Figure 1. Increased norepinephrine release by topical tyramine in ergotamine migrainous
abusers by mydriatic responsiveness – no change in phenylephrine dilatation (n = 8)

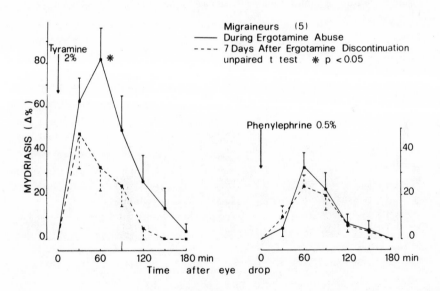

Figure 2. Decrease of norepinephrine release by topical tyramine after ergotamine discontinuation in migraine – no change in pupil dilatation from phenylephrine (n = 5)

241

of the hospital where the apparatus was not available.

One drop of tyramine was instilled into the right conjunctival sac of the three groups of migrainous patients. Baseline measurements were obtained 24 hours prior to the flunarizine administration. In the first group the tyramine test was repeated two hours after a single oral dose of flunarizine (10mg). No changes in pupil diameter nor in mydriatic response to tyramine was observed. The two

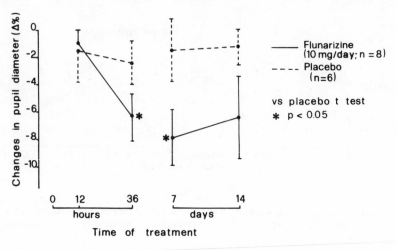

Figure 3. Decrease of pupil size during flunarizine treatment (10mg/day/14 days) in migraine

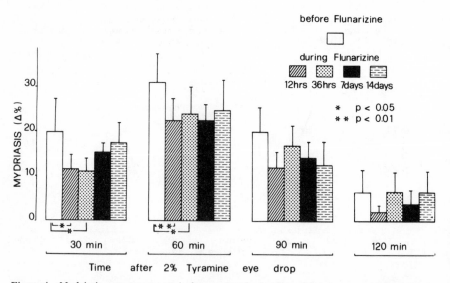

Figure 4. Mydriatic response to topical tyramine during flunarizine treatment (10mg/day/ 14 days) in eight migraine patients; 12 and 36 hours after the onset of treatment the tyramine response is reduced

242

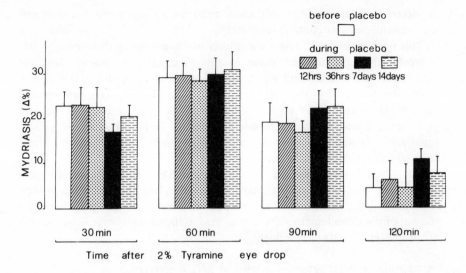

Figure 5. Unchanged mydriatic response to topical tyramine during a two week placebo treatment in six migraine patients

other groups were treated daily for two weeks with a placebo or with flunarizine (10mg) in a single administration at bedtime. The tyramine test was repeated at fixed intervals during management.

The flunarizine treated group differed from the placebo group by showing a transient reduction of pupil size during the first week of treatment with a tendency to return to pre-flunarizine pupil size at the end of the second week (Figure 3). In addition, flunarizine migrainous patients but not placebo patients showed a reduced mydriatic response after the first two doses of flunarizine (Figures 4 and 5).

Experiments with venotests

Venoconstriction and vein compliance tests

Venoconstriction and vein compliance tests represent the two main methods currently being used for studies with drugs acting on hand vein in vivo. Several years ago, the technique referred to as Venoconstriction Test was devised by Sicuteri et al [6] in order to test the action of serotonin (5-HT) on veins in man. Later it was combined with a computerised integrator [7]. The general principle was to obtain a pressure-time curve of a dorsal hand vein before and after local injection of a drug producing a venospasm. Through a needle orthodromically inserted into a superficial hand vein, drugs are administered directly into the vein and a pressure curve was obtained by means of a pressure transducer. Using an electronic integrator, the area under the pressure-time curve was measured and quantified in venoconstrictive units.

This method does not detect the effects of a venodilating drug directly, but indirectly through their inhibition of venoconstrictive substances. The vein compliance test was devised by Aellig [8] by modifying an original version where the venous diameter was determined optically [9]. This new method assesses the compliance of superficial hand veins by measuring venous diameter at a standardised congestion pressure (45mmHg). This method allows a direct registration of the effects of venoconstrictive or venodilating-acting drugs.

Essentially the device is composed of a linear variable differential transformer which is placed on the back of the hand by means of a small tripod. Its position is adjusted so that a light metal core placed in the central hole of the transformer is energised by an alternating current. The core placed over the summit of the vein alters the voltage generated in the counter coils: these changes are proportional to its displacement.

'Antiserotonin' drugs as partial agonists of 5-HT venous receptors

By using the venoconstriction test it was demonstrated for the first time in man that these antiserotonin drugs, such as methysergide, Org GC 94, ergotamine, used in migraine treatment, block the 5-HT venoconstrictor effect when administered in high doses and enhance it in low doses [10, 11]. Potentiation of venospasm was observed when the drugs were locally injected in an amount approximately similar to that obtained in plasma during therapeutic treatment.

In measuring compliance of superficial hand veins, a dose dependent reduction of venous diameter was observed after local infusion of pizotifen and methysergide [12, 13]. These results would be consistent with a partial agonist activity of these two antimigraine drugs as was previously observed with the venoconstriction test.

Propranolol blockade of venous β-adrenoceptors

By using the venoconstriction test it has been observed that propranolol, and its derivative INPEA, when given by infusion in the vein under study, potentiates the venoconstrictive effect of epinephrine, a β-receptor and α-receptor stimulant [14], thus verifying the existence of venodilating β-adrenoceptors in the human vein.

Flunarizine-induced venodilation

Migrainous volunteers received both 10mg of flunarizine orally and placebo with a three day interval between the two administrations. Placebo venous compliance remained unchanged for the entire period of observation. Flunarizine induced a venodilating effect reaching its maximum at two hours and then, though with wide individual variations, venous compliance decreased (Figure 6).

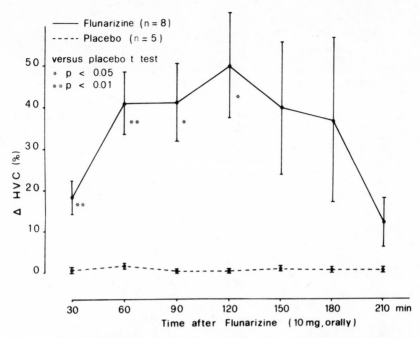

Figure 6. Increased venous compliance after a single oral dose (10mg) of flunarizine (n = number of migraine patients)

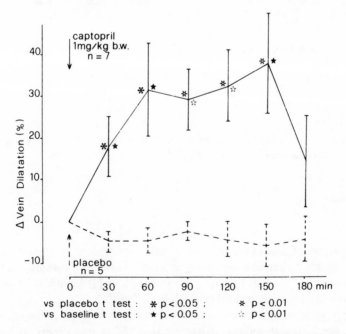

Figure 7. Increased venous compliance after a single oral dose of captopril. Each point represents the mean ± SEM of six migrainous patients; p versus pre-drug values

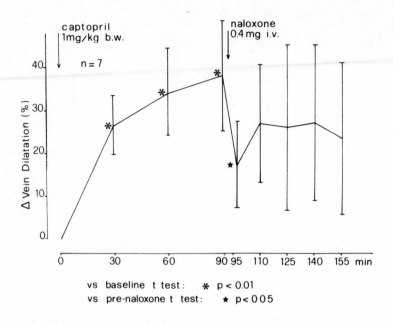

Figure 8.   Reversal of captopril-induced venodilation by naloxone. Mean ± SEM of six migrainous patients; p versus pre-captopril values

Naloxone-reversible venodilation by captopril

A group of migrainous volunteers received both a single oral dose of captopril (1mg/kg body weight) and placebo with a three day interval between the two administrations. Captopril increased venous compliance from 30–150 minutes after the drug ingestion, an effect not seen after placebo treatment (Figure 7). Naloxone (0.4mg), injected in the same vein, was able to reverse the captopril induced vein dilation (Figure 8) [15].

Discussion

Ergotamine

The symptomatic antimigraine compound, ergotamine, is known to affect monaminergic transmission by acting as a partial agonist of α-adrenoceptors and 5-HT receptors [16, 17], by inhibiting NE re-uptake [18] and also by exerting a dopaminergic action such as other ergot derivatives [19, 20].

Our pupillary findings demonstrate that chronic use of ergotamine accumulates NE in the neuronal endings thus increasing the responsiveness to tyramine. Tyramine, in fact, is taken up into the neurone by the monamine re-uptake pump and releases intraneuronal NE. The increased response to tyramine of the ergotamine abuser could be due either to an enhanced NE release, or to an iris α-adrenoceptor hypersensitivity, or even to an altered re-uptake mechanism. However, since the response to a low concentration of phenylephrine — a direct α-adrenoceptor agonist — is equal to that in a non-ergotamine abuser, a supersensitivity of post-synaptic receptors may be excluded, while an enhanced NE release is likely.

The NE storage in neuronal endings of ergotamine abusers might depend on a possible dopaminergic activity of the drug when consumed in high doses. Dopamine receptors located pre-synaptically on adrenergic terminals, inhibit NE release, thereby modulating neuronal function. Its protracted and intense activation by ergotamine abuse might render adrenergic neurone abnormally 'full' as was demonstrated by our pupillometric findings. Ergotamine withdrawal appears to decrease the intraneuronal NE content quite rapidly, thus establishing a responsiveness to tyramine equal to that of ergotamine-free migraine patients. In this respect, ergotamine might mimic the effect of endogenous opioids which also modulate pre-synaptic neuronal activity. Since poor endorphine neuronal modulation has been postulated as a mechanism of pain and other disturbances in a migraine attack [3, 4], the symptomatic effect of ergotamine might derive from the prompt but transitory correction of this impairment.

The discontinuation of ergotamine, therefore, may cause a deficient modulation which could provoke the well known post-ergotamine headache rebound [21−24]. The analgesic effect of ergotamine during a migraine attack may also depend on its action on brain serotonin receptors, which, when stimulated, inhibit central pain perception. In fact, the drug, at therapeutic doses, has a low concentration at the cellular sites, thus working as a 5-HT agonist, as results from our findings with venoconstriction test [10] confirm.

Flunarizine

Flunarizine has recently made its promising debut as a prophylactic agent in migraine treatment [25, 26].

The effects induced by flunarizine on both vein and pupil suggest a reduction of sympathetic function, which may be related to its calcium-channel blocking activity. Regarding the flunarizine-induced changes, some differences between vein and pupil responses must be noted. After a single dose, the venodilating effect corresponded to the phase of increasing concentration of the drug in plasma which occurs within two to four hours [27], while at the same time both pupil size and tyramine-induced mydriasis remained unchanged. However, since, 12 hours after the flunarizine administration, tyramine-induced mydriasis was considerably reduced, it is reasonable to infer that the drug exerts its pupillary action after peak plasma levels are achieved thereby acting on cellular sites. The decrease in pupil size occurred later than the reduction of pupillary

247

response to tyramine which likely indicates a latent adrenergic functional reduction. The pupillary effect of flunarizine disappears in several days possibly due to an adaptive mechanism.

The effectiveness of flunarizine in preventing a migraine attack is attributed to its protective action against cerebral vascular spasm and cellular damage from brain hypoxia [28, 29]. Our pupillary data suggest that Ca influx blockade may provoke other neurochemical events, not vascular in nature, which may contribute to its antimigraine action.

Our findings cannot determine if the effect obtained peripherally also reflects changes in brain centers regulating pupil and vein adrenergic neuromuscular junctions. However, it may indicate that flunarizine reduces the Ca dependent contraction of iris and vein smooth muscles, caused by the NE release induced respectively by tyramine instillation and venous congestive pressure. The possible relationship between our findings and the therapeutic action of the drug may be inferred considering that the data is compatible with a reduced response to endogenous NE during treatment. In this perspective the drug may prevent an exaggerated response to catecholaminergic stimulation probably due to a receptor supersensitivity, which seems to be an underlying mechanism of a migraine attack [30–32]. The adaptive phenomenon, which manifests itself shortly after flunarizine administration, does not seem to limit the therapeutic effect of the drug. On the contrary, the desired effect often begins several weeks after the onset of the therapy [25]. Therefore the significance of our findings in relationship to the clinical effect of the drug remain largely to be defined.

Antiserotonin drugs and β-blockers

Superficial hand vein experiments demonstrate a partial agonist activity on 5-HT receptors of antimigraine drugs of different chemical structures such as ergot compounds (ergotamine, methysergide, lisuride), pizotifen and Org GC 94. They exhibit an agonist action on 5-HT receptors in low doses corresponding to plasma therapeutic concentration, thus suggesting that the antimigraine activity, of so-called anti-5-HT receptors in low doses corresponding to plasma therapeutic concentration, thus suggesting that the antimigraine activity, of so-called anti-5-HT drugs, could paradoxically be correlated with an activation of brain 5-HT receptors which inhibit central pain perception [33]. This activation might be facilitated by the deficiency of brain 5-HT, as has been postulated in migraine [2]; in fact, the spontaneous or pharmacologically-induced deficiency of endogenous transmitter strongly sensitises its receptors to the agonistic activity of a partial agonist.

The mechanisms by which some β-blocking agents, propranolol in particular [34–36], are useful in antimigraine prophylaxis have not yet been defined. Our findings demonstrate the existence of β-adrenoceptors in the human vein and its block by propranolol treatment. Since β-receptors exert a venodilating action, propranolol may protect from this venodilating adrenergic stimulation which might contribute to the vasomotor phenomena of migraine attacks.

Captopril

Recently, it has been reported that captopril, an inhibitor of angiotensin converting enzyme and enkephalinase [37, 38], relieves migraine, suggesting that this agent should be the drug of choice in the therapy of migraine when it is associated with essential hypertension [39]. However, it is yet to be clarified whether migraine prophylactic activity is mediated by the endogenous opioid system or by other mechanisms. Naloxone reversible venodilation by captopril seems to support the former. In fact, the inhibition of endogenous opioid degradation by captopril may cause their increase in the human venous tissue where opiate receptors have been discovered [40]. Through activation of these receptors the release of NE into the synaptic cleft could be inhibited. The ability of naloxone to reverse captopril-induced venodilation is compatible with an involvement of an opioid mechanism. On the other hand, the implication of the angiotensin system in the venous effect of captopril has to be considered. Indeed, since angiotensin facilitates NE release, its inhibition might provoke a venodilation.

Final considerations

The neuroeffector junction is an apparatus implicated in a wide variety of functional human diseases such as idiopathic headaches, migraine included. The influence on neuronal junction of antimigraine drugs acquires a fundamental significance for explaining their analgesic effect on migraine. Information on the mode of action of these drugs on neuronal junction is often indirect, inadequate, and general. The main reason for that is the poor availability of suitable methods which permit its exploration with good reproducibility, patient safety and acceptability. Pupillometry and venotests, having these qualities, are sensitive detectors of the neurosynaptic and receptoral processes developed by agents used in migraine. In fact, these methods give underlying information on the influence on the synaptic transmission of the studied drugs used for migraine. Since healthy volunteers have not been investigated, it is not possible to conclude whether the observed effects are qualitatively or quantitatively peculiar to the migraine patients. Even if the exact mechanism by which these drugs improve migraine is still to be completely clear, the pupil and the vein represent two valuable indicators for a fuller understanding of the mode of action in neuroreceptor terms.

Summary

Photographic and electronic pupillometry and two venotests for measuring venoconstriction and venous compliance were used to determine the effects of various antimigraine drugs on iris and vein neuromuscular junctions in migraine patients.

Ergotamine abuse increased mydriatic response to topical tyramine, a nor-epinephrine releaser, but not to phenylephrine, an α-adrenoceptor stimulant. Thus, it may be assumed that in ergotamine abusers an accumulation of neuronal norepinephrine takes place and that this reloading may play a role in the anti-migraine effect of ergotamine.

Flunarizine, an antimigraine Ca blocker, increased vein compliance, and reduced pupil size, while also attenuating mydriatic response to topical tyramine. Due to a possible adaptive process, pupillary changes induced by flunarizine were transient. Pupillary data demonstrate that flunarizine influences not only the vascular but also other synaptic neurotransmissions which may participate in its therapeutic effectiveness, possibly by attenuating the aminergic hyper-reactivity, which seems characteristic of migraine attack. At therapeutic concentration ergot derivatives (ergotamine, methysergide, lisuride) and other migraine prophylactic agents (pizotifen, Org GC 94) demonstrated a 5-HT agonist activity, i.e. venoconstriction or a potentiation of the 5-HT-induced venoconstriction. These so-called anti-5-HT drugs could produce analgesic action during migraine by activating brain-stem 5-HT receptors involved in the antinociception process.

Propranolol blocks venodilating β-adrenoceptors, thus protecting veins from dilating stimuli which may contribute to migraine attacks.

Captopril, the inhibitor of angiotensin-converting-enzyme and possibly of enkephalinase, useful in treating migraine, provoked a reversible naloxone enhancement of venous compliance. This action may be due to an increase of opioid peptides at the venous level, which inhibit norepinephrine release, suggestive of the drugs ability to inhibit endogenous opioid degradation.

Together these observations confirm that antimigraine drugs markedly influence synaptic neurotransmission in migraine patients. These effects could play an important role in the improvement of migraine.

Acknowledgments

This work was supported by a grant for the study group 'Pain Control' of the finalised project 'Preventative Medicine' from the National Research Council of Rome (Italy).

References

1   Gardner-Medwin AR, Skelton JL. Leão's spreading depression: evidence supporting a role in the migraine aura. In Rose FC, Amery WK, eds. *Cerebral Hypoxia in the Pathogenesis of Migraine.* London: Pitman. 1982: 127–131
2   Sicuteri F, Anselmi B, Del Bianco PL. 5-Hydroxytryptamine, supersensitivity as a new theory of headache and central pain: A clinical pharmacological approach with p-chlorophenylalanine. *Psychopharmacology (Berlin) 1973; 29:* 347–356

3 Sicuteri F. Headache as the most common disease of the antinociceptive system: analogies with morphine abstinence. In Bonica JJ, Albe-Fessard D, eds. *Advances in Pain Research and Therapy Volume 3*. New York: Raven Press. 1979: 359

4 Sicuteri F, Del Bianco PL, Anselmi B. Morphine abstinence and serotonin super-sensitivity in man: analogies with the mechanism of migraine? *Psychopharmacology (Berlin) 1979; 65:* 205–209

5 Fanciullacci M, Pietrini U, Boccuni M. Disruption of iris adrenergic transmission as an index of poor endorphin modulation in headache. In Critchley M, Friedman AP, Gorini S, Sicuteri F, eds. *Advances in Neurology Volume 33*. New York: Raven Press. 1982: 365

6 Sicuteri F, Del Bianco PL, Fanciullacci M, Franchi G. Il test della venocostrizione per la misura della sensibilità alla 5-idrossitriptamina ed alle catecolamine nell'uomo. *Boll Soc Ital Biol Sper 1964; 40:* 1148–1150

7 Del Bianco PL, Sicuteri F. Computerised venospasm: a method for exploring the neurovascular junction in man. *J Pharmacol Meth 1978; 1:* 329–340

8 Aellig WH. A new technique for recording compliance of human hand veins. *Br J Clin Pharmacol 1981; 11:* 237–243

9 Nachev C, Collier JG, Robinson BF. Simplified method for measuring compliance of superficial veins. *Cardiovasc Res 1971; 5:* 147–156

10 Fanciullacci M, Franchi G, Sicuteri F. Ergotamine and methysergide as serotonin partial agonists in migraine. *Headache 1976; 16:* 185–188

11 Anselmi B, Del Bianco PL, de Vos CJ et al. Clinical and animal pharmacology of migraine: new perspectives. In Sicuteri F, Schonbaum E, eds. *Clinical Pharmacology of Serotonin. Monogr Neurol Sci Volume 3*. Basel: Karger. 1976: 45

12 Aellig WH. Clinical-Pharmacological experiments with pizotifen (Sanomigran) on superficial hand veins in man. In Greene R, ed. *Current Concepts in Migraine Research*. New York: Raven Press. 1978: 53

13 Aellig WH. Agonists and antagonists of 5-hydroxytryptamine on venomotor receptors. In Critchley M, Friedman AP, Gorini S, Sicuteri F, eds. *Advances in Neurology, Volume 33*. New York: Raven Press. 1981: 321

14 Sicuteri F, Fanciullacci M, Del Bianco PL. Alpha and beta adrenergic receptors in human vein; activity of a new beta blocking agent. *Med Pharmacol Exp 1966; 15:* 73–78

15 Fanciullacci M, Pietrini U, Salmon S, Spillantini MG. An approach to the mechanism of captopril analgesia in man. *International Work-shop on Degradation of Endogenous Opioid: Its Relevance in Human Pathology and Therapy. Abstract Book.* Rome: AISC. 1982: 27

16 Loew DM, Müller-Schweinitzer E. Alcaloides de l'ergot de seigle, recepteurs adrenergiques, serotoninergiques, et dopaminergiques. *J Pharmacol (Paris) 1979; 10:* 383–399

17 Müller-Schweinitzer E, Fanchamps A. Effect on arterial receptors of ergot derivatives used in migraine. In Critchley M, Friedman AP, Gorini S, Sicuteri F, eds. *Advances in Neurology Volume 33*. New York: Raven Press. 1982: 343

18 Berde R. New studies on the circulatory effect of ergot compounds with implication to migraine. In *Background to Migraine*. London: Heinemann. 1971: 66

19 Horowski R. Some aspects of the dopaminergic action of ergot derivatives and their role in the treatment of migraine. In Critchley M, Friedman AP, Gorini S, Sicuteri F, eds. *Advances in Neurology Volume 33*. New York: Raven Press. 1982: 325

20 Horowski R. Role of monoaminergic mechanisms in the mechanism of action of ergot derivatives used in migraine. In Rose FC, ed. *Advances in Migraine Research and Therapy*. New York: Raven Press. 1982: 190

21 Wainscott G, Volans G, Wilkinson M. Ergotamine-induced headache. *Br Med J 1974; 2:* 724

22 Anderson PG. Ergotamine headache. *Headache 1975; 15:* 118–121

23 Lippman CW. Characteristic headache resulting from prolonged use of ergot derivatives. *J Nerv Ment Dis 1955; 121:* 270–273

24 Ala-Hurula V, Myllyla V, Hokkanen D. Ergotamine abuse: results of ergotamine discontinuation, with special reference to the plasma concentrations. *Cephalalgia 1982; 2:* 189–195

25 Louis P, Spierings ELH. Comparison of flunarizine (Sibelium) and pizotifen (Sandomigran) in migraine treatment: a double-blind study. *Cephalalgia 1982; 2:* 197–203

26 Diamond S, Schenbaum H. Flunarizine, a calcium channel blocker, in the prophylactic treatment of migraine. *Headache 1983; 23:* 39–42

27 Heykants J, Wynants J, Hendrick J. *Plasma Levels of Flunarizine After Single Oral Administration of 10mg to Healthy Volunteers. Clinical Research Report.* Beerse: Janssen Pharmaceutica. 1975

28 Wauquier A, Ashton D, Clincke C, Van Reempts J. Pharmacological protection against brain hypoxia: the efficacy of flunarizine, a calcium entry blocker. In Rose FC, Amery WK, eds. *Cerebral Hypoxia in the Pathogenesis of Migraine.* London: Pitman. 1982: 139–154

29 Rose FC. Possible role for flunarizine in the prophylaxis of migraine. In Rose FC, Amery WK, eds. *Cerebral Hypoxia in the Pathogenesis of Migraine.* London: Pitman. 1982: 185

30 Fanciullacci M, Del Bianco PL, Sicuteri F. Iris and vein adrenoceptors in migraine and central panalgesia. In Szabadi E, Bradshaw CM, eds. *Recent Advances in the Pharmacology of Adrenoceptors.* Amsterdam: Elsevier. 1978: 295

31 Chose K, Coppen A, Carroll D. Studies of the interactions of tyramine in migraine patients. In Greene R, ed. *Current Concepts in Migraine Research.* New York: Raven Press. 1978; 89

32 Sicuteri F, Fanciullacci M, Michelacci S. Decentralization supersensitivity in headache and central panalgesia. In Friedman AP, Grangen ME, Critchely M, eds. *Research in Clinical Study of Headache, Volume 6.* Basel: Karger. 1978: 19

33 Basbaum A, Fields HL. Endogenous pain control mechanism: review and hypothesis. *Ann Neurol 1978; 4:* 451–462

34 Forssman B, Henriksson KG, Johannsson V et al. Propranolol for migraine prophylaxis. *Headache 1976; 16:* 238–245

35 Fozard JR. Basic mechanisms of antimigraine drugs. In Critchley M, Friedman AP, Gorini S, Sicuteri F, eds. *Advances in Neurology Volume 33.* New York: Raven Press. 1982: 295

36 Diamond S, Shapiro DB. Long-term study of propranolol in the treatment of migraine. In Rose FC, ed. *Advances in Migraine Research and Therapy.* New York: Raven Press. 1982: 217

37 Swertz JP, Perdrisot R, Macfroy B, Schwartz JC. Is enkephalinase identical with 'angiotensin-converting enzyme?' *Eur J Pharmacol 1979; 53:* 209–210

38 Bebuck M, Marks N. Co-identity of brain angiotensin-converting enzyme with a membrane bound dipeptidyl carboxypeptidase inactivating met-enkephalin. *Biomed Biophys Res Comm 1979; 88:* 215–221

39 Sicuteri F. Enkaphalinase inhibition relieves pain syndrome of central dysnociception (migraine and related headache). *Cephalalgia 1981; 1:* 229–232

40 Sicuteri F, Anselmi B, Del Bianco PL. Opiate receptors in human vein. *Int J Clin Pharm Res 1981; 1:* 145–149

Part III

PERSPECTIVES

19

IN VITRO RECEPTOR BINDING PROFILE
OF DRUGS USED IN MIGRAINE

J E Leysen, W Gommeren

Introduction

Drugs used for migraine prophylaxis, for ultimate prevention and for treating an attack and drugs used as pharmacological tools in migraine research belong to various pharmacological classes. Moreover, several of these drugs have multiple pharmacological actions.

In vitro radioligand receptor binding techniques allow direct assessment of the binding affinities of drugs for known neurotransmitter and drug receptors and receptor subtypes. Usually, there is a direct relationship between the binding affinity of a drug for a particular receptor site and the in vivo pharmacological potency of the drug in a test known to be mediated by that receptor. The advantage of the in vitro radioligand receptor binding technique is that it can be uniformly applied for a great number of different receptors and that the binding affinities of the drugs are uniformly analysed. Moreover, the in vitro assay avoids problems related to drug absorption, distribution, time of onset, time of peak effect and duration of action and drug metabolism. Assessment of the in vitro receptor binding profile of drugs, comprising binding affinities for a wide series of neurotransmitter and drug receptor sites, is a new and useful way to illustrate the potency, specificity or potential multiple actions of drugs. The ability of drugs to inhibit the in vitro uptake of neurotransmitters in synaptosomes can also be determined using a similar technique.

We studied the in vitro receptor binding profile for a variety of drugs used in migraine treatment and research; it includes the drug binding affinities for eight different neurotransmitter receptor binding sites and for the nitrendipine Ca-binding site. Also the drug potencies to inhibit in vitro uptake of serotonin and norepinephrine in synaptosomes were evaluated.

Materials and methods

Tissues were obtained from rat and guinea-pig brains. Animals were decapitated and brains immediately removed and dissected. The tissue was homogenised in

255

TABLE I. Methods for in vitro ^{3}H-ligand binding to brain membrane preparations and

Receptor	Dopamine-	Serotonin-	Serotonin-	Histamine-	ACH-MUSC
	D$_2$	S$_2$	S$_1$	H$_1$	
(references)	[1]	[2]	[3]	[4]	[5]

Tissue

species	rat	rat	rat	guinea-pig	rat
brain area	striatum	frontal cortex	hippo-campus	cerebellum	striatum
mg wet weight/ assay	12.5	10	25	10	5

^{3}H-ligand

compound	haloperidol	ketanserin	serotonin	pyrilamine	dexetimide
concentration (nM)	2	1	3	4	2
K$_D$ (nM)	1.3	0.45	11	0.85	0.65

Compounds for defining non-specific binding

compound	(+)-buta-clamol	methyser-gide	LSD	astemizole	dexetimide
concentration (nM)	2000	1000	2000	1000	200

Incubation conditions

buffer	tris-HCl	tris-HCl	tris-HCl	Na-K phosphate	Na-K phosphate
	50 nM	50 nM	50 nM	50 nM	50 nM
	pH 7.6	pH 7.7	pH 7.5	pH 7.5	pH 7.5
	salts*		4 nM CaCl$_2$		
volume per assay (ml)	1.1	4.4	2	1.1	1.2
temperature (°C)	37	37	37	25	37
time (min)	10	15	10	30	20

*   salts = 120 nM NaCl, 5 nM KCl, 2 nM MgCl$_2$, 1 nM CaCl$_2$, 0.1% ascorbic acid, 10μM
**   Krebs-Henseleit = 118.06 nM NaCl, 4.69 nM KCl, 1.8 nM MgSO$_4$, 2.51 nM CaCl$_2$,

<sup> replaced: ^{3}H-neurotransmitter uptake in synaptosome preparations

α_1- adrenergic [6]	α_2- adrenergic [6]	β- adrenergic [7]	Nitrendipine CA-site [8]	Serotonin uptake [9]	Nor-epinephrine uptake [9]
rat forebrain	rat cortex	rat cortex	rat cortex	rat cortex	rat hypo-thalamus
25	20	25	10	10	10
WB 4101	clonidine	dihydro-alprenolol	nitrendipine	serotonin	nor-epinephrine
0.5	3	1	0.1	10	10
0.29	2.1	0.88	0.65		
nor-epinephrine	nor-epinephrine	alprenolol	nifedipine	chlorimi-pramine	desimi-pramine
100 000	2000	1000	1000	1000	1000
tris-HCl	tris-HCl	tris-HCl	tris-HCl	Krebs-** Henseleit	Krebs-** Henseleit
50 nM pH 7.7	50 nM pH 7.7	50 nM pH 8.0	50 nM pH 7.7		
2.2	2.2	2.2	2.2	1.1	1.1
25	25	37	37	25	25
20	30	10	30	5	5

pargyline.
25 nM $NaHCO_3$, 1.18 nM KH_2PO_4, 5.55 nM glucose.

ice-cold buffer or sucrose and membrane fractions were prepared by successive centrifugations (references for tissue preparations are indicated in Table I). Washed membranes were suspended in the assay buffers respectively. Table I summarises the materials and assay conditions of the various in vitro radioligand receptor binding and neurotransmitter uptake models.

Incubation of both radioligand binding and neurotransmitter uptake assays were stopped by rapid filtration under vacuum of the assay mixture using Whatmann GF/B glass fibre filters. Filters were rinsed three times with 5ml ice-cold buffer. Membrane-bound radioactivity, which was retained on the filters, was counted in a ligand scintillation spectrometer.

Unlabelled drugs were tested at six to eight different concentrations in a range between 10^{-10} and 10^{-5} M for inhibition of the specific membrane labelling by the ^{3}H-ligand. IC_{50}-values, i.e. the drug concentration inhibiting 50 per cent of the specific binding of the ^{3}H-ligand, were derived from inhibition curves, generated by plotting percentage of specific ^{3}H-ligand binding versus log drug concentration.

Binding affinities were expressed as equilibrium inhibition constants: $K_i = IC_{50}/[1 + C/K_D]$ with C the concentration and K_D the equilibrium dissociation constant of the ^{3}H-ligand.

Assays were always performed in duplicate, K_i-values being mean values derived from two to four independently performed inhibition curves.

Results

The drugs used in migraine therapy investigated in this study are classified into drugs used for (a) prophylaxis (the serotonin antagonists pizotifen, cyproheptadine, methysergide; the amine re-uptake blocker amitryptiline; the α_2-adrenergic agonist clonidine; the β-blocker propranolol; the blockers of calcium transmembrane flux: nimodipine, flunarizine); (b) ultimate prevention (the peripheral dopamine antagonist domperidone), and (c) treatment of the attack (ergotamine). The equilibrium inhibition constants (K_i-values) of the drugs for binding to dopamine-D_2, serotonin-S_2, serotonin-S_1, histamine-H_1, acetylcholine muscarinic (ACH-MUSC), α_1-adrenergic, α_2-adrenergic, β-adrenergic and nitrendipine Ca-sites are presented in Table II.

Pizotifen, cyproheptadine and methysergide display, as their most potent activity, binding to serotonin-S_2 receptor sites. Methysergide shows high potency (K_i = 0.94nM) and high selectivity for this site; the potency difference for occupation of other receptor sites exceeds one hundred-fold. Pizotifen and cyproheptadine also show high binding affinity for the serotonin-S_2 receptor sites (K_i-values 0.28 and 0.44nM), but binding to histamine-H_1 receptor sites occurs only at six-fold higher concentration. Moreover, these compounds show an appreciable binding affinity for acetylcholine muscarinic receptor sites. Amitryptiline shows its highest binding affinity for histamine-H_1 receptor sites

258

TABLE II. In vitro binding affinities (K_i-value, mean ± SEM in nanomolar) for neurotransmitter and drug receptor sites of drugs used in migraine therapy

	Dopamine-D_2	Serotonin-S_2	Serotonin-S_1	Histamine-H_1	ACH-MUSC	α_1-adrenergic	α_2-adrenergic	β-adrenergic	Nitrendipine Ca-site
Prophylaxis									
pizotifen	99± 9(4)*	0.28±0.05(4)	1500± 150(2)	1.9 ± 0.3 (3)	23±7(2)	120± 30(4)	480± 50(2)	inactive	6900 (2)
cyproheptadine	31± 10(3)	0.44±0.03(2)	700 (2)	2.7 ± 0.3 (3)	19±2(2)	100± 10(5)	760±400(2)	inactive	6400±500 (3)
methysergide	200± 35(3)	0.94±0.01(4)	100± 20(4)	inactive	inactive	2300±500(4)	2600±500(2)	inactive	inactive
amitriptiline	210± 50(3)	4.2 ±0.4 (3)	1320± 80(4)	0.74± 0.04(2)	17±2(3)	30± 8(3)	6500 (2)	inactive	inactive
clonidine	inactive	inactive	4000± 900(2)	inactive	inactive	370± 80(2)	2.8± 0.4(3)	inactive	inactive
propranolol	inactive	1500± 900(2)	330± 80(2)	inactive	inactive	inactive	inactive	6.5± 1.4(3)	inactive
nimodipine	inactive	inactive	inactive	inactive	inactive	inactive	inactive	inactive	0.90±0.03(3)
flunarizine	80± 10(3)	200± 70(3)	inactive	68 ± 9 (4)	inactive	250± 80(3)	inactive	inactive	380± 70 (3)
Ultimate prevention									
domperidone	0.9±0.2(4)	80± 30(4)	7000±3000(2)	5500±600 (2)	inactive	90± 30(4)	420± 40 (4)	inactive	inactive
Treatment of attack									
ergotamine	3.2±0.7(4)	12± 2(3)	3.0± 1.3(5)	880 (2)	inactive	9.3± 2.1(2)	5.7± 1.1(5)	4200±500(2)	10,400± 50 (2)

*Values between brackets indicate the number of independently performed determinations

$(K_i = 0.74nM)$, followed by binding to serotonin-S_2 receptor sites $(K_i = 4.2nM)$. For this compound the binding to acetylcholine muscarinic and α_1-adrenergic receptor sites is also to be noted. Clonidine binds very potently and highly selectively to α_2-adrenergic receptor sites. Propranolol shows high potency and high selectivity for binding to β-adrenergic receptor sites. Nimodipine solely binds with very high affinity to ^{3}H-nitrendipine labelled Ca-sites. Flunarizine shows moderate binding affinity for five receptor sites in the following order of potency: histamine-H_1, dopamine-D_2, serotonin-S_2, α_1-adrenergic and nitrendipine Ca-sites.

The drug used for ultimate prevention of a migraine attack, domperidone, shows high potency and selectivity for binding to dopamine-D_2 receptor sites.

The drug used for treatment of a migraine attack, ergotamine, shows very high binding affinity with K_i-values of nanomolar order, for five receptor sites: serotonin-S_1, dopamine-D_2, α_2-adrenergic, α_1-adrenergic and serotonin-S_2 receptor sites.

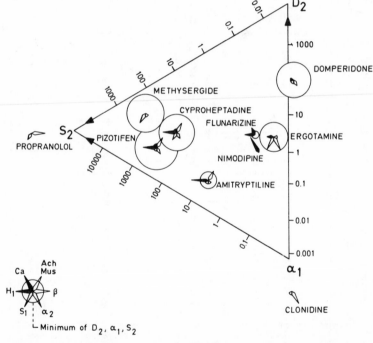

Figure 1. Triple logarithmic plot (Trilogplot^{TM}). Ratios between serotonin-S_2, dopamine-D_2 and α_1-adrenergic binding affinities are obtained by vertical projection upon the triangular axis (e.g. cyproheptadine S_2/D_2 = 70). The diameter of the circular symbol is proportional to the highest receptor binding affinity of the drug for S_2, D_2 or α_1 receptor sites. The star configuration represents the spectrum of binding affinities for serotonin-S_1, α_2-adrenergic, β-adrenergic, acetylcholine-muscarinic, nitrendipine Ca, histamine-H_1 binding sites

260

Figure 1 represents a so-called spectral map by means of which both the binding potency of the drugs and their selectivity for the receptor binding sites is visualised [10].

The potencies of the drugs for inhibiting ^{3}H-serotonin and ^{3}H-norepinephrine uptake in brain synaptosome preparations are presented in Table III. Only amitryptiline is a potent inhibitor of the uptake of both neurotransmitters. The potency of this compound to inhibit neurotransmitter uptake is of the same order of magnitude as its binding affinity for the receptor sites mentioned above.

TABLE III. Potencies of drugs used in migraine therapy for inhibition of neurotransmitter uptake in synaptosomes in vitro (IC_{50}, mean ± SEM nanomolar)

	^{3}H-serotonin uptake	^{3}H-norepinephrine uptake
Prophylaxis		
pizotifen	5700 ± 700 (2)	200 ± 60 (3)
cyproheptadine	4400 ± 1900 (2)	360 ± 40 (2)
methysergide	inactive	inactive
amitryptiline	50 ± 10 (2)	12 ± 2 (3)
clonidine	inactive	inactive
propranolol	1100 ± 500 (2)	inactive
nimodipine	inactive	inactive
flunarizine	4000 ± 2300 (2)	inactive
Ultimate prevention		
domperidone	1300 ± 400 (2)	9000 ± 1000 (2)
Treatment of attack		
ergotamine	inactive	inactive

Drugs used as pharmacological tools in migraine research (bromocriptine, apomorphine, piribedil and tyramine) were similarly studied for binding to the various receptor sites and inhibiting neurotransmitter uptake in vitro; the data being presented in Tables IV and V respectively.

Bromocriptine, apomorphine and piribedil bind primarily to dopamine-D_2 receptor sites. Bromocriptine is the most potent compound, but this agent also shows high binding affinity for the α-adrenergic and serotonin receptor sites. Apomorphine and piribedil, besides moderate binding to dopamine-D_2 receptor sites also bind to α_2-adrenergic sites. Bromocriptine, apomorphine and piribedil do not inhibit neurotransmitter uptake. Tyramine shows, as sole activity, potent inhibition of ^{3}H-norepinephrine uptake.

TABLE IV. In vitro binding affinities (K_i-value, mean ± SEM in nanomolar) for neurotransmitter and drug receptor sites of drugs used as pharmacological tools in migraine

	Dopamine-D_2	Serotonin-S_2	Serotonin-S_1	Histamine-H_1	ACH-MUSC	α_1-adrenergic	α_2-adrenergic	β-adrenergic	Nitrendipine Ca-site
bromocriptine	2.9±0.2(3)	27± 4(3)	60± 20(3)	inactive	inactive	7.3±1.0 (3)	29± 6(3)	1700±200(2)	2700(2)
apomorphine	32±4 (3)	1300±200(5)	6000±2000(3)	inactive	inactive	1200±400(2)	130 (2)	inactive	inactive
piribedil	210±60 (3)	inactive	6200	inactive	inactive	2300 (2)	1500±200(2)	inactive	inactive
tyramine	inactive	inactive	inactive	inactive	inactive	inactive	inactive	inactive	inactive

TABLE V. Potencies of drugs used as pharmacological tools in migraine, for inhibition of neurotransmitter uptake in synaptosomes in vitro (IC_{50}-value, mean ± SEM in nanomolar)

	^{3}H-serotonin uptake	^{3}H-norepinephrine uptake
bromocriptine	9000 ± 1000 (2)	inactive
apomorphine	inactive	inactive
piribedil	inactive	inactive
tyramine	2000 ± 500 (2)	56 ± 6 (2)

Discussion

The receptor binding profiles of the drugs used in migraine therapy are widely different; a common receptor binding property shared by all the drugs is not found. Five of the drugs used in migraine prophylaxis: pizotifen, cyproheptadine, methysergide, amitryptiline and flunarizine show serotonin-S_2 receptor binding and are expected to block these receptor sites at therapeutic dosages. Serotonin-S_2 receptor sites (also called 5-hydroxytryptamine$_2$ or 5-HT$_2$ receptor sites) were shown to mediate serotonin-induced vasoconstriction [2,11] and serotonin-induced platelet shape change and platelet aggregation [12,13]. In addition, it was found that the serotonin-S_2 receptor sites have a role in the amplification by serotonin of vasoconstriction induced by agents such as norepinephrine, histamine, angiotensin II and prostaglandin $F_{2\alpha}$ [14,15]. It was similarly shown that serotonin-S_2 receptor sites have a role in the amplification by serotonin of platelet aggregation induced by threshold concentrations of ADP, collagen, epinephrine and norepinephrine [13]. These findings substantiate the hypothesis that serotonin-S_2 receptor sites probably have an important role in serotonin-related impairment of microcirculation. Serotonin-S_2 receptor sites were originally detected by radioligand binding techniques in brain tissue. The sites show a typical distribution in mammalian brains, including human: the highest density is found in frontal cortical areas, followed by nucleus accumbens, tuberculum olfactorium and striatum [2,16]. In laboratory animals serotonin-S_2 receptors mediate serotonin induced behavioural excitation [2] and it has tentatively been hypothesised that the receptors may have a role in depressive illnesses [17].

Blockade of histamine-H_1 receptor sites, displayed by pizotifen, cyproheptadine, amitryptiline and flunarizine, will probably result in anti-allergic effects and may cause central sedating effects. Pizotifen, cyproheptadine and amitryptiline are also expected to produce the clinically known side effects of antimuscarinic agents.

The property of neurotransmitter uptake inhibition, such as displayed by amitryptiline, is thought to be useful for treating depression, but cardiovascular and cardiotoxic side effects can occur [18].

263

Nitrendipine binding sites, which can be occupied by flunarizine and for which nimodipine shows very high binding affinity, were suggested to be associated with sites which intervene in calcium transmembrane fluxes [19]. Preliminary investigations apparently indicate that the binding affinities of drugs for these sites correlate with the potencies of the drugs to antagonise calcium-induced vasoconstriction (unpublished observations).

The potent and selective binding of clonidine to α_2-adrenergic receptor sites probably result in an agonistic action. Stimulation of these receptor sites was reported to decrease norepinephrine release from adrenergic nerve terminals and to reduce central sympathetic outflow. Also direct α-adrenergic agonistic actions of clonidine were described [20].

Propranolol will decrease adrenergic activity at β-adrenergic receptors, owing to its potent and selective β-receptor blocking properties [21].

Domperidone, which is used for ultimate prevention of a migraine attack is primarily a potent dopamine receptor blocker which has been shown to act exclusively peripherally [22]. It was demonstrated that binding to dopamine-D_2 receptor sites correlates highly significantly with the potencies of drugs to antagonise dopamine-induced emesis in dogs [1]. Peripheral dopamine-D_2 receptor blockers were also found to promote gastric motility [23].

Ergotamine used for treating a migraine attack shows an exceptional receptor binding profile, with nanomolar binding affinities for five different neurotransmitter receptor sites. The drug probably exerts agonistic action at dopamine receptors, and presumably it acts as a mixed agonist-antagonist at serotonin receptors and α_1-adrenergic receptors [24]. The nature of its interaction with α_2-adrenergic receptors remains to be investigated.

Drugs used as pharmacological tools in migraine also display variable receptor binding profiles. The common property of bromocriptine, apomorphine and piribedil is a direct agonistic action at dopamine receptors. Also tyramine produces weak dopamine agonistic effects, probably by interfering with catecholamine stores.

It is to be noted that the receptor binding profile of both peptide ergot alkaloids, ergotamine and bromocriptine show a remarkable similarity, yet the first drug is used for treating an attack whereas the second one is used in migraine research for detecting particular reactivity (e.g. blood pressure changes) during the headache-free interval. Subtle differences, probably in the balance of the multiple pharmacological effects may result in a different clinical profile. In contrast to the two peptide ergot alkaloids, the lysergic acid amide, methysergide, is a potent prophylactic agent for migraine and shows a very selective receptor binding profile. It interacts only with serotonin receptors but mixed serotonin agonist-antagonist actions were described.

In conclusion, antimigraine drugs and drugs used as pharmacological tools in migraine research, show widely differing receptor binding profiles.

The question emerges whether improvement of impaired microcirculation

264

is the eventual result of serotonin-S_2 receptor blockade, interference with sympathetic tone through stimulation of α_2-adrenergic receptors and blockade of Ca^{++}-transmembrane fluxes, and whether this is the basis of a prophylactic effect against migraine. However, drugs not displaying one of the above properties, such as the selective peripheral dopamine antagonist, domperidone, were found to be active as well. These drugs are likely to interfere at another level in the chain of events leading to a migraine attack. The common dopamine receptor stimulating effect of drugs used as pharmacological tools seems to point to a potential role of (peripheral?) dopamine-D_2 receptors in the pathogenesis of migraine.

Summary

Drugs used for migraine prophylaxis (pizotifen, cyproheptadine, methysergide, amitryptiline, clonidine, propranolol, nimodipine, flunarizine), for ultimate prevention (domperidone), for treatment of the migraine attack (ergotamine) and drugs used in migraine research (bromocriptine, apomorphine, piribedil, tyramine) were investigated in vitro for binding to various neurotransmitter and drug receptor sites and for inhibition of neurotransmitter uptake in synaptosomes. We report the in vitro receptor binding profiles of the drugs, consisting of the binding affinities (expressed as K_i-values, i.e. equilibrium inhibition constants) of the drugs for dopamine-D_2, serotonin-S_2, serotonin-S_1, histamine-H_1, acetylcholine muscarinic, α_1-adrenergic, α_2-adrenergic, β-adrenergic and nitrendipine binding sites. We also report the potencies of the drugs to inhibit in vitro serotonin and norepinephrine uptake.

The drugs show widely differing receptor binding profiles, several of them displaying potent interaction with multiple receptor sites and others showing selectivity for a particular receptor. A common receptor binding property shared by all the drugs is not found. The implications of the receptor binding properties of the drugs for clinical effects and side-effects are discussed.

Acknowledgment

Part of this work was supported by a grant from I.W.O.N.L. The authors are indebted to Dr Paul Lewi, Information Science Department, for providing the spectral map represented in Figure 1. Sincere thanks to Dr Willem Amery for advice and helpful discussions.

References

1   Leysen J, Tollenaere JP, Koch MHJ, Laduron P. Differentiation of opiate and neuroleptic receptor binding in rat brain. *Eur J Pharmacol 1977; 43:* 253–267
2   Leysen JE, Niemegeers CJE, Van Nueten JM, Laduron P. [^{3}H] Ketanserin (R 41 468), a selective ^{3}H-ligand for serotonin$_2$ receptor binding sites. Binding properties, brain distribution and functional role. *Mol Pharmacol 1982; 21:* 301–314

265

3   Leysen JE. Serotonergic receptors in brain tissue: properties and identification of various ^{3}H-ligand binding sites in vitro. *J Physiol (Paris) 1981; 77:* 351–362

4   Laduron PM, Janssen PFM, Gommeren W, Leysen JE. In vitro and in vivo binding characteristics of a new long-acting histamine-H_1 antagonist, astemizole. *Mol Pharmacol 1982; 21:* 294–300

5   Laduron PM, Verwimp M, Leysen JE. Stereospecific in vitro binding of [3H] dexetimide to brain muscarinic receptors. *J Neurochem 1979; 32:* 421–427

6   Greenberg DA, U'Prichard DC, Snyder SH. α-Noradrenergic receptor binding in mammalian brain differential labelling of agonist and antagonist states. *Life Sci 1976; 19:* 69–76

7   Bylund DB, Snyder SH. Beta adrenergic receptor binding in membrane preparations from mammalian brain. *Mol Pharmacol 1976; 12:* 568–580

8   Leysen JE, Gommeren W. Receptor binding profile of flunarizine. *Janssen Research Products Information Services, Preclinical Research Report, March 1983.* Serial Number R 14 950/24

9   Leysen J, Gommeren W, Laduron P. Inhibition by tetramisole and Imafen of biogenic amine uptake. *Janssen Research Products Information Services, Preclinical Research Report,March 1976.* Serial Numbers R 12 564/14, R 25 540/2

10   Lewi PJ. The use of multivariate statistics in industrial pharmacology. *Pharmac Ther 1978; 3:* 481–537

11   Van Nueten JM, Janssen PAJ, Van Beek J et al. Vascular effects of ketanserin (R 41 468), a novel antagonist of 5-HT_2 serotonergic receptors. *J Pharmacol Exp Ther 1981; 218:* 217–230

12   Leysen JE, Gommeren W, De Clerck F. Demonstration of S_2-receptor binding sites on cat blood platelets using ^{3}H-ketanserin. *Eur J Pharmacol 1983; 88:* 125–130

13   De Clerck F, David JL, Janssen PAJ. Inhibition of 5-hydroxytryptamine-induced and -amplified human platelet aggregation by ketanserin (R 41 468), a selective 5-HT_2 receptor antagonist. *Agents and Actions 1982; 12:* 388–397

14   Van Nueten JM, Vanhoutte PM. Selectivity of calcium-antagonism and serotonin-antagonism with respect to venous and arterial tissues. *Angiology 1981; 32:* 476–484

15   Van Nueten JM, Janssen PAJ, De Ridder W, Vanhoutte PM. Interaction between 5-hydroxytryptamine and other vasoconstrictor substances in the isolated femoral artery of the rabbit; effect of ketanserin (R 41 468). *Eur J Pharmacol 1982; 77:* 281–287

16   Schotte A, Maloteaux JM, Laduron PM. Characterisation and regional distribution of serotonin S_2-receptors in human brain. *Brain Res 1983.* In press

17   Peroutka SJ, Snyder SH. Regulation of serotonin$_2$ (5-HT)$_2$ receptors labelled with [3H] spiroperidol by chronic treatment with the antidepressant amitryptiline. *J Pharmacol Exp Ther 1980; 215:* 582–587

18   Risch SC, Groom GP, Janowsky DS. The effects of psychotropic durgs on the cardiovascular system. *J Clin Psychiat 1982; 43:* 16–31

19   Murphy KMM, Gould RJ, Largent BL, Snyder SH. A unitary mechanism of calcium antagonist drug action. *Proc Natl Acad Sci USA 1983; 80:* 860–864

20   Lal H, Fielding S. Psychopharmacology of clonidine. *Progress in Clinical and Biological Research Vol 71.* New York: Alan R Liss. 1981

21   Heinsiner JA, Lefkowitz RJ. Adrenergic receptors: biochemistry, regulation, molecular mechanism and clinical implications. *J Lab Clin Med 1982; 100:* 641–658

22   Laduron PM, Leysen JE. Domperidone, a specific in vitro dopamine antagonist, devoid of in vivo central dopaminergic activity. *Biochem Pharmacol 1979; 28:* 2161–2165

23   Schuurkes JAJ, Helsen LFM, Van Nueten JM. Improved gastroduodenal co-ordination by the peripheral dopamine-antagonist domperidone. In Wienbeck M, ed. *Motility of the Digestive Tract.* New York: Raven Press. 1982: 565–572

24   Berde B, Schild HO. Ergot alkaloids and related compounds. *Handbook of Experimental Pharmacology Vol 49.* Berlin, Heidelberg, New York: Springer-Verlag 1978

20

THE PATHOMECHANISM OF MIGRAINE AS A BASIS FOR PHARMACOTHERAPY: A Clinician's Epilogue

G W Bruyn

In accordance with the explicit wish of the editors of this volume, this epilogue should reflect the data presented by the invited contributors against a clinical background, synthetise them and, if possible, indicate promising, pathogenetically based, strategies for future drug research in migraine.

For those participants, whom the national strike in this country did not succeed in preventing full-time attendance, the meeting which gave rise to the present book will remain in their memories as a milestone, marking the transition from traditional concepts about the pathogenesis of migraine to a new era.

The first four papers in this book proceed from the traditional tenet that migraine is a syndrome produced by pathological changes in cerebrovascular dynamics, be it either vasoconstriction or A-V shunting.

Olesen, utilising the ^{133}Xe procedure to analyse cortical blood flow (CoBF) changes during the migraine attack, made a few points unequivocally clear:

1. Common and classic migraine not only differ clinically, but also pathophysiologically, inasmuch as common migraine is not preceded by, or associated with, CoBF changes and classic migraine is, with reduced CoBF in the aura-phase spreading from occipital to rostral areas disrespecting the arterial supply territories, with reduced CO_2-response but with normal autoregulation.

2. The development of reduced CoBF ('oligaemia') may precede the aura (scintillating scotoma or other neurological deficit) and persist long after the neurological signs have disappeared. Therefore, oligaemia cannot be considered the single factor producing neurological dysfunction in classic migraine.

3. The headache develops when cortical hypoperfusion is still present. Headache, accordingly, is not due to vasodilatation.

One can draw from Olesen's contribution two important conclusions: 1) vasoconstriction can be discarded from further discussions on the pathogenesis of migraine, and 2) there is no strictly time-tied or causal relationship to be recognised between neurological deficit, pain, and reduced CoBF in classic migraine, the 'oligaemia' possibly being just as much an epiphenomenon of the mysterious underlying process as the neurological signs or the pain.

Olesen had among his cases, two mavericks. They showed the usual ^{133}Xe-CoBF changes indicative of classic migraine. One suffered from the common type, however (so that the common and classic types perhaps do not differ too much after all), and the other had no migraine at all, which clearly shows the absence of any relationship between 'oligaemia', pain, and neurological deficit. This seems all the more plausible, inasmuch as the CoBF-reduction in the patient material of the Danish group was said to average 36 per cent (15–60%). Regrettably, digital data on CBF were not immediately accessible (to be derived from the technicolour slides) but even at a reduction of 60 per cent, CoBF reduction seemed well above the whole brain tolerance limit of $18ml/min^{-1}/100gr^{-1}$. In most of Olesen's patients normal CoBF seemed to be as high as $105ml/100gr^{-1}/min^{-1}$. The normal CoBF is $\pm80ml/100gr^{-1}/min^{-1}$. Carlier [1] also found CoBF averages of $90-100ml/100gr^{-1}/min^{-1}$ in patients with migraine, hypertension, or nervousness; he considered a CoBF below $40ml/100gr^{-1}/min^{-1}$ as the tolerance limit.

For the clinician it became clear that the use of antimigraine drugs on the basis of their supposedly vasospasmolytic virtue means doing well for the wrong reasons.

Cerebral vasoconstriction remained the subject of Dr van Nueten's paper, as caused by vasoactive substances and their amplifiers. The vasodynamic effects of adrenaline, serotonin and transmembranous Ca^{2+}-shift, combined with the state of dopamine hypersensitivity in migraine were reviewed. The complexitiy of the actions of various substances both in time and in space are such that the clinician called upon to prescribe an effective treatment gets easily lost in the pharmacological domain. Blockers of Ca^{2++}-entry into vascular smooth muscle cells certainly seem helpful. Intriguingly, in his Table I, cyproheptadine and flunarizine are equipotent (and most potent) in inhibiting Ca^{2++} induced arterial contractions, and pizotifen and chlorpromazine are most potent in thwarting 5-HT and NA to induce arterial constrictions.

The Rotterdam-school of migrainology critically reviewed the late Hartwig Heyck's A-V shunting theory from their pharmacological-experimental results obtained in the cat and pig. The A-V shunts seem to be shut by serotonin, opened by cholinergic and purinergic substances, and either opened or shut by adrenergic activators. The importance, attached by Saxena and Spierings to the presence or absence of A-V shunts in the frontal and temporal regions is curious, in that these areas are *not* the typical seat of migrainous headache but rather the retro-orbital, occipital and temporoparietal areas. Anyway, though a single observation, viz that of reduced A-V-O_2 difference noted by Heyck remains an unexplained relic, erect amidst the ruins, the experimental results contradict the the A-V pathomechanism. Accordingly, the A-V-theory should be laid to rest along its vasoconstriction fellow in the Cemetery of Speculations.

Why ergot-alkaloids are effective, as well as the 5-HT antagonist methysergide, whereas the specific 5-HT_2 antagonist ketanserin is not, the clinician still does not understand.

The haematological experts De Clerck and David then tackled the ungentlemanlike behaviour of the platelet in its biochemical intercourse with biogenic amines, vasoactive substances, and enzymes, in three successive stages: induction (receptor activation), transmission (shift from membranous Ca^{2++} into the cytoplasm), and execution (shape change, aggregation, release). They stressed that intracellular redistribution rather than transmembrane Ca^{2+} entry during the first two stages is taking place (with one exception however: epinephrine-induced primary platelet aggregation). Consequently, it seems to transpire that Ca^{2+}-entry blockers may well exert their beneficial effect in migraine by quite a different mechanism than preventing the calcium ion getting into the cell. Why the non-selective β-blocker propranolol is effective in migraine cannot be satisfactorily explained in terms of platelet-activation stages.

The clinical perspective of the fascinating tale of the platelet demeanour apparently shows it to be a marker for migraine, but nothing more. It seems a haematological epiphenomenon, just as are the pain, the neurological and vegetative symptoms, and the spreading CoBF reduction.

Johnson reviewed the reported evidence indicative of adrenergic hyperactivity in migraineurs just prior to the attack (and in all probability between attacks). The central adrenergic coeruleic fibres contacting intracerebral arterioles provide the basis for a central neuronal theory of migraine. By virtue of this, one would theoretically expect a post-synaptic α-blocker to be effective in preventing or mitigating the attack. Reality did not bear this out, although, as far as the writer is aware, no trial with prazosin has yet been reported. Curiously, clonidine, an α_2-agonist, has only a limited and erratic effect, although it should have an effect, because it pre-synaptically activates NA re-uptake. Again no explanation can be given why propranolol as a non-selective β-blocker beats its α fellow-travellers.

Edvinsson enlarged upon the theme broached by Johnson. The cerebral blood vessels show β_1- rather than β_2-adrenoceptors, leaving the propranolol effect unexplained. If one realises that destruction of the blood brain barrier with hypertonic urea with resultant CBF-increase and increased oxygen/glucose metabolism, is blocked by β_2-antagonists, clearly, propranolol may act on endothelial rather than neural receptors. The cerebrovascular innervation is extremely complex, as shown by Owman's group over the last few years: cholinergic fibres lie next to adrenergic; substance P is present in sensory meningeal fibres, and recently a new NA-potentiating neuropeptide Y has been revealed in adrenergic nerves surrounding the blood vessels [2]. Edvinsson presented new data on intracerebral vascular noradrenergic (locus coeruleus) and serotonergic (nucleus raphes) innervation, quite apart from the well known post-ganglionic sympathetic

269

innervation (carotid plexus!) of the extracerebral arteries.

Intriguing in this context are, to the present writer, the experiments by Lance on the coeruleic fibres in monkeys (to explain the unilaterality of migraine). The central systems indicated by Edvinsson partly run in the central forebrain bundles to innervate the intracerebral capillaries and arterioles, and partly must leave the neuraxis via the facial nerve, greater superficial petrosal nerve and tympanic nerve to get at the pial arteries. Edvinsson stressed that 80 per cent of the cerebral blood volume is in the venous and 20 per cent in the arterial compartment, a ratio which is also governed by tissue pH.

In the clinical perspective, the feasibility of central neurogenic coeruleic and dorsal raphe nucleic influence on microvascular permeability (blood brain barrier) stands out as the salient feature in Edvinsson's presentation.

The next section starts with Amery's critical review of an impressive wealth of literature data, marshalling arguments in support of a fourth pathogenetic alternative, viz an attack-initiating episode of focal cerebral anoxia. In a tripartite approach, Amery

1. Reasoned by analogy (comparing Leão's spreading depression with the migraine attack, having $[K^+]$ changes as common root);

2. Surveyed seven factors potentially causing hypoxia (and retained no candidate as a winner);

3. Synthetised reported evidence of increased CVA risk in migraine.

However, no element of the reviewed material could, to Amery's full satisfaction, be made to fit comfortably the requirements for the hypothetic episodic focal anoxia.

Wauquier put the postulated pivotal points of ischaemia and/or hypoxia to the test by examining the effect of seven antimigraine drugs on: a) ischaemic hypoxia (bilateral carotid ligatured mice); b) hypoxic hypoxia (rats put in a 100% N_2 environment); and c) hypoxic hippocampal sections in vitro. In these three test situations the following drugs came out best: a) methysergide and flunarizine; b) ergotamine, clonidine and flunarizine; c) flunarizine. The mechanism of the protective action of these drugs has not been defined precisely.

At this point of the conference the traditional, rather threadbare theories of vasospasm, A-V-shunting, platelet serotonin, and hypoxia had all been collected into the garbage-van, leaving a tidy scene for a fresh wind that came from the North.

The Scandinavian workers enlarged upon an alternative mechanism that seems most promising in the view of the present writer, viz a neuronal pathogenesis. In 1972, Sjaastad and I were the only advocates of a CNS origin of migraine, but ours was a *vox clamans in deserto.*

Lauritzen convincingly argued that Leão's spreading depression (SD) is the most likely candidate for migraine's pathogenesis. It is an animal model of migraine. The 'spreading oligaemia' associated with it as a sequel is the consequence rather than the cause of neuronal dysfunction. Clearly, this nailed the lid on the coffin of the H G Wolff paradigm. Lauritzen confirmed and in detail enlarged upon the data presented by Olesen over the last years. The many features shared by migraine and SD, mentioned by Olesen and Amery (this volume), were extended by Lauritzen, as well as the differences between the two. Interestingly, again underlining the absence of a strictly linear relationship between CoBF changes and symptoms, Lauritzen had three patients with classic attacks but normal flow maps! The dissociation of neural signs and SD has been noted in the experimental animal [3].

Hansen's presentation pursued the SD hypothesis and made a strong case for it. In view of the opening-up of non-specific 6.6 Å ion-channels, the enormous shifts of $[K^+]$ (from 3 to 30–60mM), $[Na^+]_e$ (from 150 to 50), $[Cl^-]_e$ (from 130–75) and $[Ca^{2+}]_e$ (from 1.2 to 0.1), it is no surprise that neither flunarizine, nor methysergide, nor propranolol block SD, though flunarizine shortens recovery time and reduces the slow DC potential wave. Flunarizine has shown to be active in muscle cells and in all probability in the intracellular redistribution of Ca^{2+}; as to the neurone, its effect upon Ca^{2+} is unknown. Yet, divalent cations (Mg^{2+}, Mn^{2+}) as well as high CO_2-air inhalation block SD. Tetradotoxin, a Na-ionophore blocker, does not block it.

The Danish data clearly herald a new era in migraine research, to be focused on substances that block the event initiating the neuronal firing burst, the slow DC potential wave, the 250 per cent hyperperfusion, cellular K^+ release and Na^+, Cl^-, Ca^{2+} entry, followed by hypoperfusion, reduced CO_2- and metabolic (pH) vasomotor response, with intact autoregulation, spreading across the cortex irrespective of arterial territories but respecting architectonic boundaries.

The Mediterranean (or should one say Occitanean?) migrainologists adduced further detail. Sicuteri, like a modern pharmacological alchemist, enlarged upon three simple clinical tests, indicating a state of exhausted adrenergic neurones, peripheral DA hypersensitivity, and central endorphinergic deficiency. For the clinician, this means that effective medication in migraine should include haloperidol/domperidone (anti-DA), thiorphan, and captopril (anti-enkephalinase/ ACE). Fanciullaci pursued the value of these neuro-effector junction tests as sensitive methods for pharmacological management of migraine. The Tolosa-group enlarged upon the DA-agonist piribedil test as a marker, and domperidone as an effective drug.

Ghose advocated the use of the tyramine-pressor test to monitor pharmacotherapy in migraine.

Clifford Rose's review of migraine-markers pressed home the basic truth that an unequivocally defined operational programme for migraine is illusory as long as no single cause or pathognomonic specific change has been identified. If the diagnostician errs, the patient writes off medical science as a loss and turns to mystic alternatives, which is what we actually see happen nowadays.

271

Oosterveld, finally, surveyed the knotty aspect of vestibular derangement in migraine and the anti-vertiginous activity of antimigraine drugs. These drugs do reduce labyrinthine irritability, which, however, appears to be a migrainous epiphenomenon in his case-series, and was not influenced by flunarizine.

From the clinical perspective, the pharmacological manipulation of provoking certain signs in migraineurs may well, if substantiated in larger series or simplified in protocolled form, turn out to be of help to the diagnostician.

This conference clarified considerably future approaches to the puzzle, by clearing away the time-worn concepts of vasoconstriction/dilatation, A-V-shunts, ischaemia/hypoxia, etc., and positioning as a central item the spreading depression/ hypoperfusion [4], in which the vascular and neuronal facets seem to have gone to a happy wedding.

The idea that migraine, SD and epilepsy might have a basic mechanism in common certainly is not new [5—13] and was intimated as early as 1941 by Lashley [14], but acquired reality only since advanced techniques of clinical examination became available.

Of course, the differences between SD and cortical migrainous events are not negligible and it is as yet conjecture to identify the two on the basis of similarities (Table I). The similarities are such however, as to promise a new road towards understanding of what really happens and, perhaps, an effective treatment. Therefore I should like to close this epilogue by proposing my own speculative view on the pathomechanism of migraine.

In man's brain, sets of millions of neurones are constantly firing, particularly in the areas that are at the receiving end of sensory input (tactile, visual, acoustic). These constantly active neurone-masses release their K^+ into an intercellular space of $\pm$ 200 Å, by a factor 50 the narrowest of any organ in our body and totalling $\pm$ 12 per cent of volume mass (the figure of 20% as derived from the wet weight/dry weight difference seems too high). The extrusion of K^+ into the gel of this intercellular space would prevent repolarisation of the neurone, if nothing happened. Surprisingly, until recent years, it was tacitly assumed that re-uptake, and interstitial diffusional redistribution of K^+ took place. Amazingly, nobody wondered why the number of astrocytes in the CNS exceeds by a factor 10 the number of neurones, enveloping them in their entirety [15]. Thanks to the recent work of Gardner-Medwin from London, it has been established that the redistribution of K^+ over the relatively large neuronal IS distances of $100-200\mu$ (i.e. 10,000 times as long as the width of the intercellular space) is mainly done by the glia cells, who account for at least 80 per cent of the cortical K^+-flux. The astrocytes are selectively avid for K^+ and they are the K^+-transport cells par excellence, in their low-resistance coupled enormous network forming the so-called spatial buffer, cytoplasmically redistributing K^+ and effectively controlling $[K^+]_e$. The K^+ released into the intercellular space and taken up by glia, takes H_2O with it, in this way narrowing the IS by 50 per cent [16] because it

TABLE I

	Spreading depression	Classic migrainous symptoms
	Differences	
Species	Lower mammals	Man
Site	Superficial layers lissencephalic cortex	Convoluted cortex? [10]
		Hippocampus
		Striatum [26]
Cortical neuronal/ glia ratio	High	Low [15]
Origin	Pathological physicochemical stimulus	? ('spontaneous')
Features	Spreading DC negative wave, 1–2 min	?
	250% ↑ CoBF, 1–2 min	Possible
	Hypoperfusion (−25%), 1 hour	4–5 hours
	Refractory period, 1–15 min	Hours
	Cortical pO_2 ↓ [8]	?
	Creat. phosph. ↓ [27]	?
	Phosphate ↑ [28]	?
	Co met. rate O_2 ↑ [29]	?
	Co met. rate glucose ↑ [30]	?
	Lactic acid ↑, cAMP ↑ [31]	↑
	GABA ↑	
	HCO_3^- ↑	↑
	NADH → NAD 25% ↓ [32]	?
	$[K^+]_e$ 3mMol → > 20mMol	
	$[Na^+]_e$ 150mMol → 55mMol	?
	$[Cl^-]_e$ 130mMol → 70mMol	
	$[Ca^{2++}]_e$ 1.3mMol → 0.1mMol	
Blocked by	High CO_2-inhalation	±
	Cocaine [18], Mg, Mn, Co	?
	Similarities	
Not blocked by	Anaesthesia, anoxia [33]	–
VER	↓	↓
SSEP	↓	↓ ?
Arterial supply territories	No barrier	No barrier
Anatomical boundaries	Form barrier	?

makes the glia swell. The glial spatial K^+ buffer system keeps the $[K^+]_e$ constant at a value of 2.7–3.2mMol, with a cortical 'ceiling' of 12mMol.

It logically follows, that if a certain event at a certain cortical locus (whether that be intense stimulation of a limited set of neurones in a few cortical columns igniting them in a firing burst with high depolarisational K^+ release, or a break in the blood-brain-barrier with seepage of serous fluid, containing high K^+, between the astrocyte's feet directly into the IS) causes the cortical astrocyte population to fail suddenly in its major task (viz the redistribution of K^+) while the princely neurones all the time merrily continue their business as usual throwing out K^+. As a consequence the ceiling of 12mMol is trespassed, and the scene is set, primed, and triggered for the self-sustained and propagating electronegative DC potential. This slow DC potential shift is caused by the glial-depolarisation of ±20mV, caused by the intraglial K^+. The SD may occur without neuronal discharge [17]. The neurones stay depolarised, $[Na]_o$ drops 100mMol, $[Ca^{++}]_o$ drops by a factor 12, $[Cl^-]_o$ drops 70mMol, all disappearing into the neurones, water disappears from the IS into the swelling glia. In this view, it is not the continuous, or even increased, neuronal K^+-release, but the glial failure to spatially buffer the K^+ that causes the igniting event of the neuronal dysfunction in classic migraine. Note that ischaemia and hypoxia are not required in this model of SD. For the differences and similarities of SD and ischaemia, see [18–20].

How can one conceive of such a sudden, if transient, failure on the part of the mass of silent glial slaves? That one is easy to answer: 1) It may be caused by glial inability to cope with an overload of K^+ released from intensely firing neurones (in some patients intense light may induce an attack). 2) Or it may occur at those loci where the numerical ratio of astrocytes to neurones is tipped in favour of the latter (migraine disappears in senility *a pari passu* the senile neuronal depletion); over the range of lower vertebrates with increasing brain weight, glial density remains constant but neuronal density falls gradually by a factor 7, resulting in an increasing astrocyte/neurone ratio. In other words, in lower animals there are less astrocytes per neurone, which explains why SD is more readily elicited in them [21]. 3) Or, the most likely, it originates from the blood vessels the glia is so intimately connected with. Astrocytes swell easily. Any neurosurgeon faced with the task of getting the bone-flap again in position over an acutely oedematous brain mushrooming like tooth-paste out of the trepanned skull can testify to that. So can any neuropathologist trying to define the very perimeters of glia cells with a H&E or a PTAH stain. The photographs of retinal SD actually depict the swelling of the retinal tissue spiralling and advancing like a rolling wave. Osler called migraine 'hives of the brain', i.e. cerebral 'urticaria'.

If anything disrupts the endothelial (whether structural or enzymatic) blood-brain-barrier [22, 23], e.g. by hypertonic urea, by slight injury or platelet microthrombus, or allergy to food substances, serous fluid leaks into the cortical parenchyma. The colloid osmotic pressure of the IS rises locally, with grave consequences, viz rising pressure of the IS and therefore interstitial oedema, with disruption of the normal neuronoglial relationship.

A short digression will clarify this. Four pressure forces control the exchange of fluid between the capillary and the tissue: a) the colloid osmotic pressure of the blood, drawing the fluid from the tissue into the vascular lumen (pCO = 28mmHg); b) the hydrostatic blood pressure in the capillary, driving fluid from the blood into the tissue (at the arterial end of the capillary 25mmHg, at its venous end 10mmHg), pCap = 25 or 10mmHg; c) the negative interstitial gel pressure, sucking fluid out of the capillary into the tissue (pIG = 6.3mmHg) (Figure 1); d) the interstitial colloid pressure, having the same effect as (c), pIC = 5mmHg.

Normally, the forces driving fluid from the blood into the tissue at the arterial end, are pCap + pIC + pIG = 36.3mmHg countered by pCO, resulting
          25   5   6.3   28
in a net force of 8.3mmHg, driving 0.3 per cent of the plasma into the tissue. In the brain this net driving force is only 2mmHg.

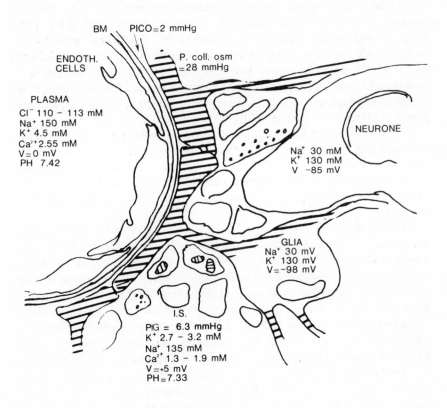

Figure 1

275

At the venous end of the capillary the values are $10 + 5 + 6.3 = 21.3 - 28$, resulting in a net reabsorption pressure driving fluid from the tissue back into the blood. The mean Starling equilibrium indicates a net filtration pressure of 0.3mmHg. As soon as the hydrostatic capillary pressure ($\simeq$ the arterial blood pressure) rises more than 17mmHg above normal, to say ±40mmHg, the net filtration pressure increases from 0.3 to 20.3mmHg, i.e. 70 times, and interstitial oedema develops.

This is what may happen in effort migraine (runner's migraine, weight-lifter's migraine) or coital migraine. As soon as the plasma colloid osmotic pressure falls from 28 to ±10, the same happens, because the safety factor is 17−18mmHg. As soon as capillary permeability increases, oedema will again develop. (In this survey the effect of the negative intracranial pressure in standing man is left out of consideration for purposes of simplicity).

When this happens, the glial network has to cope not only on the neuronal front, but on the vascular and intimal fronts as well. Precisely here, at the vascular barrier, the whole gamut of factors of innervation and receptors repeatedly discussed in the pertinent literature come into play: NA, 5-HT, DA, substance P, CCK-8, VIP, SS, enkephalin, histamine, kinins, ACE, β-TG, TxA2, FFA, prostaglandins, leukotrienes, arachidonate, Ca^{2+}, and phosphatidyl-inositol [24]. For all we know, even the as yet unidentified Serotonin Releasing Factor with a molecular weight below 50,000 daltons, may either change the blood-brain barrier or activate the central nervous cell and fibre systems that put the migraine attack into motion. After all, the actual attack usually follows quite a period of preparation often sensed by the migraineur as impending.

Precisely here, the local blood-brain-barrier permeability may be changed neurogenically via the adrenergic (locus coeruleus) or serotonergic (nuclear raphes) innervation of the capillaries, as Edvinsson so convincingly showed. The astrocyte as the link between neurone and endothelial cell, occupies the position of supreme intermediary, both literally and in any concept of pathomechanisms in migraine.

To characterise this personal view as the proposition of a pathogenetic theory, called 'Migraine as Glial Failure' would be wrong. Indeed, the sketched chain of events would account for the migrainous cheiro oral syndrome, for scintillating scotoma, perhaps even for dysphrenic migrainous syndromes such as transient global amnesia or confusion. It does not explain the specific stereotyped train of events of prodromes, aura, pain, vegetative symptoms (typifying what is called a migraine attack), triggered by a wide gamut of non-specific precipitating events, even though it is known that hypoglycaemia, mechanical head injury, over-hydration (menstrual cycle), etc., may provoke a migraine attack and SD alike.

The sketched view, as yet, only accounts for certain phenomena in classical migraine, but puts the pathomechanism of a restricted series of events in a larger frame, potentially capable of accommodating more aspects of the migraine attack. It has the virtue of being open to test and may explain the remarkably rapid restorative effect of naloxone on migrainous neurological deficit [25] in the presence of continued hypoperfusion.

References

1   Carlier. Cerebrographie: [133]Xenon inhalation method. Experience after 650 tests. In Bès A, Géraud G, Jauzac Ph, Guëll A, eds. *Cerebral Circulation and Neurotransmitters. Proc Int Congr Cerebral Circulation, Toulouse, 1979*. Amsterdam: Excerpta Medica. 1980: 139–143

2   Tatemoto K. Neuropeptide Y: complete amino acid sequence of the brain peptide. *Proc Natl Acad Sci USA 1982; 79:* 5485–5489

3   Carew TJ, Crow TJ, Petrinovich LF. Lack of coincidence between neural and behavioral manifestations of cortical spreading depression. *Science 1970; 169:* 1339–1341

4   Lauritzen M, Jørgensen MB, Diemer HD, Gjedde A, Hansen AJ. Persistent oligemia of rat cerebral cortex in the wake of spreading depression. *Ann Neurol 1982; 12:* 469–474

5   Leão AAP. Pial circulation and spreading depression of activity in the cerebral cortex. *J Neurophysiol 1944; 7:* 391–396
     Leão AAP. Spreading depression of activity in the cerebral cortex. *J Neurophysiol 1944; 7:* 359–390

6   Leão AAP. Spreading depression. In Purpura DP et al, eds. *Experimental Models of Epilepsy*. New York: Raven Press. 1972: 174–196

7   Milner PM. Note on a possible correspondence between the scotomas of migraine and spreading depression of Leão. *EEG Clin Neurophysiol 1958; 10:* 705

8   Marshall WH. Spreading cortical depression of Leão. *Physiol Rev 1959; 39:* 239–279

9   Basser LS. The relation of migraine and epilepsy. *Brain 1969; 92:* 285–300

10   Oka H, Kako M, Matsushima M, Ando K. Traumatic spreading depression syndrome. *Brain 1977; 100:* 287–298

11   Gardner-Medwin AR. Possible roles of vertebrate neuroglia in potassium dynamics, spreading depression and migraine. *J Exp Biol 1981; 95:* 111–127
     Gardner-Medwin AR. The effect of carbon dioxide and oxygen on Leão's spreading depression: evidence supporting a relationship to migraine. *J Physiol 1981; 316:* 23P–24P

12   Gardner-Medwin AR, Skelton JL. The relation between depression and migraine. *Neuroscience 1982; 7:* S77
     Gardner-Medwin AR, Skelton JL. Leão's spreading depression: evidence supporting a role in the migraine aura. In Clifford Rose F, Amery WK, eds. *Cerebral Hypoxia in the Pathogenesis of Migraine*. London: Pitman. 1982: 127–131

13   Lauritzen M, Olsen T, Lassen NA, Paulson OB. Changes in regional cerebral blood flow during the course of classic migraine attacks. *Ann Neurol 1983; 13:* 633–641

14   Lashley KS. Patterns of cerebral integration indicated by migrainous scotoma. *Arch Neurol Psychiat 1941; 46:* 331–339

15   Phillis JW, Ochs S. Excitation and depression of cortical neurones during spreading depression. *Exp Brain Res 1971; 12:* 132–149

16   Hansen AJ, Olsen CE. Brain extracellular space during spreading depression and ischemia. *Acta Physiol Scand 1980; 108:* 355–365

17   Sugaya E, Takato M, Noda Y. Neuronal and glial activity during spreading depression in cerebral cortex of cat. *J Neurophysiol 1975; 38:* 822–841

18   Leão AAP. Further observations on the spreading depression of activity in the cerebral cortex. *J Neurophysiol 1947; 10:* 409–414

19   Hansen AJ, Zeuthen Th. Extracellular ion concentrations during spreading depression and ischemia in the rat brain cortex. *Acta Physiol Scand 1981; 113:* 437–445

277

20   Hansen AJ. Extracellular potassium concentration in juvenile and adult rat brain cortex during anoxia. *Acta Physiol Scand 1977; 99:* 412–420

21   Tower DB, Young OM. The activities of butyrylcholinesterase and carbonic anhydrase, the rate of anaerobic glycolysis, and the question of a constant density of glial cells in cerebral cortices of various mammalian species from mouse to whale. *J Neurochem 1973; 20:* 269–278

22   Harper AM, MacKenzie ET, McCulloch J, Pickard JD. Migraine and the blood-brain-barrier. *Lancet 1977; iii:* 1034–1036

23   van Rossum JM. Migraine als uiting van een gestoorde cerebrale vaatregulatie. *Actua Sandoz 1982; 2:* 57–60

24   Downes CP. Inositol phospholipids and neurotransmitter-receptor signalling mechanisms. *TINS 1983; 6:* 313–316

25   Sicuteri F, Boccuni M, Fanciullacci M, Gatto G. Naloxone effectiveness on spontaneous and induced perceptive disorders in migraine. *Headache 1983; 23:* 179–183

26   Sramka M, Brozek G, Bures J, Nadvornik P. Functional ablation by spreading depression: possible use in human stereotactic neurosurgery. *Appl Neurophysiol 1977/78; 40:* 48–61

27   Krivanek J. Changes of brain glycogen in the spreading EEG depression of Leão. *J Neurochem 1958; 2:* 337–343

28   Krivanek J. Some metabolic changes accompanying Leão's spreading cortical depression in the rat. *J Neurochem 1961; 6:* 183–189

29   Gjedde A, Hansen AJ, Questorff B. Blood-brain glucose transfer in spreading depression. *J Neurochem 1981; 37(4):* 807–812

30   Shinohari M, Dollinger B, Brown G, Rapoport S, Sokoloff L. Cerebral glucose utilization: local changes during and after recovery from spreading cortical depression. *Science 1979; 203:* 188–190

31   Krivanek J. Brain cyclic adenosine 3'; 5'-monophosphate during depolarization of the cerebral cortical cells in vivo. *Brain Res 1977; 120:* 493–505

32   Mayevsky A, Zeuthen Th, Chance B. Measurements of extracellular potassium, ECoG and pyridine nucleotide levels during cortical spreading depression in rats. *Brain Res 1974; 76:* 347–349

33   Grafstein B. Mechanism of spreading cortical depression. *J Neurophysiol 1956; 19:* 154–171

INDEX

carbon monoxide poisoning and
headache, 124
catecholamines *see* adrenaline; dopamine;
isoprenaline; noradrenaline
cerebral anoxia *see* cerebral hypoxia
cerebral atrophy, in migraine patients,
121–122
cerebral blood flow
autoregulation,
abnormal, 12–13, 14, 121–122, 156
normal, 7, 156
dopaminergic effects, 203–204
functional activation, 14, 156
increase *see* hyperaemia
measurement, 9–10
in migraine, 11–15, 19, 154–156,
158, 267
noradrenergic effects, 108
and propranolol, 115
reduction *see* oligaemia
regional, 8
assessment, 9–11
functional depression vs spasm and
ischaemia, 8
serotonergic effects, 23
cerebral hypoxia
animal models, 136–146
ion changes, 146, 162, 164, 167
in migraine pathogenesis, 118–133,
134, 164, 194, 248, 270, 272, 274
cerebral ischaemia
animal models, 134–136
in migraine, 7, 30, 38, 69, 134, 150,
194, 272, 274
pathophysiology, 8
cerebral metabolism
assessment, 11
and cerebral blood flow, 7, 152
and cerebral function, 8
in migraine pathogenesis, 123–124
and propranolol, 115
cerebral oxygen uptake
assessment, 11
and cerebral blood flow, 7, 12, 152
cerebral vasoconstriction, assessment,
9–11
cerebrospinal fluid (CSF), changes in
migraine, 15
cerebrovascular complication(s) *see* stroke;
transient ischaemic attacks; transient
global amnesia

chlorpromazine, pharmacological effects,
268
cholecystokinin, in migraine
pathogenesis, 276
cinnarizine, pharmacological effects, 21
citrus fruit (juice), in migraine
pathogenesis, 196
clonidine
in migraine, 185, 269
pharmacological effects, 21, 27, 63,
86, 91, 110, 111, 135, 137, 140,
260, 264, 269, 270
and tyramine effects, 224
vascular effects, 111–113
vestibular effects, 233
cluster headache
changes in cranial circulation, 38
pathogenesis, 173–174, 198
and platelet enzymes, 195
and pupil changes, 198
and vestibular abnormalities, 230–231
cobalt, and spreading depression, 164
cocaine, instillation into the eye, 198
cocoa, in migraine pathogenesis, 196
coffee, in migraine pathogenesis, 196
collagen, effect on platelets, 70, 263
consciousness, loss of, 174
contraceptive pills
and migraine, 75, 104, 197, 226
and platelets, 75
and tyramine effects, 225
cortical membrane(s), in spreading
depression, 151
corynanthine, pharmacological effects,
110
CT scanning, in migraine, 12, 127
cyclic AMP
and beta-receptors, 111, 114
in migraine patients, 108
in platelets, 90–91
cyclic GMP, and alpha-adrenoceptors,
111
cyproheptadine
pharmacological effects, 21, 25, 27,
54, 61, 258, 263, 268
vestibular effects, 231

decompression, headache caused by, 124
depression
and migraine pathogenesis, 226
spreading *see* spreading depression

glial cells *(continued)*
function, 272–274, 276
in spreading depression, 168
glyceryl trinitrate, in migraine
pathogenesis, 105
GMP cyclic *see* cyclic GMP
guanfacin, pharmacological effects,
113

haloperidol
and dopaminergic effects, 180
in migraine treatment, 185, 202, 210,
271
headache
see also migraine, headache
cluster, 38, 173–174, 195, 198
due to hypertension, 182
idiopathic, 171, 202
tension, 195
head injury, in migraine pathogenesis,
276
heparin, in migraine pathogenesis, 73
histamine
induction of headache, 175
in migraine pathogenesis, 276
receptor(s) blockade, 258, 260, 263
vascular effects, 263
Horner's syndrome, in migraine, 198
5-HT *see* serotonin
l-5-hydroxytryptophan, in migraine
treatment, 184
hyperaemia
focal, 14, 15, 152
global, 15
reactive, 13, 100, 194
hyperventilation, response in migraine,
12
hypoglycaemia
in migraine pathogenesis, 124, 276
ion changes, 162
hypotension, orthostatic, 174, 205, 206
hypoxia
cerebral *see* cerebral hypoxia
effect on vasomotor function, 27

indomethacin, pharmacological effects,
63, 91
indoramin and tyramine effects, 195,
216, 224

INPEA and venoconstriction, 244
insulin, in migraine treatment, 184
ion shifts, in spreading depression,
119, 151
ischaemia
see also oligaemia
cerebral *see* cerebral ischaemia
isometheptene, mechanism of action,
62–63
isoprenaline
effect on arteriovenous shunts, 53
effect on cerebral blood flow, 16
effect on platelets, 90

ketanserin
in migraine treatment, 25, 269
and serotonin receptors, 83
kinins, in migraine pathogenesis, 276

lactate
in CSF, 15
in spreading depression, 152, 164
leukotrienes, in migraine pathogenesis,
276
levodopa *see* L-dopa
linoleic acid, in migraine pathogenesis,
192
lisuride
mechanism of action, 210, 211, 244
treatment, 176, 210, 211
lithium, and tyramine effects, 225
LSD-25, mechanism of action, 180

magnesium, and spreading depression,
164
manganese, and spreading depression,
164
mechanical stimulation of brain tissue,
150, 163
Ménière's disease
and headache, 230, 231
treatment, 197, 235
menopause and migraine, 104
menstrual cycle
and migraine, 104, 168, 192, 226, 276
and platelet MAO, 72
and tyramine effects, 218–219
methergoline, vestibular effects, 231

283

noradrenaline *(continued)*
  in migraine pathogenesis, 16, 20, 70,
    75, 99, 100, 101, 102, 103, 104,
    108, 174, 178, 192, 211, 214, 219
  neuronal uptake, 261
  and platelets, 75, 84, 263
  release, 109, 264
  vascular effects, 111, 263
norepinephrine *see* noradrenaline

octopamine, in migraine pathogenesis,
    214, 220
oedema formation, in brain, 275–276
oestrogens
  in migraine pathogenesis, 226
  and platelets, 75
  and tyramine effects, 219, 225
oligaemia
  focal, 13, 14, 15
  global, 14, 15, 156
  spreading, 14, 152, 155, 267, 268,
    271, 272
opiates, in migraine treatment, 177
opioid(s)
  and antimigraine drugs, 247
  deficiency in migraine, 176–180
Org GC 94
  mechanism of action, 248
  and venoconstriction, 244
overhydration, in migraine pathogenesis,
    276

pain
  in migraine *see* migraine, headache
  and spreading depression, 152
  threshold, 150
paracetamol, and tyramine effects, 222
pentobarbital, pharmacological effects,
    135
PET scanning
  brain, 8, 9, 10, 11
  in migraine, 9, 11, 12, 121
phenelzine, and tyramine effects, 225
phenols, dietary, 72, 196
phenolsulphotransferase (PST), platelet,
    72, 196
phenoxybenzamine, pharmacological
    effects, 113
phentolamine, pharmacological effects,
    114

d-phenylalanine, in migraine treatment,
    182
phenylephrine
  conjunctival instillation test, 174, 240
  pharmacological effects, 110
  and platelets, 86
phenylethylamine, in migraine
    pathogenesis, 71, 105
phosphodiesterase, cyclic; inhibition of,
    90–91
pimozide, vestibular effects, 234
piribedil
  in migraine, 13, 193, 203–205
  pharmacological effects, 261, 264, 271
  vestibular effects, 234
pizotifen
  mechanism of action, 21, 25, 27, 58,
    62, 83, 91, 135, 136, 140, 180,
    248, 258, 263, 268
  and tyramine effects, 224
  and venous compliance, 244
  in vertigo treatment 197
  vestibular effects, 232
placebo, in migraine treatment, 184
plasma factor(s), in migraine, 70, 72,
    75–76
platelet(s)
  activation, 73–74
  aggregation, 72–74, 74, 75, 76, 90
  aggregation inhibitors, 185, 263
  behaviour and function, 81–82
  in cerebral ischaemia, 69
  in hypoxia, 19
  inhibition of function, 81–98, 263
  MAO content, 71–72, 213, 214, 220
  membrane changes, 70, 74–75
  in migraine pathogenesis, 20, 27, 69–80,
    81, 122–123, 194, 195–196
  PST content, 72
  release of serotonin, 70–71, 71, 74, 75
  taurine content, 71
  uptake of serotonin, 69–71, 75, 76
platelet factor 4, release by platelets,
    73, 74
pO_2, in cerebral venous blood, 8, 9
potassium
  extracellular rise, 119, 146, 150, 151,
    162, 163, 164, 165, 168, 271,
    272–274
  and glial cells, 272
potentials, evoked, 124, 151, 196–197

285

practolol
  in migraine, 115
  and platelets, 87
prazosin
  in migraine, 269
  pharmacological effects, 110, 113
  and platelets, 86
pregnancy
  and migraine, 104
  and migraine pathogenesis, 226
pretonine, in migraine treatment, 211
progesterone, in migraine pathogenesis,
  225, 226
propranolol
  effects on spreading depression,
    165–167
  mechanism of action, 63, 87, 88, 91,
    135, 248–249, 260, 264, 269, 271
  in migraine, 109, 115
  and venoconstriction, 244
  in vertigo treatment, 197, 233
prostacyclin
  in migraine pathogenesis, 195
  and platelets, 90
prostaglandins
  and arteriovenous shunts, 63
  and ergotamine, 84
  in migraine pathogenesis, 19, 81, 192,
    194, 214, 276
  and platelets, 90, 91
  vascular effects, 263
psychometric tests, in migraine patients,
  127
puberty, and migraine pathogenesis, 226
pupillometry, in migraineurs, 197–198,
  239–243, 249

rauwolscine, pharmacological effects, 110
receptor binding profile, of antimigraine
  drugs, 255–266
reserpine
  induction of headache, 55, 175, 191
  and migraine pathogenesis, 104

sensorial stimuli, in migraine
  pathogenesis, 123, 197, 272
serotonin
  amplifying effects, 27, 70, 73, 83, 263
  blood level, 16, 27

serotonin *(continued)*
  cerebrovascular innervation, 269, 276
  effect on arteriovenous shunts, 53–55
  effect on veins, 22–23, 202, 243
  and microcirculation, 263
  in migraine pathogenesis, 16, 19,
    22–27, 55, 69, 70, 73, 76, 81,
    180, 191–192, 202, 211, 214, 276
  neuronal uptake, 261
  and platelets, 16, 19, 27, 69–71, 73,
    74, 75, 83, 195
  receptor activation, 264
  receptor binding, 69, 258, 260, 261
  receptor blockade, 25, 83, 88,
    231–232, 258, 260, 263, 264, 265
  tachyphylaxis, 177, 180
  and vasospasm, 15–16, 20, 22–23, 27,
    178
sex, and tyramine effects, 216, 226
sex hormones, in migraine pathogenesis,
  104–105
single photon emission tomography,
  brain, 9, 11
smoking, and migraine, 105
somatostatin tachyphylaxis, 179, 180
spreading depression
  cortical, 46, 119, 149–160, 161–170,
    270, 271, 272, 274
  and migraine, 272, 276
stress, in migraine pathogenesis, 75, 123,
  192
stroke
  and headache, 120
  in migraine patients, 12, 15, 126–129
study of cerebral vasoconstriction,
  methods, 9–11
substance P
  cerebrovascular innervation, 269
  in migraine pathogenesis, 269
sulpiride
  effect on prolactin, 207
  in migraine treatment, 210
sympathetic nervous system
  see also autonomic nervous system
  and vasospasm, 7, 121
systemic lupus erythematosus, and
  migraine, 76, 77

taurine, and migraine, 71
tension headache, and platelet MAO, 195